Current Therapy Series

Bayless, Brain, and Cherniack:
Current Therapy in Internal Medicine 1984-1985
Brain and McCulloch:
Current Therapy in Hematology-Oncology 1983-1984
Cameron:
Current Surgical Therapy 1984-1985
Cherniack:
Current Therapy of Respiratory Disease 1984-1985
Dubovsky:
Current Therapy in Psychiatry 1985-1986
Fortuin:
Current Therapy in Cardiovascular Disease 1984-1985
Garcia, Mastroianni, Amelar, and Dubin:
Current Therapy of Infertility — 2 1984-1985
Gates:
Current Therapy in Otolaryngology —
Head and Neck Surgery 1982-1983
Glassock:
Current Therapy in Nephrology and Hypertension 1984-1985
Johnson:
Current Therapy in Neurologic Disease 1985-1986
Kass and Platt:
Current Therapy in Infectious Disease 1983-1984
Krieger and Bardin:
Current Therapy in Endocrinology 1983-1984
Lichtenstein and Fauci:
Current Therapy in Allergy and Immunology 1983-1984
Long:
Current Therapy in Neurological Surgery 1985-1986
Nelson:
Current Therapy in Neonatal—Perinatal Medicine 1984-1985
Provost and Farmer:
Current Therapy in Dermatology 1984-1985
Trunkey and Lewis:
Current Therapy of Trauma 1984-1985
Welsh and Shephard:
Current Therapy in Sports Medicine 1984-1985

CURRENT THERAPY OF TRAUMA 1984-1985

DONALD D. TRUNKEY, M.D.

Chief of Surgery
San Francisco General Hospital;
Professor and Vice-Chairman
Department of Surgery
University of California
School of Medicine
San Francisco, California

FRANK R. LEWIS, M.D.

Chief of Emergency Services
San Francisco General Hospital;
Professor
Department of Surgery
University of California
School of Medicine
San Francisco, California

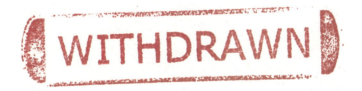

1984

B.C. DECKER INC. • Philadelphia • Toronto
The C.V. MOSBY COMPANY • Saint Louis • Toronto • London

Publisher: **B.C. Decker Inc.**
3228 South Service Road
Burlington, Ontario L7N 3H8

B.C. Decker Inc.
Six Penn Center Plaza, Suite 305
Philadelphia, Pennsylvania 19103

North American and worldwide sales and distribution:
The C.V. Mosby Company
11830 Westline Industrial Drive
Saint Louis, Missouri 63141

In Canada: **The C.V. Mosby Company, Ltd.**
120 Melford Drive
Toronto, Ontario M1B 2X5

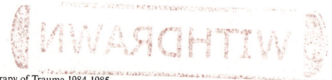

Current Therapy of Trauma 1984-1985   ISBN 0-941158-12-8

Library of Congress catalog number: 83-72756

10 9 8 7 6 5 4 3 2 1

CONTRIBUTORS

HENRY M. BARTKOWSKI, M.D., Ph.D.

Assistant Chief of Neurosurgery, San Francisco General Hospital; Assistant Professor of Neurosurgery, University of California, San Francisco, California
Neurologic Injury

JURIS BUNKIS, M.D.

Assistant Clinical Professor of Surgery, University of California, San Francisco, California
Wound Management
Maxillofacial Trauma
Burns

H. BARRIE FAIRLEY, M.B., B.S.

Chief of Anesthesia, San Francisco General Hospital; Professor and Vice-Chairman of Anesthesia, University of California, San Francisco, California
Anesthetic Management

FRANK R. LEWIS, M.D.

Assistant Chief of Surgery, San Francisco General Hospital; Professor of Surgery, University of California, San Francisco, California
Prehospital Trauma Care
Emergency Department Care
Special Problems

ROBERT E. MARKISON, M.D.

Chief of Hand Surgery, San Francisco General Hospital; Assistant Professor of Surgery, University of California, San Francisco, California
Trauma to the Extremities

JUDITH J. PETRY, M.D.

Assistant Professor of Plastic Surgery, University of Massachusetts Medical Center, Worcester, Massachusetts
Maxillofacial Trauma

LAWRENCE H. PITTS, M.D.

Chief of Neurosurgery, San Francisco General Hospital; Associate Professor, Vice-Chairman of Neurosurgery, University of California, San Francisco, California
Neurologic Injury

PETER TRAFTON, M.D.

Assistant Professor of Orthopaedic Surgery, University of California, San Francisco, California
Fractures

DONALD D. TRUNKEY, M.D.

Chief of Surgery, San Francisco General Hospital; Professor and Vice-Chairman of Surgery, University of California, San Francisco, California
Emergency Department Care
Trauma Principles and Penetrating Neck Trauma
Thoracic Trauma
Abdominal Trauma

ROBERT L. WALTON, M.D.

Associate Professor and Chairman, Division of Plastic Surgery, University of Massachusetts Medical Center, Worcester, Massachusetts
Wound Management
Maxillofacial Trauma
Burns

RICHARD WEISKOPF, M.D.

Associate Professor of Anesthesia, University of California, San Francisco, California
Anesthetic Management

v

PREFACE

In 1984 trauma remains the most important health and social issue in the United States. More people between the ages of one and forty die traumatically than from any other cause; and for every death there are at least two disabilities resulting from traumatic injury. The staggering health care costs in administering to trauma victims exceeds the combined costs of treating patients with heart disease and those with cancer.

An entire literature is devoted to efforts aimed at reducing trauma or minimizing its toll. Our focus in this volume is entirely on therapy, and our purpose is to provide the surgeon with practical, proven guidelines for managing trauma. The work is based solely on the authors' experience at the San Francisco General Hospital. It is neither a review of trauma surgery nor an eclectic look at a variety of approaches to management. We have eschewed alternative treatments in favor of current practices which in our hands have produced good results over time.

Unlike other trauma management books, we have waived the use of illustrations. Few if any wholly new procedures or techniques are described herein; we assume the reader has access to the periodical and book literature that abounds with illustration. Instead, we provide the nuances of care—patient selection, timing of therapy, medical care, follow-up treatment—that influence greatly the outcome of trauma surgery. Also conspicuous by their absence are reference citations in support of the text. We do not expect the reader to accept our every statement as *ex cathedra*; rather, we have looked inward upon our own practices in putting the work together, and we feel a bibliography citing principally our own publications would be fatuous. Please do not brand us self-indulgent for the result; our objective is the most direct means of describing our approach to trauma management.

We gratefully acknowledge the cooperation and forbearance of the publisher in bringing this book to fruition. We wish to thank our coauthors, who are colleagues and members of the "trauma team"; they have been willing collaborators both in the production of this book and in the care of patients over several years. Particular thanks are due the many surgical residents with whom we have worked. Not only do they provide most of the direct care involved in managing severely injured patients at our institutions, they also lead us to improved therapy by questioning and scepticism of established practices.

Donald D. Trunkey, M.D.
Frank R. Lewis, M.D.

CONTENTS

PREHOSPITAL TRAUMA CARE

Frank R. Lewis, M.D.

Views regarding the appropriate level of care for traumatized patients in the prehospital setting are currently in a state of ferment, with considerable debate and controversy regarding what is effective and justifiable. There is no uniform set of practices in the different states, and in California, which has evolved a system with autonomy at the county rather than the state level, practices are markedly variable even within the State. The controversy that prevails is a result of the nearly total lack of clinically relevant studies regarding paramedic practices in trauma. There is virtually no advanced life-support modality advocated for care of the trauma patient—field stabilization, intravenous lines, MAST suits, endotracheal intubation, esophageal obturator airways (EOA), McSwain darts, or any of the myriad drugs—for which a study exists showing the overall efficacy of that modality. There is no area of medicine which is practiced today on a less scientific basis than prehospital care for trauma. It seems that most advanced life-support (ALS) practices have been adopted with the faith that doing something to the patient is better than doing nothing, and that even if they are ineffective, most interventions are at least not harmful. In light of recent experience, both of these assumptions have to be questioned.

Prehospital care for cardiac arrest victims is fortunately on firmer ground, and there have been excellent studies from the greater Seattle area as well as elsewhere which document the advantages of advanced life-support practices for cardiac arrest or major arrhythmias. The most recent data from the Seattle area show that paramedic field care improves net survival after cardiac arrest from 8 percent to 18 percent. Because of the demonstrated value of paramedic services for cardiac patients, a tacit assumption seems to have been made that comparable benefit will obtain for trauma victims. As a result, similar practices have evolved, and field assessment, at-the-scene stabilization, and multiple interventions have become the standard. In the last 2 years, articles have begun to appear questioning the value of these practices and, in some instances, documenting poorer outcomes in trauma patients when paramedic interventions are attempted. It is not that the interventions themselves are normally harmful, although that is certainly possible for some, but rather that the time taken to provide them results in clinical deterioration. Exsanguination is the most common cause of preventable mortality in the first 2 hours after traumatic injury, and it is rare that it can be controlled in the field. Therefore, time works strongly against the paramedic, as it will be difficult for him to do anything for the exsanguinating patient that will compensate for the additional blood loss that occurs with prolonged field time.

Skepticism is also developing regarding the effectiveness of many of the modalities that are routinely used. In the last year, studies of EOA use in the field have shown that it does not provide effective ventilation for as many as 70 percent of patients in whom it is used. Pneumatic antishock garment (PASG) usage has shown that old beliefs regarding its autotransfusion effect are invalid, and that it raises blood pressure principally by increasing cardiac afterload, because perfusion is interrupted to the lower half of the body. Harmful effects of PASG usage have been well documented, and somewhat belatedly we have realized that there is no study in the literature showing that, overall, PASG usage has net beneficial effects. In San Francisco, we attempted such a study during the last 2 years, and after examining 250 traumatized patients randomly treated with or without the PASG, we could show no effect on patient outcome, despite the fact that patients were stratified objectively according to severity of injury. We point this out not because we are convinced that the PASG has been proved to have no value, but rather to let the reader understand how barren this area is in regard to clinical studies. It is a triumph of politics over science that approximately one-third of the states have legislation requiring PASGs to be carried by ambulances where there are as yet no studies available documenting their benefit.

As a result of this paucity of data in the area of prehospital care for trauma, few measures can be said to have proven benefit. This chapter must therefore present my opinions, based on my experience and analysis of the problem. In the next few years, however, as additional studies are done, this field is likely to change rapidly. It should be clearly understood that the points to be made are not held unanimously among emergency physicians and trauma surgeons, nor even perhaps among a majority.

BASIC SKILLS

The skills for which there is seemingly no disagreement are those that are simplest, quickest, and most effective—extrication, spinal protection, splinting, control of external bleeding, and basic cardiopulmonary resuscitation. We will briefly touch on each of these.

Extrication is a complex subject, requiring a variety of devices and techniques and considerable ingenuity in the face of unpredictable situations. Most of the heavy equipment used in automobile extrication is provided by fire departments, which respond jointly with paramedics to accident scenes. The area of specific paramedic expertise is in the handling of the patient. The principal objectives during extrication are to provoke as little extraneous movement as possible and to provide immobilization of extremities and spine until fractures are defined. Whenever possible, rigid immobilizing devices, such as short or long spine boards, should be used, and the patient should be either fastened to these in situ, or moved as gently as possible onto them. During any movement careful attention should be paid to extremities, to keep them in anatomic positions and prevent any flailing or distortion.

Spinal protection has been heavily emphasized in paramedic training, because of the disastrous and irreversible consequences if an unstable fracture, particularly of the cervical spine, produces spinal cord injury which was not already present. The actual frequency with which this might occur is not well documented. One might intuitively think that cord injury would be most likely at the moment of impact, when the fracture actually occurs. It would seem that the forces and displacement of the fracture site would be greatest at this moment, and that subsequent displacement would normally be slight by comparison. The literature tends to show that this is indeed correct, and that most cord damage does occur at the time of the injury. Nevertheless, there are well-documented cases in which cord damage was clearly not present initially, but was produced by patient movement either in the ambulance or in the hospital before adequate immobilization was provided. Although rare, such cases have emphasized the tremendous hazard of this injury and have made most paramedics and emergency physicians extremely careful in their handling of patients prior to obtaining spinal radiographs. This caution is generally appropriate, but the paranoia regarding possible cervical spine injury has reached such proportions that other more life-threatening injuries are often treated inadequately rather than risk cervical spine movement. Many deaths have unquestionably resulted, and in my opinion, the pendulum needs to swing back a bit the other way. If the patient has an obstructed airway, for example, and is becoming asphyxiated in spite of the usual attempts to treat it, it makes no sense to prohibit cervical spine extension to open the airway because of the possibility of a cervical injury. It should be recognized that statistically the chance of damaging the spine is slight, and that it is far more important to treat immediately life-threatening airway problems in the most effective manner, rather than let the patient arrest from hypoxia. Although no good data have been presented on this point, it is my impression that airway obstruction is at least 100 times more common than cervical spine injury as a cause of death or major disability. Treating the greatest threat to life at each moment should therefore be the governing principle. Under nearly all circumstances, this will allow appropriate spinal protection to be given, but occasionally it must be ignored.

The actual means of spinal immobilization for cervical fractures has been debated extensively, and it appears that the best method is to use a spinal board or other rigid device, with the head and thorax secured to it. When the patient is on a stretcher, sandbags on each side of the head may be used, with tape across the forehead, secured to each side of the sandbags. Cervical collars alone are of little value and do not effectively stabilize the neck. As soon as possible, of course, the patient with a cervical fracture should be placed in axial traction, using a halo and tong arrangement secured to the skull.

Immobilization of extremities for possible fracture is a time-honored principle and continues to be one of the most important field treatments. Effective immobilization will prevent further damage to vessels, nerves, and soft tissues, and is thought by some to reduce the extent of hemorrhage surrounding a fracture. Fractures of the forearm and of the leg below the knee can be effectively splinted either with inflatable tubular splints, which are commonly available today, or with splints made of a rigid material and secured to the extremity by wrapping with gauze or other soft material. For fractures of the femur, the most effective immobilization is via a Thomas splint or equivalent with distal traction applied to the ankle and foot. Convenient mechanized splints (Hare traction splint) are commercially available today to accomplish this. Obviously, one must ascertain that lower leg fractures are not present before applying traction to the ankle for a femur fracture. Fractures of the upper arm are best splinted by strapping the arm to the trunk with circumferential wrapping, with sling support of the forearm, so that the elbow is at approximately 90°.

External bleeding may be arterial or venous, the source usually being indicated by the pressure and color of the blood. In either case, direct compression over the bleeding site is the best method of control. This is usually done with sterile gauze placed directly over the wound and the fingers or palm applied firmly over it. Occasionally, when the bleeding is from a relatively proximal artery, control is difficult and pressure must be more focal or intense. Tourniquets are rarely necessary and should be avoided if at all possible. If they are used, they must be released at least hourly to allow reperfusion of the extremity for a few minutes. Pressure dressings often are utilized, with either gauze rolls or elastic rolls wrapped around the extremity to generate pressure over the wound. Although these can be effective in some cases, direct manual pressure is usually more effective and should be used preferentially. Inflatable tubular splints or the legs of the pneumatic antishock garment (PASG) can also be used to tamponade extremity bleeding, particularly if it is coming from a large area, as with an extensively avulsed skin flap. They are most effective with venous bleeding, but if inflated above arterial pressure, they may be used to control that as well. The same precautions as with tourniquets apply if such high pressures are used.

The final basic skills which should be discussed involve cardiopulmonary resuscitation. Of the two elements involved—ventilation and cardiac massage—ventilation is by far the more valuable one to emphasize in trauma victims. External cardiac massage in the hypovolemic patient who has arrested due to exsanguination is ineffective and rarely successful. Ventilation, however, is frequently compromised and can be effectively treated, particularly in cases of head injury and coma, or of aspiration. A knowledge of how to clear the oropharynx, open the airway, and provide effective ventilation, either by mouth-to-mouth or bag and mask techniques, should be essential skills for all EMTs, from the most basic level to paramedics. Objective assessment suggests that this frequently is not the case, and that this fundamental skill deserves greater emphasis, training, and testing in most programs. External cardiac massage should also be attempted in all trauma patients in cardiac arrest, but should never delay transport, unlike myocardial infarct and arrhythmia victims. Unless the arrest is due to hypoxia which has been corrected, or the patient in arrest can be delivered within 5 to 10 minutes to a facility where definitive care is provided, survival is unlikely. Patients who arrest in the field after blunt trauma are virtually never resuscitatable. Those who arrest after penetrating trauma have salvage rates as high as 40 percent with emergency room thoracotomy, but only when transport is extremely rapid and definitive care is immediately available on arrival at the hospital.

ADVANCED SKILLS

The items to be discussed here encompass the ALS skills which have already been mentioned in the introduction, but rather than basing the discussion around each of the skills, we would like to present a different perspective. If prehospital trauma care is to save lives, it must specifically address the causes of early mortality in trauma victims and provide effective treatment for these.

Trauma patients, for purposes of analysis, may be divided retrospectively into three categories of severity: (1) rapidly fatal, (2) urgent and life-threatening, and (3) stable. The first group encompasses injuries in which rapid exsanguination, massive head injury, cervical cord transection, or major airway disruption are present and produce inevitable death in less than 10 minutes. Approximately 5 percent of all injuries and 50 percent of trauma deaths fall into this category. For the foreseeable future, we have no way of improving salvage in this group, other than through prevention or environmental modification.

The third group, which accounts for 80 percent of all trauma, includes those in whom injuries are minor and those whose injuries are confined to soft tissues or isolated extremity fractures. Rarely does this group have major injury within the thorax or abdomen. For this group, urgent treatment is not essential, as they will survive without significant disability, even with a delay in treatment of 2 hours or more.

We wish to focus on the second group—those who are potentially salvageable if the medical care system is operating competently and efficiently—and to examine the specific paramedic skills that may affect survival.

Three types of injury account for most prehospital trauma mortality. Direct cerebral and high spinal cord injuries cause approximately 50 to 55 percent of deaths. Exsanguination due to thoracic, abdominal, and major vascular injuries, or severe pelvic and long bone fractures, accounts for 30 to 40 percent of deaths. Airway obstruction, open or tension pneumothorax, and hypoxia from other causes account for 10 to 15 percent of the total. Obviously, many of these injuries fall into the first group described and are unsalvageable with present therapies. The remainder, however, fall into group 2. How can they be benefited by advanced life-support skills?

In potentially salvageable patients with head injuries who die, the usual cause of death is airway obstruction or aspiration causing acute hypoxia. This is true, of course, only when prompt neurosurgical care is provided, so that avoidable neurologic death does not occur. Patients with massive cerebral injury or brain stem herniation in the first hour or two are generally not salvageable, unless an acute epidural or subdural hematoma is present and can be decompressed. In the potentially salvageable group, cerebral edema causing significant elevation in intracranial pressure usually does not occur for at least 30 to 60 minutes, if not longer. Preventable death in the field is therefore mostly due to airway problems that occur with unconsciousness, not to the head injury directly. The most essential skill the paramedic can provide is therefore endotracheal intubation, which at once provides ventilation and airway protection. The neurologic lesion itself cannot be treated in the field and is best handled by rapid transport to definitive neurosurgical care. Spinal protection, in appropriate cases, is also an essential maneuver which can be quickly accomplished in patients requiring it. Since edema does not usually develop for 30 to 60 minutes, mannitol given in the field is unlikely to be of benefit and might aggravate coexisting hypovolemia.

The second most common cause of death is exsanguination. What can the paramedic offer? For isolated sources of external bleeding, direct pressure to control it is the obvious answer. The majority of patients who exsanguinate, however, do so from internal bleeding, which is not controllable without surgical intervention. The only treatments that are potentially beneficial are the establishment of an intravenous (IV) line with rapid fluid administration and the use of the pneumatic antishock garment (PASG). At first, each of these would seem to be noncontroversial. However, when the time taken for establishment of an IV is considered, it is more questionable. There are minimal data on the success rate or the realistic time it takes to start an IV in the field in trauma patients. In a study of 100 arrested patients by McSwain et al., the average time for starting an IV was 11 minutes. Given the suboptimal conditions under which the paramedic is working, this seems like an appropriate figure.

In a patient who will potentially exsanguinate in 15 to 40 minutes, the bleeding rate is in the range of 60 to 200 ml/minute, as it requires a loss of 40 to 50 percent of the blood volume to cause hypovolemic arrest. An average delay of 11 minutes to start an IV (plus an unknown failure rate, but probably at least 20 to 30 percent) will therefore lead to blood loss of 700 to 1800 ml while the attempt is being made, plus additional losses before and after. Given the fact that the paramedic cannot normally infuse more than 1,000 to 2,000 ml of IV solution in the usual 10 to 20 minutes between establishment of the IV and arrival at a hospital, it seems that the trade-off is not a good one. Under the best of circumstances, the loss of blood will have been offset by an equal volume of asanguineous, non-oxygen-carrying solution. Under more usual circumstances, the replacement volume will not even equal the lost volume. When one further considers that the balanced salt solutions normally used for IV administration have only one-third the intravascular filling effect of a comparable volume of blood, the trade-off is further worsened. The patient threatened with exsanguination in less than 40 minutes therefore loses more circulating blood volume during the average IV attempt than can be given subsequently to make up for it. If the failure rate involved in starting field IVs is considered, it only tips the balance further in favor of not starting the IV.

One might argue that the IV does not have to be started prior to transport and could be attempted en route. This is theoretically true, but the additional practical problem of starting an IV in a moving, bouncing ambulance are well known to paramedics, and they are prone to delay transport until the IV is established.

If total field times in excess of 40 to 60 minutes are encountered, the foregoing analysis does not apply, and the benefits of an IV might outweigh its disadvantages. This would occur with prolonged extrication or long transport distances; in the average urban setting where paramedic services are provided, these are not common problems. Where transport times of 5 to 20 minutes are more usual, it is clear that starting IVs in trauma patients is illogical: Patients who are bleeding rapidly and urgently need volume replacement will be harmed by the delay in starting the IV, and those who are not bleeding rapidly do not need the volume replacement.

What of the pneumatic antishock garment, which has enjoyed widespread usage in civilian systems since its introduction in Vietnam? It is clear that arterial hypotension can often be partially corrected by pneumatic antishock garment application. Originally this was thought to be due to autotransfusion of blood from the legs and lower abdomen. More recently it has been shown that only 200 ml of blood is autotransfused and that the major effects are due to increased peripheral resistance due to the tourniquet effect below the waist.

The beneficial effects of the pneumatic antishock garment are a rise in proximal aortic pressure, and potential tamponade of bleeding sources which lie within the garment itself, such as a badly fractured pelvis. Potential negative effects are increased bleeding from sources above the level of garment application, compromise of ventilation due to restriction of rib cage expansion and elevation of the diaphragm, and ischemic damage to tissues within the garment if it is kept inflated too long. In addition, there is a profound hypotensive effect when the PASG is deflated, which has been responsible for precipitating many cardiac arrests in emergency departments, and a concurrent washout of lactic acid from ischemic tissues analogous to that which occurs with aortic declamping.

It seems impossible in the abstract to weigh the negative and positive effects of the PASG application and decide whether there is net benefit; a randomized clinical trial is the only way we are going to learn if it is useful or not. We would advocate such a trial, preferably multicenter, to develop data as rapidly as possible. As noted in the opening paragraphs, we have done a preliminary study in San Francisco, and after examining 250 patients, we could find no difference in survival with or without PASG usage. A study to answer the question posed would therefore probably require 2,000 to 3,000 patients. In the interim, it seems reasonable to continue pneumatic antishock garment usage as is the current practice.

To summarize, in the patients who will potentially die of exsanguination in the first 40 minutes after injury, paramedics have little to offer other than direct control of bleeding where possible and rapid transport to a trauma center where definitive surgical care is available. Intravenous line placement appears to be counterproductive and pneumatic antishock garments will elevate blood pressure, but have not been proven to have more positive than negative effects.

Finally, what of the acute airway problems that are lethal? The great majority of these are effectively treated by endotracheal intubation, as it protects from aspiration and provides a closed pneumatic system for ventilation. It has been thought to the present time that the esophageal obturator airway (EOA) was an effective alternative to endotracheal intubation that did not require as high a level of skills training. It has now been shown in two different systems that the EOA does not function as well as thought, and that the incidence of inadequate ventilation when utilizing it is unacceptably high. It therefore appears that endotracheal intubation, though more demanding in training time and skill required, is sufficiently superior in results to justify this investment. When the benefits described earlier in comatose patients are also considered, the benefits seem overriding.

For the remainder of the acute, potentially lethal chest problems, there seems little that can be done in the field. Placement of McSwain darts for relief of pneumothorax has been advocated, but given the difficulty of making this diagnosis on clinical grounds, it seems unlikely that field use of these devices will ever be practical. The harm resulting from placement in a large number of patients with respiratory distress of other origin would almost certainly outstrip the benefits in the small number of patients with tension pneumothorax. Rapid transport is also again an essential factor in obtaining good results with major airway problems, since it is only in an emergency department or surgical suite that adequate facilities for diagnostic evaluation, tube thoracostomy placement, and possibly thoracotomy will be provided.

SUMMARY

Trauma patients are fundamentally different from cardiac arrest victims, who are customarily resuscitated and stabilized before transport. The difference is that cardiac patients already have an arrested circulation, and transport without resuscitation will only guarantee irreversibility. The trauma patient, in constrast, begins with a normal circulatory system and is progressively worsening with time. Attempts at "stabilization," other than for airway control and basic care, will only use up time and allow deterioration through progressive hypovolemia. Stabilization of the exsanguinating patient can only be achieved in an operating room by a surgeon trained to deal with traumatic injuries. In the patient who is bleeding rapidly enough to have his life threatened, time is critical, and wasting minutes in the field with ineffectual therapeutic maneuvers should not be tolerated.

The value of rapid transport has been shown in several studies, but seems not to have had the impact it should have had on paramedic practice. Military experience, from World War II through Vietnam, shows clearly that survival is inversely proportional to time of injury to effective treatment. McSwain has shown, in both trauma and cardiac arrest patients, that rapid transport leads to improved survival. Most recently, Gervin and Fischer have shown that delayed transport due to paramedic field interventions *decreases* survival in patients with cardiac injuries. The conclusion of all these studies is in agreement with my analysis.

It appears that a reorientation of paramedic field care for trauma patients needs to occur, and the skills and services that are actually beneficial need to be emphasized and taught. The overriding benefits will be from endotracheal intubation and rapid transport, with spinal and extremity immobilization when indicated. Intravenous lines seem counterproductive other than in prolonged transports or delayed extrication, and the pneumatic antishock garment is possibly useful, but needs to be objectively evaluated. Use of EOAs should probably be phased out and replaced by training for direct endotracheal intubation. Use of drugs is rarely, if ever, indicated. By focusing paramedic training on fewer skills which are truly beneficial, and ensuring that those skills are developed and maintained, the large investment in paramedic services will produce more effective benefits in the trauma patient than is currently the case.

EMERGENCY DEPARTMENT CARE

Frank R. Lewis, M.D.
Donald D. Trunkey, M.D.

The majority of trauma patients present to the Emergency Department without life-threatening injuries and may be assessed in the orderly manner to which physicians are traditionally accustomed. Roughly 10 percent of patients, however, will have life-threatening injuries; speed in assessment, diagnosis, and therapy becomes crucial to their survival. If the emergency physician or surgeon who initially sees such patients has not developed a logical and sequential plan for their management, then when confronted with the problem, he will almost surely function poorly and inefficiently. In contrast, the experienced physician who is able to quickly discern the critical areas of injury and deal with them appropriately can provide immediate treatment and can supervise and direct the multiple casualty situation with relatively inexperienced personnel. Disaster or triage situations only heighten the need for such expertise.

Although nothing can take the place of extensive experience in seeing and treating a variety of complex injuries, we have found that the following plan provides a framework which allows the most critical injuries to be dealt with first, but prevents minor injuries from being overlooked in the multiple trauma situation. With use, it becomes second nature whenever a trauma patient is encountered and rapidly allows the inexperienced physician to gain confidence.

In addition to expertise, it should perhaps be noted that the demeanor of the physician in charge of the resuscitation situation is also important. A calm and deliberate manner is essential, and instructions to other medical and paramedical personnel must be given clearly and unambiguously. Vacillation, indecision, and overt anxiety will alarm the patient, as well as everyone else in the vicinity.

The sequential steps in rapidly assessing and treating the patient are the following:

1. Airway and pulmonary evaluation
2. Estimation of blood volume loss and cardiac status
3. Brief history and physical
4. Initial treatment
5. Definitive diagnosis and care

In the following pages these will be discussed in detail. One should bear in mind that it should be possible to complete the first 3 items in the above list in less than three minutes. A relatively good picture of the patient's injuries, status, and prognosis will then be apparent, and one can return to any area that demands urgent attention or can proceed with diagnostic studies or surgical intervention, as indicated. It is absolutely essential that the responsible physician take the time to make this assessment when he first sees the patient, and not to take the word of anyone else for the findings that are present. We commonly see instances of over- and undertreatment of patients because this principle is ignored, and therapy is instituted for the most obvious injury without evaluating all systems. There is virtually never a reason not to take the brief time necessary for a thorough assessment.

AIRWAY AND PULMONARY EVALUATION

Airway obstruction is generally recognized as the most rapidly fatal problem seen in the emergency setting; not so well recognized are the injuries to the lung or chest wall, which impair ventilation almost as severely as an obstructed airway, and which can also be rapidly fatal: open pneumothorax (sucking chest wound), tension pneumothorax, and flail chest. These entities should always be considered in any patient with severe respiratory distress.

An initial look at the patient after he or she has been completely undressed should give the examiner several pieces of information about respiratory status: Is the patient making respiratory efforts? How strongly and how rapidly? Is he awake and able to protect his airway from aspiration? Is air actually exchanging via the nose and mouth? Is respiratory noise present—gasping, stridor, or wheezing? Is the chest wall moving symmetrically on both sides, or is there splinting or paradoxical movement? Are there any surface markings, wounds, abrasions, or ecchymoses indicative of the area and extent of trauma? Is the patient breathing easily, or are the accessory muscles being used? What are the relative durations of inspiration and expiration? Is the patient comfortable lying supine, or does he need to sit upright or in some other position to maximize ventilation?

If the foregoing assessment indicates that the patient is apneic, or if the airway is totally obstructed, immediate attention must be directed to it. One should first open the mouth and suction the back of the throat. If a "cafe coronary" is a possibility, and the patient is unconscious, insertion of two fingers over the tongue to the area of the glottis will usually disclose a foreign body if present and allow its easy removal. In the awake patient in respiratory distress, insertion of anything into the nose or mouth will usually exacerbate the distress and should be avoided unless a specific therapeutic maneuver, such as endotracheal intubation, is being carried out.

Once secretions or foreign body have been excluded, one should displace the jaw anteriorly, either by grasping the symphysis and lifting or by using both hands and lifting forward on the mandibular angles. If the airway can be opened, a well-fitting mask can then be used to ventilate the patient with positive pressure and 100 percent oxygen for 2 to 3 minutes. If it is not possible to establish ventilation with a mask, one should move immediately to intubate the patient via the oral route with either a No. 6 or No. 7 cuffed endotracheal tube. For the nonanesthetist physician who intubates patients infrequently, we prefer a large straight blade for the laryngoscope (Miller or Wisconsin blades) rather than the curved MacIntosh blade.

In more than 99 percent of patients, airway access via oral intubation of the trachea is successful in the emergency department. The occasional patient, however, because of severe maxillofacial injury, bleeding, distortion of anatomy, or foreign body, will require emergency tracheostomy. When necessary, a cricothyroidotomy should be done between the laryngeal cartilage and the cricoid, rather than a classic tracheostomy through the second or third tracheal rings. Access to the cricothyroid membrane is much faster and easier, as it lies nearer the surface and requires minimal retraction for exposure. Concern about subglottic stenosis or vocal cord dysfunction following this procedure has been shown in recent series not to be a significant problem. A transverse incision 2 to 3 cm long is made transversely directly over the cricothyroid membrane, with the patient's neck extended. The membrane is incised transversely over the anterior third of the tracheal circumference, and a curved clamp is inserted and spread to define the opening. A No. 5 to No. 7 curved (60°) tracheostomy tube is then inserted, and the cuff is inflated. The tube should be immediately secured around the neck with umbilical tape.

We are often asked whether endotracheal intubation or tracheostomy, both of which require neck extension, should be attempted in the unconscious patient when a cervical spine fracture is a possibility and x-ray studies have not been obtained. In such circumstances, one must decide which is the greater threat to the patient—the obstructed airway or the possible cervical spine fracture. In our opinion, the airway virtually always has priority, as the possibility of cervical cord injury is relatively remote. If circumstances allow, however, and the patient is not facing a life-threatening situation, cervical spine injury should certainly be excluded first.

We might parenthetically comment on the value of oxygen administration in the acutely traumatized patient with airway or pulmonary problems: it rarely provides significant benefit, as most of the life-threatening problems are due to inadequate ventilation of the alveoli, and are mechanical in nature. While increased inspired concentrations of oxygen are unlikely to be harmful, and should be used if readily available, one should not waste time in the acute emergency looking for a source of oxygen when what the patient really needs is effective definition and correction of his ventilatory inadequacy.

Let us return now to the completion of the pulmonary assessment, assuming that the degree of airway impairment is not such as to require immediate intervention. After a careful visual inspection, as already described, one should palpate the entire thorax for crepitus or rib instability, or (if the patient is awake) to see whether pressure in any area causes pain. This is most easily done by compression of the sternum toward the spine, followed by compression with the examiner's hands on each side of the chest. Rib fractures are the most common injury seen after blunt trauma, and their diagnosis is predominantly clinical. When a rib is fractured, there is point tenderness at the fracture site, and pressure on the rib at a distant location will reproduce the pain. X-ray examination should be used to define multiple rib fractures, but multiple views to rule out all possible fracture sites are not necessary. It should also be remembered that costochondral fractures do not show on x-ray films. The trachea should be palpated and its position relative to the sternal notch carefully noted. The clavicles and scapula should also be palpated for tenderness or deformity.

If respiratory distress is present, one should auscultate the chest to see whether breath sounds are reduced on one side. If the patient is not in any respiratory distress, we do not waste time with auscultation at this point in the assessment. It should be noted that although physical diagnosis books describe marked differences in breath sounds on the two sides as the diagnostic criteria for pneumothorax, the practical usefulness of this observation is limited. The differences may be quite subtle and, in a noisy trauma room, impossible to distinguish. Thus auscultation should be recognized as of limited value and should never be the sole determinant of treatment or of nontreatment of pneumothorax.

At this point one should have a fairly good idea of the thoracic pathology present, based on the examination and the mechanism of injury. If the trauma is penetrating, is it confined to one hemithorax, or does it cross the midline, with the concomitant risk of major vascular or cardiac injury and perforation of the esophagus or trachea? Is there subcutaneous emphysema, suggesting tracheal or bronchial disruption? Are there obvious rib fractures, and if so, approximately how extensive are they? Is there good reason to suspect that there is a pneumo- or hemothorax? The final decision on many of these points must often await the chest roentgenogram, as physical diagnosis is at best inexact. In the compromised patient, however, one may not have time to get the roentgeno-

gram, and therapy must be undertaken on the basis of the physical findings and likely injury. The patient in severe respiratory distress, who is not relieved by tracheal intubation, should have chest tubes placed prior to any x-ray examination, as they may be lifesaving. If injuries appear confined to one side, then initially a unilateral chest tube should be placed; if lateralization is not possible, bilateral tubes should be inserted. The actual technique of insertion will be addressed later in this chapter.

ESTIMATION OF BLOOD VOLUME LOSS AND CARDIAC STATUS

The next priority is to assess the degree of shock and decide how much intravascular volume replacement the patient is likely to need, how rapidly, and what size and type of intravenous catheters are needed. A judgment about degree of shock must always be considered in light of the time since injury. If, for example, the injury occurred 15 minutes before and the patient is in profound shock, massive bleeding is occurring and several large-bore IV access lines are needed. Conversely, if the injury occurred 2 hours before and the degree of shock is mild, the rate of bleeding is not immediately life-threatening, and less aggressive volume restitution is called for.

The indicators that are commonly used for assessment of shock in the emergency setting are the following:

1. Blood pressure
2. Pulse rate
3. Skin perfusion (color, temperature, moisture)
4. Urine output
5. Mental status
6. Central venous pressure

We would like to discuss each of these and indicate its sensitivity and accuracy in the assessment of shock.

Although blood pressure is the time-honored parameter that is used to define volume loss, we feel it is less accurate and sensitive than items 2, 3, and 4 above. The response of the blood pressure to intravascular depletion is nonlinear, as compensatory mechanisms of increased cardiac rate and contractility, and venous and arteriolar vasoconstriction provide excellent compensation for the first 15 to 20 percent of intravascular volume loss in the healthy young adult. After about 20 percent volume loss, the blood pressure begins to decline, and in the average patient, it will be in the 60 to 80 mmHg range with 30 percent volume loss and the 30 to 50 mmHg range with 40 percent volume loss. As volume loss becomes more severe, therefore, the decline in blood pressure is more precipitous. In the elderly patient who cannot compensate as well by the aforementioned mechanisms, the decline in blood pressure begins at 10 to 15 percent volume loss and will proceed to the point of arrest by 40 percent loss. The nonlinear behavior of blood pressure has two disadvantages: Declines in blood pressure are a relatively insensitive sign of early shock, and in the infrequently monitored patient, blood pressure may appear stable for an initial period, and then rather suddenly appear to "crash." We often hear the inexperienced observer speculate about how a bleeding source must have suddenly appeared to explain this behavior; in reality the patient was bleeding all the time and finally reached the point of decompensation.

The other obvious deficiency with blood pressure monitoring is the lack of an absolute "normal." A patient who is normally hypertensive may be in profound shock when his systolic blood pressure is 120 mmHg, whereas the healthy young athlete may be entirely normal with a systolic pressure of 90 mmHg.

Pulse rate is the second commonly used indicator and, indeed, is more sensitive than blood pressure. Its value is significantly limited by its lack of specificity, as the emotionalism, pain, and excitement surrounding the usual trauma situation may result in tachycardia without hypovolemia. However, if tachycardia is sustained above levels of 120/min, it should be considered an indicator of hypovolemia until proven otherwise. In young patients, the heart rate may accelerate to 160 to 180/min with severe volume depletion. The older patient is unable to accelerate to this degree and rarely will sustain rates greater than 140/min.

Skin perfusion is, we feel, a greatly underappreciated indicator of hypovolemia, but it is the observation we place most confidence in when initially evaluating the patient. The early physiologic compensation to volume loss is to vasoconstrict vessels to the skin and muscle, and this is manifested by paleness and coolness of the skin, which develops quite rapidly. The release of epinephrine, which also accompanies hypovolemia, causes

sweating, and on palpating the patient's trunk in such a situation one will be immediately struck by the coolness and moisture. The lower extremities are the first to manifest the vasoconstriction, and palpation over the kneecaps or the feet provides the best "early warning" of impending shock. We routinely use these findings with confidence in all age groups and all types of injuries, and have yet to find them unreliable.

The fourth indicator is urine output, and any patient with significant trauma should always have an indwelling urinary bladder catheter inserted as soon as possible to monitor urine volumes every 15 minutes. This is the second most reliable indicator of volume loss, after skin perfusion, and is only slightly less sensitive than that. The second level of compensation of the body to hypovolemia is visceral vasoconstriction, and this results in decreased flow to the gut, liver, and kidney. Urine output will immediately reflect decreases in renal blood flow; hence its value as an indicator. A minimally adequate urine volume is 0.5 ml/kg/hr, and resuscitative fluids should be administered rapidly until this level is reached. If urine output exceeds 1 ml/kg/hr, the fluid administration rate can be cut back. On an ongoing basis during resuscitation or surgery, the urine output is overall the best indicator of adequacy of volume restitution.

The fifth indicator of hypovolemia, alteration in mental status, is rarely seen because it is present only with preterminal degrees of hypovolemia. Compensatory mechanisms maintain flow to the myocardium and brain with great tenacity; hence one does not see cerebral hypoperfusion until blood pressure is in the 30 to 60 mmHg systolic range or below. The alteration usually seen is agitation and mental confusion, so that the patient becomes irrational, anxious, and uncooperative. Such states are also commonly produced by alcohol or other drugs in the emergency setting; hence it may be hard to distinguish alterations due to hypovolemia from those due to drugs, particularly when both may be present. There is no sure way to resolve this problem, other than to retain a high degree of suspicion and to be aware that the agitated patient must immediately be checked carefully to exclude hypovolemia as a cause for his behavior.

The last parameter, central venous pressure, is not a very good indicator of hypovolemia, since the normal levels of 3 to 8 mmHg are relatively hard to distinguish from hypovolemic levels of 0 to 5 mmHg, particularly when one is initially estimating the pressure only by inspection of external jugular neck veins. The importance of this indicator, rather, is to distinguish hypovolemia from cardiogenic shock due to tamponade, tension pneumothorax, or cardiac contusion. In the trauma patient who is in shock, only two diagnostic possibilities are likely: (1) he has lost significant intravascular volume, or (2) he has some interference with cardiac function. When the injury is a stab or gunshot wound over the precordial area, one has no way of knowing from external inspection which of these is present, yet rapid and correct treatment is absolutely dependent on making the distinction. In this setting, the central venous pressure, as judged by inspection of the neck veins or by actual measurement if a central venous catheter is inserted, is the only test that will provide immediate and unambiguous discrimination of the two conditions. With hypovolemia the CVP is less than 5 mmHg in the shocky patient. To produce a similar degree of cardiogenic shock, the CVP must be 25 mmHg or above. It is very easy to distinguish these two ranges on external inspection, and it should be the next observation one makes after determining that a patient is in shock.

BRIEF HISTORY AND PHYSICAL EXAMINATION

After determining that the patient is not in imminent danger from airway or circulatory problems, a quick but comprehensive survey should be undertaken. This begins with a brief history, followed by a "head to toe" physical, in which the areas of major injury are defined and plans are formulated for continuing diagnosis and therapy.

During the early phases, histories are kept to a minimum, but some information needs to be obtained if at all possible. The mechanism of injury should be defined, and any information available from patient or paramedics regarding circumstances of the accident and energy dissipation should be considered. This might include speed of automobiles, height of falls, and such associated findings as a collapsed steering wheel, ejection from an automobile, and whether the victim was a passenger or pedestrian. With penetrating trauma, the caliber of a gun or the size of a knife is important information, but not often known. If the patient is conscious, the examiner should determine where the major symptoms are and focus the examination there. Although internal thoracic

and abdominal injuries do not produce reliable physical findings, injuries to extremities, spine, and chest wall virtually always do. A clear statement by the patient that there is no pain or tenderness in the neck or back, and none in the arms or legs either at rest or with movement, can immediately eliminate the need for extensive and time-consuming x-ray studies. One should also obtain a medical history in regard to allergies, medications, pre-existent disease, and prior surgery.

Initial Neurologic Evaluation

The neurologic assessment of the patient overlaps with the history and really begins during the initial contact with the patient, as it immediately becomes evident whether the patient is conscious or comatose, and if conscious whether there is alteration of the normal mental state. Decisions about respiratory and circulatory status, already discussed, are not greatly affected by the mental state, as they depend on objective signs and require immediate therapy no matter what the mental state. Attempts to take the history also define the patient's mental status, and usually only a few questions are required to tell whether the patient is normal, confused, agitated, or inappropriate. If the patient is significantly obtunded or unconscious, the history is bypassed and one moves immediately to specific neurologic assessment.

The dominant element of CNS assessment in the trauma patient, both initially and on a continuing basis, is level of consciousness. There are multiple ways of defining this, but we find it most useful to use five levels: normal, obtunded, appropriately responsive to pain, inappropriately responsive to pain, and unresponsive. The first of these is self-explanatory and defines the awake, alert patient who answers questions appropriately. The second category is broad, but generally defines the patient who is responsive to verbal stimuli, but in whom the responses are inappropriate or mentation is sluggish. The third category defines one who does not respond to verbal stimuli, but will withdraw from a painful stimulus. The fourth category defines patients who do not attempt to withdraw from the source of pain, but do respond by movement of some type, either of another part of the body, or by extensor posturing. The last group are those who make no movement in response to pain but who retain brain stem functions.

An important point to mention at this point is that CNS injury does not cause hypotension until brain stem function is lost, and by the time this occurs the patient is universally unsalvageable. One should therefore never blame hypotension on neurologic injury, but rather should assume there is a source of blood loss in addition to the neurologic injury. The only exception to this occurs in patients with spinal cord injuries and paraplegia, who may develop postural hypotension because of a failure of sympathetic tone peripherally. In these patients the hypotension is usually readily corrected by intravascular volume administration.

In the patient with any degree of mental impairment, it is essential that mental status be initially documented and then repeatedly assessed at 15 to 30-minute intervals. Most of the treatable intracranial lesions produce deteriorating levels of consciousness during the first 1 or 2 hours of observation; failure to detect these may lead to delay in treatment with associated poorer outcome. Patients who have altered mental status due to drugs will usually improve during the first few hours of observation; thus the ongoing assessment is critical to distinguish those with organic disease from those with pharmacologic alterations.

The second part of the neurologic assessment is the definition of lateralizing signs. These are sought most commonly in the pupillary reflexes, because increased intracranial pressure is usually manifested first by sluggishness or loss of the pupillary response to light. Less commonly, the extraocular movements are impaired. Lateralization should be further defined by examining the extremities and determining whether movement and strength of arms and legs are full and equal. One has to be careful that movements are not attempted when fractures may be present, but in the awake patient the pain at the fracture site will prevent any attempt to move that area.

Scalp and Face

These areas should be inspected and palpated for evidence of lacerations, bleeding, hematoma, tenderness, or deformity.

Often there is brisk bleeding from the scalp or face, which is best controlled by closing the bleeding lacerations with monofilament suture. Compressive wrapping is usually ineffective with arterial pumpers. Sutures are placed rapidly, without attempting to obtain the best cosmetic result; the wounds can be reclosed later with more attention to plastic technique. Brisk bleeding from the nasopharynx can be slowed by inserting a No. 20 Fr Foley catheter with a 30-ml balloon through one of the nostrils into the nasopharynx. When the balloon is inflated and traction applied to the catheter, the inflated balloon lodges in the nasopharynx, thus tamponading the bleeding.

Once brisk bleeding is controlled, the face and scalp are inspected and palpated for hematomas, nonbleeding lacerations, and bony deformities. Inspection of the scalp under matted bloody hair takes extra effort, but it is worthwhile to expose the skin in all areas in the search for lacerations.

Palpation of the facial bony prominences will detect most major facial fractures. The physician should palpate the orbital rims, zygomatic arches, mandible, and nose, and examine the maxilla for unstable fractures by grasping the upper incisors and attempting to rock the maxilla back and forth. Inspection of the face and skull in a patient with injuries more than 24 hours old may reveal a Battle's sign, or raccoon eyes, presumptive evidence for a basilar skull fracture.

Ears, Eyes, Nose, and Throat

The ears are examined for blood in the external canal, again presumptive evidence for a basilar skull fracture, whereas blood behind the tympanic membrane is pathognomonic evidence for a basilar skull fracture. Hearing can be roughly evaluated while talking to the patient.

The eyes are checked for extraocular movements: Limitation of upward gaze suggests a blowout fracture of the orbit; disconjugate gaze suggests neurologic damage. Pupils are checked for size and reactivity, both ipsilateral and conjugate. Fundoscopic examination should detect trauma to the lens, reveal retinal bleeding, and establish the presence or absence of retinal venous pulsations. Increasing intracranial pressure is presumed if pulsations are present initially and disappear during the observation period. Binocular vision can be checked by asking the patient to state the number of fingers displayed to him. Visual acuity can be assessed by asking the patient to read the label on a bottle of intravenous fluid.

The nose and throat are examined for adequacy of airway. Blood issuing from the nose or a retropharyngeal hematoma warns of possible airway obstruction. Clear fluid draining from the nose should make one suspect a cerebrospinal fluid leak, which, if present, is a pathognomonic sign of a basilar skull fracture. Fluid from the nose is determined to be cerebral spinal fluid and not merely catarrhal exudate if its glucose concentration approximates blood glucose levels.

The Neck

Distended neck veins suggest a cardiac cause of shock; flat veins suggest hypovolemia, and swelling indicates bleeding into one of the fascial planes of the neck. Such bleeding can obstruct the airway, and intubation may become difficult if the hematoma displaces the larynx; it is best to intubate these patients early, before laryngeal anatomy becomes excessively distorted.

Palpations may reveal a shifted trachea, suggesting a tension pneumothorax. Subcutaneous emphysema indicates a rupture somewhere in the tracheobronchial tree or, less likely, somewhere in the esophagus. Tenderness over the cervical spine suggests a fracture, especially if the patient has associated major maxillofacial trauma.

The Chest

We have previously addressed the initial chest examination, performed when the patient is first seen. As one is going through the "head to toe" assessment, any areas that were not checked previously should be evaluated. In particular, relative motion of the two hemithoraces should be noted. The paradox present with multiple rib fractures may be quite subtle and confined to a small area of the chest wall. Splinting should be carefully noted, as it will markedly restrict vital capacity if present. Any surface trauma should lead to careful palpation of the area to determine whether rib fractures are present. As noted previously, their diagnosis is predominantly clinical, not radiologic. The trachea should be carefully palpated relative to the sternal notch, and both hemithoraces should be percussed for a hyperresonant note denoting pneumothorax. Auscultation should be done briefly, and the heart tones particularly noted. In early tamponade, distant or muffled heart tones may be an early clue, and the apical beat will be reduced.

Abdomen and Lower Chest

The abdomen and lower chest should be considered as a single unit in the trauma patient. Some of the most commonly injured organs in blunt trauma, including the spleen, liver, and kidneys, lie in part under the lower ribs. Penetrating injuries of the lower chest can easily damage intra-abdominal organs, and perhaps the easiest injury to miss is retroperitoneal penetration of the colon from posterior or flank wounds.

Inspection is again most important; ecchymosis and abrasions suggest underlying organ damage. The location of penetrating injuries should be noted, but characterization of the nature of the injury should be tempered with the knowledge that it may be in error. Knife wounds large enough to admit the tip of a gloved finger should be gently explored with the finger, but the physician must remember that if the patient's muscles were in a different position at the time of injury they may cover up a penetrating tract, thus leading the physician to underestimate the depth of the wound. Gunshot wounds should be described but not labeled as exit or entrance wounds, since this is best left to the forensic pathologist to determine.

The contour of the abdomen and movement of the abdominal musculature in response to voluntary coughing or spontaneous ventilation are observed. Abdominal distention indicates intra-abdominal gas or bleeding. Muscle splinting indicates pain from muscular trauma or from irritation of the parietal peritoneum.

Percussion of the abdomen is mainly useful in detecting gastric distention, a condition that should be promptly treated by passage of a nasogastric tube. It also confirms irritation of the parietal peritoneum if the patient's muscles tighten in response to a light tap. A dull percussion note suggests intra-abdominal fluid—usually blood, occasionally urine.

Palpation of the abdomen can detect hematomas in the abdominal wall. Involuntary guarding indicates irritation of the parietal peritoneum.

Auscultation of the abdomen offers little in the trauma patient. A silent abdomen may only represent a temporary ileus after extra-abdominal trauma. Conversely, bowel sounds may be heard even in the presence of a ruptured or perforated viscus.

Pelvis and Rectum

If during initial resuscitation the patient was in deep shock and required passage of a Foley catheter, the perineum, genitalia, and rectum will have been examined quickly then. If not, they should be examined at this time. The perineum is inspected for lacerations and hematomas, the urethral meatus for blood, and the scrotum for hematomas, an indication of a retroperitoneal hematoma. Inspection of the vagina with a speculum is impractical in most trauma patients; however, the vagina can be palpated for deep lacerations, and blood in the vagina will be detected on the glove of the examining hand. Blood in the rectal vault will similarly be detected during rectal examination, which also allows assessment of sphincter tone and position of the prostate.

Vascular System

The neck, supraclavicular spaces, groin, and all four extremities are inspected. Large expanding hematomas, in conjunction with either a nearby penetrating injury or a broken bone, often indicate disruption of a major artery. All four extremities are inspected for adequacy of skin perfusion and temperature. Poor perfusion of all extremities suggests shock; poor perfusion of one with good perfusion of the others suggests an arterial injury.

The carotid, subclavian, brachial, radial, femoral, popliteal, dorsalis pedis, and posterior tibial pulses are palpated. Blood pressures are obtained in both arms to assess the subclavian arteries. The area around any penetrating injury is auscultated for the continuous to-and-fro bruit of an arteriovenous fistula. The presence of distal pulses does not rule out vascular injury.

Musculoskeletal System

In addition to noting gross deformities and hematomas, the skin overlying the musculoskeletal system is inspected for ecchymosis, abrasions, and lacerations. Grossly deformed limbs should be gently straightened and placed in a splint or in traction, especially if the limb is ischemic.

The purpose of palpation is to elicit tenderness or instability. The large bones are palpated first, paying particular attention to those underlying or near any abnormality detected by inspection (the head, cervical spine, and ribs have already been examined). The pelvis is palpated by pressing down on the pubis and by compressing the iliac wings toward one another; the clavicles and the bones of the extremities are palpated last.

Abnormalities will prompt the physician to obtain appropriate x-ray studies and, in some instances, initiate treatment. For example, continued movement of unstable fractures of large bones can cause pain, major tissue damage, major blood loss, and, occasionally, damage to adjacent neurovascular structures; such fractures should be immobilized to minimize these sequelae. Open fractures should be cultured, to pave the way for subsequent antibiotic administration as indicated, and temporarily covered with sterile dressings. Dislocations and fractures that have compromised the neurovascular supply to an extremity should be manipulated into better alignment in an attempt to reestablish flow.

Neurologic Re-evaluation

The second neurologic examination expands on the first. The character and adequacy of the patient's ventilation are noted. The patient's mental status is described by using the categories of the Glasgow coma scale. The eyes are described as opening spontaneously, to speech, to pain, or not at all. Verbal response is described as oriented, confused, frankly inappropriate, incomprehensible, or none.

The necessary cranial nerve information is extrapolated from the ears, eyes, nose, and throat examination, but particular note is made of the presence or absence of vision, pupil size and activity, and extraocular movements.

The patient is assessed for spontaneous purposeful motor function, purposeful reaction to voice command, purposeful response to pain, withdrawal from pain, nonpurposeful flexion to pain, nonpurposeful extension to pain, and no response. Deep tendon reflexes and a sensory examination are not usually necessary at this time, unless the preceding examination indicates spinal cord injury, in which case they should be evaluated.

As with the initial neurologic examination, the primary purpose here is to establish baselines for later evaluations. Any deterioration in neurologic status should prompt a more thorough evaluation, including computerized tomography of the head.

A secondary purpose is to recognize symptoms and signs of increasing intracranial pressures so that treatment can begin. The intubated patient should be hyperventilated to an arterial PCO_2 of approximately 30 mmHg. Mannitol may be given after consultation with the neurosurgeon.

INITIAL TREATMENT

We have already outlined several points in patient assessment where a critical injury might necessitate immediate therapy. These principally relate to major airway or ventilatory problems, or significant external bleeding. If these are not present, the examiner has now completed a thorough but brief evaluation, taking no more than 2 to 3 minutes, and should institute appropriate therapy.

Airway problems that are not severe enough to require immediate intubation, but nevertheless are significant, should be reassessed every few minutes. In general, the tendency is to wait too long to intubate patients, and it is generally true that when they are in obvious distress or when respiratory rates exceed 35/minute, intubation is indicated. Injuries that result in swelling or hematoma in the tongue and floor of the mouth are particularly hazardous, as they cause airway obstruction early and render the patient extremely difficult if not impossible to intubate. It is our strong preference to obtain continuous presence of an anesthesiologist with any patient who exhibits any respiratory distress or major thoracic injury, even if the patient is not thought to need intubation at the time. The initial 1 to 2 hours after injury provide many surprises, and failure to closely monitor airway problems frequently leads to preventable mortality, particularly when patients get sequestered in radiology suites for extended periods.

The second major intervention needed for respiratory problems is tube thoracostomy. Occasionally, unilateral or bilateral chest tubes should be inserted prior to chest roentgenography if the patient is in marked distress and is likely to have a pneumothorax or hemothorax. Normally, however, there is time to get the chest roentgenogram, which should be upright if possible to better define intrapleural fluid. If this shows hemo- or pneumothorax, a large-bore (No. 36 or No. 40 Fr) straight siliconized tube should be inserted on the appropriate side(s). In trauma patients, the tube should *always* be inserted at or above the nipple level between the anterior and posterior axillary folds, and as it is inserted, it should be directed posteriorly and superiorly until it contacts the posterior mediastinum. Insertion of the tube below the nipple line will occasionally lead to transdiaphragmatic insertion into the spleen or liver, as the dome of the diaphragm at end expiration is only a couple of centimeters below nipple level. Insertion of chest tubes in the second anterior interspace should also be condemned. One of the most persistent myths in medicine is that an anterior chest tube is necessary for the evacuation of pneumothoraces. This is totally false, as the lung retracts equally from anterior and posterior surfaces when a pneumothorax is present; hence, a posteriorly placed tube will evacuate air and blood and is universally effective in trauma. In addition, the anterior second interspace tube is difficult to place, as it traverses breast and pectoralis major muscle, whereas the lateral tube traverses only the serratus anterior and intercostals, and enters the chest where the ribs are most easily spread.

The third therapeutic intervention is placement of intravenous catheters. The urgency, size, and number of lines is dictated by the degree of shock and apparent rate of bleeding. Patients who are hemodynamically stable, with no signs of shock and apparently minimal injury, need only a percutaneous catheter of approximately 18 gauge size. If they are hemodynamically stable, but more major injury is suspected, a large-bore percutaneous line, either No. 16 or No. 14, is started. If shock is present to any degree, a large-bore percutaneous catheter plus a cutdown is placed. If shock is profound and injuries are massive, two or three cutdowns are placed.

When doing cutdowns, we prefer the saphenous vein at the ankle for rapid access, and use a No. 8 feeding tube or cut-off IV extension tubing as the intravenous catheter. The second most favored site is the antecubital crease, where either the basilic or cephalic vein is available and also accepts large catheters. As a third choice, we would use the saphenous vein at the fossa ovalis, and thread the catheter into the femoral vein. The latter two sites offer the advantage that the catheter can be threaded centrally to obtain central venous pressure readings, but they are more time-consuming to place.

We prefer not to use percutaneous puncture of central veins, such as the internal jugular and subclavian, as there are several disadvantages.

First, they are usually collapsed in the hypovolemic patient and therefore harder to puncture blindly. Second, the size of the catheter that can be introduced is smaller than one that is introduced via cutdown. Finally, the risk of pneumothorax is significant—probably at least 10 percent—and the last thing one needs in a critically ill patient is an unnecessary iatrogenic complication.

The need for multiple large-bore IV access in the rapidly bleeding patient cannot be overemphasized. Once the patient is on the operating table with drapes in place, it is too late to get rapid access. If the patient has a massive bleeding site in the abdomen, he will predictably "crash" when the abdomen is initially opened and decompressed, and it usually takes a few minutes to identify and control the bleeding site. Unless the anesthetist can pump rapidly during this time (~ 1000 ml every 5 minutes), the patient may arrest from hypovolemia, no matter how controllable the injury may ultimately be. This problem must be anticipated in advance, as it is too late to start putting in lines after the abdomen is opened. One of our residents recently summed up our point of view in this area with the statement: "No one ever died of too many lines."

The next question to be addressed is what resuscitative fluid to use after the IV lines are placed. Initial choices, prior to blood availability, are balanced salt solutions alone or in conjunction with colloid solutions. Either can be used to adequately resuscitate patients if given in appropriate quantity. A great deal of debate has revolved around the potential detrimental effects of one or the other on pulmonary function. Based on our experience and a thorough review of the literature, we do not feel that there is any difference in the pulmonary effects of balanced salt solutions vs. colloids, as long as each is given to the same hemodynamic end point.

The major difference in these solutions is economic, as balanced salt solutions typically cost about $2.00 per liter, while plasma or a plasmalike substitute typically costs well over $100.00 per liter. If both produce equivalent effects, it makes little sense to use the much more expensive product.

There is a difference in resuscitation effects of the solutions, which has been shown in multiple studies. This relates to relative intravascular filling effects, which is greater with the colloid solution. Balanced salt solutions equilibrate rapidly with the interstitial space and hence have a greater volume of distribution than colloids. As a result, it requires about 2 to 3 times as much balanced salt solution as colloid solution for equivalent intravascular filling. If one gives this extra amount, however, the hemodynamic effects are equivalent, and there are no ill effects from the extra salt solution other than increased peripheral edema. As mentioned before, it has been well shown in clinical studies that there are no harmful effects on the lung.

Whichever fluid is chosen, it should be administered to the patient in sufficient quantity to rapidly correct his intravascular volume status to normal. This will be evidenced by the disappearance of any signs of shock, the return of vital signs to normal, and a urine output of 0.5 to 1 ml/kg/hr. In the initial therapy of the trauma patient, aggressive fluid administration is mandatory to restore physiology to normal. The correction of shock should not require more than 10 to 15 minutes after the patient's arrival at the Emergency Department. If shock cannot be immediately corrected, or if it recurs after initial correction, this is the best evidence one has for ongoing blood loss and the need for definitive surgery.

The second major component needed is, of course, red cells, to provide oxygen-carrying capacity. We prefer to give sufficient red cells to maintain hematocrit around 30 percent, though much lower levels are usually well tolerated in previously healthy young patients. Either packed cells or whole blood can be used for this, but our preference is for whole blood, since it has much lower viscosity and is more easily and quickly transfused in the acute emergency. When crossmatching is not possible, we prefer type-specific blood, though O-positive or O-negative universal donor blood is also used in many centers and appears to have minimal risk.

One situation should be noted that calls for maintenance of hematocrit at near-normal levels, and certainly above 35 percent. This is the patient who has a low relatively fixed cardiac output because of prior disease or myocardial injury. The major physiologic compensation for anemia is increased cardiac output; if a patient is unable to accomplish this, he is at special risk from a low hematocrit. This must be considered in the elderly patient, the patient with known heart disease, or the patient with a major myocardial contusion.

Emergency department management related to specific organ systems will not be further discussed here, but will be covered in the individual chapters.

DEFINITIVE DIAGNOSIS AND CARE

The principal diagnostic studies in the Emergency Department are radiographic; laboratory testing has relatively little to contribute other than arterial blood gases to assess respiratory dysfunction, hematocrit to assess blood loss, and serum amylase to assess pancreatic injury. Unless there is a prior history to suggest a problem, electrolytes, liver function studies, and clotting studies are rarely abnormal and, in most situations, are not indicated.

The Chest

The most common radiographic study done, and the one that is essential in all patients, is the chest roentgenogram. There is virtually never a reason to delay or bypass this, short of cardiac arrest and emergency department thoracotomy.

The reasons are obvious: The chest roentgenogram gives the greatest immediate information about intrathoracic injury and allows pneumothorax, hemothorax, rib fractures, mediastinal injury, and sometimes diaphragmatic injury to be quickly defined.

The patient who is in shock, but has no external source of bleeding, must be bleeding into fracture sites, or into the chest, or into the abdomen. Examination will disclose any fractures and associated hematomas, and so these can be directly assessed. The chest film provides a reliable guide to intrathoracic blood loss. If the chest film is normal and there are no fractures, but the patient is hypovolemic, one knows that the bleeding source is in the abdomen.

The Abdomen

In contrast to the chest roentgenogram, a plain film of the abdomen usually does not contribute much to the therapeutic management of trauma patients. On the other hand, intravenous pyelography, excretory urography, cystography, and urethrography are the mainstays for preliminary evaluation of injuries to the genitourinary tract.

An intravenous pyelogram should be obtained in any stable patient with hematuria defined as more than 100 red blood cells per high-powered field in an unspun specimen or, even in the absence of hematuria, in a stable patient with severe blunt trauma or with penetrating injuries near a kidney or ureter. The film is taken by intravenously administering to the adult patient 100 ml of contrast material early during the course of resuscitation. The first plain film of the abdomen usually gives most of the information that will be needed.

A cystogram should be obtained in any patient with hematuria or severe lower abdominal or pelvic trauma, particularly the inebriated patient with lower abdominal blunt trauma. The procedure is done by infusing by gravity 150 ml of contrast material through a Foley catheter into the bladder, after which an anteroposterior view and either an oblique or lateral view of the bladder are taken.

A urethrogram should be taken in any patient with a suspected urethral tear, or in any male patient with severe pelvic trauma. The urethrogram is obtained by gently injecting 30 ml of contrast material into the urethral meatus. If a Foley catheter is already in place, some detail of the urethra can be obtained by injecting contrast material into the urethra around the catheter.

Lower Chest and Abdomen

Computerized tomography (CT) of the abdomen can help to evaluate hemodynamically stable patients who have been subjected to blunt trauma to the lower chest or abdomen, especially patients with equivocal indications for celiotomy or patients who are difficult to evaluate because of obtundation or spinal cord damage. CT not only detects intra- and retroperitoneal bleeding, but also identifies the damaged organ. CT is most accurate in assessing the organs most likely to be damaged with blunt trauma, i.e., liver, spleen, kidneys, and pancreas. It is also accurate in detecting retroduodenal air or edema associated with duodenal disruptions and in detecting free intraperitoneal air associated with rupture of the small or large intestine.

The indications for peritoneal lavage in the stable patient are the same as those for computerized tomography of the abdomen: equivocal findings on abdominal examination or neurologic abnormalities that preclude abdominal examination. To perform a lavage, the bladder is first emptied by passing a Foley catheter. The skin below the umbilicus is infiltrated with a local anesthetic, and an incision is made through the skin and down to fascia; a catheter should be inserted through the fascia into the peritoneal cavity. Some 1000 ml of normal saline is infused into the peritoneal cavity, allowed to equilibrate, and then drained off. The lavage is considered technically adequate if more than 500 ml is recovered. A red blood cell count greater than $50,000/mm^3$ or a white blood cell count greater than $500/mm^3$ suggests injury to the abdominal viscera.

The Head

CT of the head should be obtained in any hemodynamically stable patient with a suspected depressed skull fracture or severe neurologic deficit and in any stable or even moderately unstable patient whose neurologic status is worsening. It is definitive for diagnosis of depressed fractures, epidural hematomas, subdural hematomas, intracerebral hematomas, and cerebral edema.

Not every obtunded inebriated patient needs computerized tomography, so long as no other neurologic deficit is noted. However, if obtundation persists for more than a few hours, CT should be done—drunkenness should lighten with time, not remain the same, and it should certainly not worsen.

The Spine

All hemodynamically stable patients with major craniofacial trauma or with physical signs of a cervical spine injury should also have x-ray studies of the cervical spine. The most important film to obtain is the lateral view (the seventh cervical vertebra must be visualized, since it is involved in many cervical fractures), which will demonstrate misalignment in most patients with an unstable spine. The anterior or posterior borders of the spinal canal may be out of line, the atlas and odontoid may be displaced, or the vertebral bodies may be compressed or fractured. The lateral film may also indicate the need for more views, such as odontoid, arteroposterior, oblique, or flexion-extension films.

In any patient with major deceleration injury or significant findings near the spine, x-ray examination of the thoracic and lumbar spine must also be considered. Particularly if there are calcaneal fractures, a compression fracture of the lumbar spine should be ruled out.

Vascular System

A thoracic aortogram should be obtained in any hemodynamically stable patient who has a suspected disruption of the thoracic aorta or of the great vessels. Suspicion should be aroused by a decreased blood pressure in the left arm, by a wide mediastinum, or by obliteration of the aortic knob on chest roentgenogram.

In the stable patient, selective arteriograms may be used to evaluate suspected arterial injuries in the neck and extremities. Suspicion should be aroused by a penetrating injury near an artery or by a hematoma, bruit, decreased distal pulses, diminished peripheral perfusion, or compromised neurologic function associated with a penetrating injury. Patients with severe blunt trauma to the region of the knee dislocation are also suspect. If arteriograms are not obtained in patients with suspected injuries to large arteries (carotids, brachials, femoropopliteals), the vessels should be explored. Presence of distal pulses in no way rules out the need for arteriography when arterial injury is suspected. Approximately 15 percent of patients with repairable arterial injury have relatively normal distal pulses.

FURTHER CARE

After patients have been evaluated according to the foregoing sequence, one should have a complete picture of their knowns or probable injuries. At this point definitive management, either in the operating room or by other means, can be planned. As we have frequently noted, acute emergencies may develop during the course of evaluation, necessitating immediate therapy of one type or another. The first few hours after arrival are always the most critical, and patient monitoring must be intensive until stability and lack of serious injury are proved. As patients are evaluated, one should always try to match the known sources of blood loss with the degree of hypovolemia or need for volume replacement manifested by the patient. If these do not match, one should retain a high index of suspicion for intra-abdominal bleeding, as large volumes may be hidden there without evident external signs.

Finally, it should be emphasized that whenever one can reasonably conclude that there is a high likelihood of intra-abdominal bleeding, the patient should immediately be taken to the operating room for laparotomy, and should not undergo more tests. There is a strong tendency to do excessive testing to document the need for surgery, when adequate indications are already present clinically. The patient with unexplained volume loss or peritoneal signs needs a laparotomy, not a CT scan or peritoneal lavage, to document the problem further.

The major preventable mortality which occurs in trauma today is related to failure to aggressively evaluate and treat the patient. It is safe to say that far more patients have died unnecessarily because of the lack of a laparotomy than have died because of it. As a result, we believe it is an appropriate closing note to emphasize the need for laparotomy whenever there is probable injury. Delay in treating most intra-abdominal conditions substantially increases the morbidity. Doing the occasional negative laparotomy should not be a cause for criticism, but unnecessary death due to failure or delay in doing so should always be.

ANESTHETIC MANAGEMENT

Richard B. Weiskopf, M.D.
H. Barrie Fairley, M.B., B.S.

The purpose of this chapter is to familiarize the reader with the role of the anesthesiologist as it is practiced in our trauma center, to acquaint the non-anesthetist clinician with the clinical problems and therapeutic options faced on the "other side of the screen," and to provide a brief framework for anesthetists who only occasionally are required to anesthetize trauma victims.

ANESTHESIA FOR MINOR TRAUMA

Trauma that does not require surgery of a major body cavity (abdomen, thorax, cranium) and has neither caused significant blood loss nor created other major alterations of systemic physiologic function may be considered to be minor from surgical and physiologic perspectives. Occasionally, the risks attendant with the administration of an anesthetic may be substantial. These risks include the management of the patient's airway and the consequences of any important coincidental disease(s), particularly if inadequately treated. The required anesthetic techniques and agents differ between the elective (prepared) patient and the emergency patient with, for example, uncontrolled hypertension, cardiac failure, or fluid and electrolyte disturbance. Therefore, the risks of proceeding immediately with administration of an anesthetic must be balanced with the urgency of the need for surgical correction. There will be times when an interim period is inappropriate (e.g., severe, multiple trauma), and there may be occasions when surgery may be forgone (e.g., minor tendon laceration in a respiratory or cardiac cripple).

Problems surrounding airway management are the single largest cause of anesthetic morbidity and mortality. All anesthetic and surgical plans must take full cognizance of this problem. Trauma patients must be regarded as having a "full stom-ach," i.e., the stomach may contain significant amounts of food or fluid, or both. Patients who have been traumatized frequently give unreliable histories with respect to most recent alimentation. In addition, trauma may decelerate or halt gastrointestinal processes. Options for handling this problem are discussed later in this chapter. The risk inherent in proceeding with anesthesia and surgery with a patient with a "full stomach" may vary with the patient and the injury; no rule can be given, other than the need for careful evaluation of the relative merits of delaying or proceeding with surgery. *The option of regional anesthesia* (to be discussed) *does not guarantee airway protection, and thus does not solve the problem.*

Choice of Anesthesia for Minor Trauma

The surgical site of many minor injuries may be adequately anesthetized by local infiltration, a regional anesthetic, or block of peripheral nerves with a local anesthetic; or by a general anesthetic. Available data fail to show a difference in mortality between recipients of general and regional anesthesia. Other considerations frequently narrow the options.

Airway

Regional anesthesia is not a satisfactory solution for dealing with the hazard of the full stomach. Accidental intravascular injection of local anesthetics, cuff failure during an intravenous regional anesthetic (Bier block), or the use of excessive amounts of local anesthetic (to be discussed) may cause unconsciousness and convulsions with resultant emesis or regurgitation and subsequent aspiration.

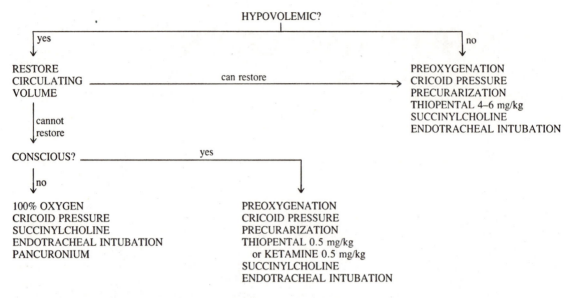

Figure 1 Scheme for induction of anesthesia in victims of major trauma.

Because of the potential for airway infringement, with the exception of the smallest, most superficial lacerations, no injury of the face or neck that requires surgical correction should be regarded as a "minor" anesthetic procedure (to be discussed).

Use of Local Anesthetics

All local anesthetics can achieve toxic blood concentrations. The plasma concentration achieved depends on the site of injection, the amount of drug injected, the presence or absence of a vasoconstrictor mixed with the local anesthetic, and the patient's size, blood volume, hepatic function, and general physical status. Table 1 lists commonly used local anesthetics and their maximal doses in an otherwise healthy, fit patient. *As a patient's physical state deteriorates, the maximal safe dose of local anesthetic decreases.* The table must be considered a *guideline.* Following various types of regional anesthesia, plasma concentrations of local anesthetics vary, in descending order, after intercostal nerve block, epidural block, axillary block, and subcutaneous infiltration. In general, toxicity of local anesthetics is additive; as maximal dosage is neared, switching to the use of another local anesthetic does not offer any advantage. The ad-

dition of a potent vasoconstrictor (epinephrine 1:200,000) decreases blood flow to the site of injection and, thereby, uptake by the blood of the anesthetic, thus decreasing plasma concentration and prolonging the neural blockade. Table 1 assumes that epinephrine 1:200,000 is added to the local anesthetic. However, it is pointed out that as relatively large volumes of solution are injected, the patient may exhibit signs and symptoms of excessive epinephrine administration. If a vasoconstrictor is not added to the local anesthetic (for example, because of concern of resultant tachycardia or hypertension in a patient with heart disease), the maximal amount of local anesthetic agent should be reduced by at least one third. The addition of epinephrine to the local anesthetic is also valuable as a diagnostic tool providing early indication of an intravascular injection. Three milliliters of the local anesthetic containing 1:200,000 epinephrine are injected. Failure to increase the heart rate and an absence of manifestations of intravenous administration of anesthetic in the ensuing 1 to 2 minutes signify that the drugs were not administered intravascularly, and the remainder of the injection at that site may proceed. The practitioner is referred to texts of regional anesthesia for descriptions of techniques and complications of individual nerve blocks, blocks of plexi, and major regional blocks.

TABLE 1   Commonly Used Local Anesthetics*

Local Anesthetic	Maximal Safe Dose (mg/kg)	Adequate Concentration for Subcutaneous Infiltration (%)	Maximal ml of Adequate Concentration in 70-kg Patient†
Chloroprocaine	20	1	140
Cocaine‡	2	0.25	84
Bupivacaine	3	1	105
Procaine	15	0.5	100
Lidocaine	7	0.1	140
Tetracaine	2		

Amounts assume a healthy fit patient and addition of epinephrine 1:200,000 to local anesthetic (except cocaine).

†Each 20 ml of these solutions contain 0.1 mg epinephrine; subcutaneous infiltration of 60 ml of solution may result in signs and symptoms of administration of excessive quantities of epinephrine.

‡Cocaine is not recommended for subcutaneous infiltration. It is included in this table because of its usefulness as a topical mucosal anesthetic.

ANESTHESIA FOR MAJOR TRAUMA

Initial Evaluation and Management

Airway and Gas Exchange

All seriously traumatized patients should receive oxygen during transport to, and upon arrival in, the emergency room, because many physiologic sequelae of trauma result in arterial hypoxemia while the patient is breathing air. The chest should be auscultated bilaterally, and if there is any question of a possible chest injury, radiographs should be obtained immediately. Hemothoraces or pneumothoraces should be relieved by placement of large-bore chest tubes. If systemic arterial blood pressure is unobtainable, the trachea should be intubated immediately and the lungs ventilated with 100 percent oxygen as part of the initial emergency room resuscitation sequence (rapid intravenous fluid administration and, if necessary, thoracotomy and aortic cross-clamping). Fixed, dilated pupils do not necessarily indicate irreversible central nervous system damage and do not contraindicate early aggressive management. If an esophageal obturator airway has been previously inserted, it should not be removed until the airway is protected with a cuffed endotracheal tube, because of the likelihood of regurgitation of gastric contents and the possibility of subsequent aspiration. Masks attached to esophageal obturators may be removed by squeezing components at the mask orifice. Patients who are markedly hypotensive despite rapid intravenous infusion also require early intubation to support gas exchange and protect the airway, since cerebral ischemia commonly causes muscular flaccidity and regur-gitation of gastric contents. It is difficult to time endotracheal intubation of an awake, hypotensive patient in the emergency room; the decision requires experience and judgment. Intubation frequently can be accomplished without drugs, or with the aid of topical anesthesia alone. If anesthesia is necessary for intubation of the trachea, we use a ketamine-succinylcholine sequence (to be described).

Facial Fractures and Upper Airway Injuries

Airway assessment is the first priority in this group of patients. Massive facial injuries may result in nasal obstruction, oropharyngeal edema, or hematomas of such magnitude that immediate tracheotomy or cricothyroidotomy is necessary in the emergency room. In all other cases, the rate of swelling in the upper airway must be evaluated. The principle is to ensure the maintenance of a patent airway and to avoid limitation of available techniques by "sudden" airway obstruction. In patients with major fractures of the mandible and maxilla (LeFort III) in whom massive edema has yet to occur, oral intubation is preferred and, if required, is usually easily accomplished. In the most obtunded, the trachea may be intubated without anesthesia. If this situation is misjudged, vomiting may occur and strong suction with a large-bore sucker must be immediately available. Blind nasal intubation following major facial injury is discouraged because of the hazard of potential false passages into nasal sinuses and the cranial vault and the possibility of dislodging loose bone and tissue. It is unusual for an alert, cooperative patient with facial injuries to require intubation in the emergency department. However, if endotracheal intubation is necessary, the options for its accomplishment following direct laryngoscopy are (1) topical anesthesia of the tongue and hypopharynx by alternately spraying with a local anesthetic and advancing the laryngoscope; or (2) general anesthesia preceded by preoxygenation, cricoid pressure, thiopental or ketamine, and succinylcholine. Fractures of the mandible alone usually do not cause airway or intubation difficulties when the larynx is normal.

Injuries of the larynx may cause rapid respiratory obstruction and require immediate tracheotomy. In less urgent situations, a history of trauma to the head and neck, stridor, hoarseness, and crepitus in the neck are all suggestive of a possibility of laryngeal injury. Deceleration is the most frequent cause of a fractured larynx, which is often associated with a fracture of C6 or C7. Three useful tests for evaluation of laryngeal fracture are (1) a check of the ability of the patient to make a high-pitched "e" sound, which requires mobile cricoarytenoid joints, normal tense cords, and functioning intrinsic laryngeal neuromuscular mechanisms; (2) indirect laryngoscopy; and (3) radiography of the larynx, especially a computerized tomographic (CT) scan. If uncertainty exists, fiberoptic laryngoscopy may be performed under topical anesthesia. If laryngeal injury is suspected, all possible information should be accumulated prior to induction of general anesthesia. Attempts at endotracheal intubation may cause mucosal stripping and bleeding, displacement of fractured cartilage into the airway lumen, and laryngeal obstruction.

When a fractured larynx is present, laryngofissure and repair of mucosal lacerations and cartilage fractures are frequently carried out. Classically, a tracheotomy under local anesthesia is performed first. Alternatively, endotracheal intubation through the glottis may be attempted, but only in the presence of the most benign preoperative findings and when laryngeal visualization is excellent. If a tracheotomy is necessary in an uncooperative child, a small dose of ketamine may be used as a supplement to local anesthesia; however, airway obstruction may ensue.

In all cases of possible airway compromise, when it is uncertain whether a patent airway can be maintained, that is, if airway obstruction could occur, the procedures should be carried out in an operating room with equipment and personnel ready for immediate tracheotomy.

Head Injuries

A high percentage of unconscious patients with recent head injuries require intubation for one or more of the following indications: (1) to alleviate airway obstruction, (2) to prevent aspiration, or (3) to ensure hyperventilation for the purpose of minimizing intracranial pressure. If it is decided not to intubate the trachea of a patient who has a fresh head injury, this individual must be observed closely; personnel able to intubate the patient's trachea must be readily available. Sudden rapid deterioration occurs commonly within the first few hours and therefore a single evaluation is not sufficient. When possible, cervical films should be obtained prior to intubation, although, in our experience, cervical fractures are quite rare in patients who require intubation for a head injury. If it is suspected that the neck is unstable, a cervical collar is placed, and oral intubation may be attempted using an endotracheal tube with the distal 3 to 5 cm bent in the shape of a "hockey stick," by means of a lubricated stylet. If oral intubation appears technically straightforward, we do not hesitate to use muscle relaxants with application of cricoid pressure, following a period of preoxygenation. During laryngoscopy and intubation, the surgeon should hold the patient's head applying axial traction, and warn of any impending excessive extension. Alternatives to direct laryngoscopy are blind nasal intubation (which may be easy in the hyperventilating patient) or, if the former cannot be accomplished, and time permits, intubation over a fiberoptic laryngoscope or fiberoptic bronchoscope. If all else fails, tracheotomy may be necessary.

Barbiturates, other hypnotics, or muscle relaxants may be required to control restlessness, either to permit CT scanning or angiography or to prevent an increase in intracranial pressure owing to straining caused by the irritation of an endotracheal tube. The resultant decreased ability to conduct a neurologic assessment should not be an overriding consideration. Either a surgical decompression is indicated by the radiologic findings or, if not, a catheter may be inserted to accurately monitor intracranial pressure.

Fluid Resuscitation

In any patient in whom a major injury is suspected, at least two large-bore intravenous cannulae should be inserted, one of which should be located centrally (superior vena cava or right atrium). These cannulae should be at least 16 gauge and preferably larger. It is not unusual to need 3 or 4 large-bore cannulae to rapidly and adequately restore circulating blood volume of a major trauma victim. One should not depend on lower extremity lines for infusion in patients in whom disruption of iliac veins or the inferior vena cava is a possibility. Placement of a central venous catheter is essential to properly manage the fluid volume resuscitation. A catheter should be placed in the bladder in all patients; however, for many reasons, urine output should not be the primary guide for fluid management. Patients who have decreased skin perfusion with resultant pallor and coolness, narrow pulse pressure, tachycardia, and orthostatic hypotension, are likely to have lost in excess of 20 to 25 percent of their blood volume (normal blood volume in the adult is approximately 75 ml per kg body weight). Cardiac output will have decreased in approximate proportion to blood loss. Deterioration of mental status indicates a more severe loss of blood volume, usually in excess of 40 percent. Vigorous fluid resuscitation must be started. To help keep track of infused volume, it is useful to sequentially number each new bag of fluid. Blood volume should be restored so that central venous pressure measures several millimeters of mercury. We use a balanced salt solution for this purpose. Three or more liters may be required if the previously described signs are present. If a pneumatic suit (G or MAST suit) has been inflated around the victim's abdomen and lower limbs, a variable but potentially large amount of intravascular volume may have been shifted centrally. The measured central venous pressure then is not an accurate reflection of total intravascular volume. With careful observation of hemodynamic status, the suit should be deflated one compartment at a time, only after volume replacement has started and the central pressure is at least 6 mm Hg, and when immediate surgery can be performed if necessary.

Premedication Agents

Premedication should not be used routinely. Sedatives, hypnotics, and narcotics should be administered to hypovolemic patients only with extreme caution. Agents without effective antidotes should be avoided. Although narcotics are effective in relieving pain and anxiety, they dilate peripheral blood vessels and may produce further hypotension with resultant cerebral ischemia, adding to the sedative effect of the narcotic. This may result in regurgitation of gastric contents and aspiration. Intramuscular cimetidine is sometimes advocated as a means of decreasing gastric acidity in emergency surgery patients. This is not universal practice and we do not rely on this approach; nor do we rely on metoclopramide to speed gastric emptying.

Operating Room Management

Preparation of Equipment

In order to provide expeditious care for major trauma at a moment's notice, a completely ready operating room should be available at all times. The anesthesiologist should have the following recently checked equipment in place: (1) anesthesia machine; (2) volume-controlled ventilator, with appropriate values preset; (3) suction; (4) laryngoscope with spare blades and endotracheal tubes with stylets; (5) appropriate drugs (pancuronium, succinylcholine, intravenous induction agent) drawn into labeled syringes; (6) two intravenous infusion sets with pumps and blood warmers, filled with balanced salt solutions; (7) material required for placement of an arterial line; (8) warming blanket and a device to provide heated humidified inspired gases; (9) defibrillator with internal and external paddles; (10) calibrated equipment to monitor arterial blood pressure, central venous pressure, neuromuscular blockade, temperature, and electrocardiograph.

Choice of Anesthetic (Regional or General)

For the more major injuries, particularly in the presence of cardiovascular instability or injuries of the abdomen or thorax, we prefer general anesthesia to regional. Spinal anesthesia does not permit control of ventilation, and the resultant sympathetic block abolishes important homeostatic responses to hypovolemia. Additionally, in patients with abdominal injuries, preoperative uncertainty regarding the extent of the necessary exploration and procedures precludes limited block levels. On the other hand, infiltration anesthesia or regional blocks can be extremely useful for the management of the more minor peripheral injuries, provided attention is paid to the maximum safe dose of the selected local anesthetic agent relative to the patient's body size and physical status (already discussed).

Induction and Maintenance of General Anesthesia (see Fig. 1)

During induction of anesthesia, aspiration of gastric contents into the lungs may follow passive regurgitation or active vomiting. When diaphragmatic relaxation occurs secondary to cerebral ischemia, heavy sedation, or anesthesia, passive regurgitation may occur as a result of the difference in pressure between the abdomen and the thorax. Several hours of delay in scheduling surgery, and administration of metoclopramide may decrease the probability of food remaining in the stomach, but this is never totally reliable and may be contraindicated by the urgency of the injury. A low gastric acidity and/or an empty stomach cannot be assumed for extended periods following trauma. To prevent gastric contents from reaching the pharynx and resulting in aspiration, the following steps should be taken:

1. In all cases of intestinal obstruction, ileus, or gastroduodenal perforation or bleeding, a nasogastric sump tube should be placed and the stomach aspirated immediately prior to induction (although this does not ensure an empty stomach).

2. The probable ease of laryngoscopy and oral intubation should be assessed. If an extraordinarily difficult laryngoscopy and endotracheal intubation are anticipated, alternative approaches should be considered (to be discussed).

3. Prior to proceeding further, powerful suction must be available.

4. To minimize the increase in intragastric pressure subsequent to administration of succinylcholine, a small dose of a nondepolarizing muscle relaxant is administered (e.g., 4.5 mg d-tubocurarine chloride, or 1.5 mg pancuronium) 3 to 5 minutes before the succinylcholine. The patient is given 100 percent oxygen to breathe by use of a tight-fitting face mask. This preoxygenation is carried out for at least 3 minutes of quiet breathing, time permitting. If time does not permit, four or five maximum inspirations may suffice. Anteroposterior pressure is then applied with two fingers on the cricoid cartilage (compressing the upper esophagus against the cervical vertebral column) (Sellick maneuver), and a rapidly acting hypnotic and muscle relaxant (usually succinylcholine) are administered intravenously.

Laryngoscopy, tracheal intubation, cuff inflation, and checks of tube location are carried out before cricoid pressure is removed. Endotracheal tube placement is confirmed by observation and auscultation of the chest, by absence of sounds in the stomach in response to positive pressure ventilation, and by palpation of the endotracheal tube cuff between the cricoid and the suprasternal notch upon injection into the cuff of an additional 5 to 10 ml of air. If intubation cannot be accomplished following the aforementioned sequence of full preoxygenation, precurarization, cricoid pressure, a single induction dose of an appropriate intravenous induction agent, and succinylcholine, and if the patient is not grossly hypotensive, the actions of the intravenous agent and succinylcholine should be allowed to terminate (approximately 5 minutes) and the patient allowed to awaken. Alternate approaches can then be considered. If laryngoscopy and intubation are expected to be difficult, other options are, in order of preference, awake intubation (nasally or orally) following topical anesthesia (if necessary with a fiberoptic laryngoscope) or a tracheotomy under local anesthesia. In many acute injuries of the jaw and neck, in which the state of the pharynx is in doubt, we prefer direct laryngoscopy and oral intubation as a first step. Then, if nasal intubation is required, a nasal tube may be advanced under direct vision, with the larynx in full view and the airway protected. This permits full evaluation of the injury prior to nasal intubation.

Whenever possible, hypovolemia is corrected before the patient is transported to the operating room and anesthesia is induced. If correction is not possible because of the nature and extent of the injuries (that is, the rate of hemorrhage exceeds maximal capability to restore intravascular volume), it may be necessary to induce "anesthesia" in the hypovolemic patient. If the patient is unconscious or severely obtunded, intubation of the trachea should be accomplished without drugs or with neuromuscular blocking agents alone. If the patient is conscious despite being uncorrectably hypovolemic, some mode of anesthesia should be provided prior to initiation of surgery.

In the presence of hemorrhagic hypotension and decreased venous return, no anesthetic technique or agent reliably maintains homeostatic mechanisms and hemodynamic function. This is true not only of those anesthetic agents which during normovolemia result in cardiovascular depression, but also those agents which during normovolemia may result in cardiovascular stimulation (e.g., ketamine). Very small doses of ketamine (0.35 to 0.7 mg per kg intravenously) can be useful for inducing "anesthesia" in hypovolemic, hypotensive conscious patients. In a hypovolemic patient, the indirect stimulatory responses may not be elicited, and ketamine's direct action of myocardial depression may result in cardiovascular decompensation. The maximal depressant effect is seen 5 minutes after administration. The anesthetist should expect cardiovascular decompensation following administration of any anesthetic agent to a hypovolemic patient. Once intubated, the patient should be mechanically ventilated to free the anesthesiologist's hands. Evidence is lacking that either respiratory acidosis or alkalosis is beneficial during massive hypovolemia. We therefore attempt to maintain normocapnia, which has the added advantage of not confusing interpretation of acid-base status.

Following induction of anesthesia, only oxygen and neuromuscular blocking agents are administered until the hemodynamic situation is stabilized and systemic blood pressure rises to a mean of 50 torr. At that point cerebral perfusion should be adequate, and it is then appropriate to consider the administration of other anesthetic agents. The goal is to provide analgesia or amnesia with minimal cardiovascular disturbance. Since the clinical situation is still in great flux and conditions may deteriorate, in principle, agents that are easily removed or whose actions are readily terminated should be used. Cyclopropane and ether are contraindicated because of the risk of explosion in a setting with a multiplicity of personnel and electrical equipment. Furthermore, cyclopropane decreases survival time in shocked dogs. Halothane, enflurane, or isoflurane may be cautiously added in very small concentrations (for example, 0.1 percent) to the background of 100 percent oxygen and the cardiovascular effects noted. All the inhalation agents are direct myocardial depressants and may result in significantly decreased myocardial performance and hypotension if added too rapidly or in too great a concentration. Recent data suggest that isoflurane and halothane may provide better tissue oxygenation than enflurane during hypovolemia. However, because isoflurane normally causes hypotension and tachycardia, its use in a patient with large fluid volume shifts may lead to a diagnostic dilemma; we therefore avoid its use in these circumstances. Thus our anesthetic vapor of choice is halothane. The anesthetist must pay extremely close attention to the variable clinical situation and be prepared to cease administration of all inhalation agents should hypotension ensue.

Nitrous oxide should not be used for these patients. Although nitrous oxide is a superior analgesic, it is frequently depressant in the hypotensive, hypovolemic patient. Since it must be used in relatively high concentrations, this adds to the potential for hypoxia because of decreased inspired oxygen concentration. Furthermore, nitrous oxide increases the volume of any previously unrelieved pneumothorax and increases bowel distention, potentially adding technical difficulty to the surgery. We avoid the use of narcotics here, because once given they cannot be removed as can the inhalation agents. The use of naloxone to reverse narcotic action may be only partially successful because of hypoperfusion at the site(s) of action and because of shorter duration of action of the antagonist than of the agonist. Using this approach, some patients may recall some intraoperative events, especially if anesthesia is not instituted as mean systemic arterial pressure rises to 50 torr.

In selecting a muscle relaxant for continued use during the procedure, d-tubocurarine is avoided because of its propensity to release histamine, resulting in further hypotension. Pancuronium is preferred to gallamine because of its greater vagolytic properties and its lesser obligatory dependence on renal excretion. Metocurine and vecuronium (not yet clinically available) have the least cardiovascular actions of nondepolarizing muscle relaxants.

Hemodynamic Management

After the airway has been secured and ventilation has been established, the hemodynamic status of the patient remains the primary issue. The hemodynamic status of the patient changes rapidly because of the rapidity and intensity of physiologic response to hemorrhage (increased sympathetic system activity, increased renin-angiotension system activity, increased vasopressin secretion, peripheral circulatory effects, actions of acidic metabolites, direct hypoxic effects, and fluid shifts) and the multiplicity of therapeutic manuevers in the acute situation. Anesthetic agents alter all these processes and thereby further complicate the physiologic response, diagnosis, and therapy.

Accordingly, accurate beat-to-beat blood pressure monitoring is an important aspect of the acute management of the major trauma victim. For this reason and to allow repeated, rapid sampling of arterial blood for measurement of Po_2, Pco_2, and pH, an indwelling arterial cannula should be placed as early as feasible in the operating room sequence and connected to a pressure transducer for continuous measurement of blood pressure. Percutaneous insertion may be difficult in a patient whose systemic arterial blood pressure is unobtainable or is very low; a surgical cut-down may be required. The arterial line should be placed in the upper extremity because it may be necessary to cross-clamp the thoracic aorta. A central venous (superior vena cava or right atrial) cannula should be placed, time permitting, while the patient is in the emergency room. If the patient arrives in the operating room without a centrally located catheter, its placement is a high priority, and should be accomplished soon thereafter. In the operating room, introduction through an internal jugular vein is favored over the approach from an antecubital or subclavian vein, both because of the ease and rapidity of insertion through the former and because of the accessibility of this route while surgery proceeds. To permit continuous accurate assessment of central venous pressure, and for rapid verification of position, the cannula should be connected to a pressure transducer and the wave-form visually displayed. Measurements obtained by the use of hydraulic manometers are unreliable. It is essential to obtain accurate reference of zero pressure for the CVP. This is conveniently accomplished by placing a length of intravenous line connecting tubing, filled with saline, from the transducer to a point on the patient's midaxillary line. Opening the transducer to this line, while it is closed to all other ports, will establish a correct zero point. It will not be necessary to alter the height of the transducer should patient position or operating room table height be altered. The correct zero reference may be re-established by again opening the transducer to the "zero-line" with other ports closed. The preponderance of victims of major trauma are young and without heart disease, thus central venous pressure usually is an adequate reflection of left-sided cardiac filling pressure. Placement of a pulmonary arterial line in the early care of the massively injured patient is neither necessary nor advisable; time is better spent tending to issues of higher priority.

If need arises for intraoperative assessment of left-sided filling pressure, a left atrial catheter may be inserted directly if thoracotomy has been performed. Direct observation of filling of the heart is also useful in the evaluation of the patient's volume status. The early stages of resuscitation of the massively bleeding patient require continuous communication between the surgeons and the anesthetists as to the nature and extent of the injuries and the hemodynamic indices. If it is necessary to cross-clamp the aorta to provide adequate blood flow to the brain and heart in the presence of massive hypovolemia and marked hypotension, sub-

sequent removal of the clamp may result in hypotension, owing to circulating volume filling a previously empty, acidotic vascular tree. Consequently, reperfusion should be established gradually by partial unclamping as hemodynamics permit, with addition of volume or base (to be discussed), or both, as required.

Intraoperative Fluid Resuscitation

The amount of fluid volume to administer is guided by the systemic blood pressure and cardiac filling. Fluids are administered as rapidly as possible until the central venous pressure is in the normal range for an anesthetized patient (8 to 10 torr) or the systemic blood pressure is in the normal range.

Much research and discussion have surrounded the issue of which fluid to administer. The clinician may currently choose from whole blood, red blood cell suspensions (packed, washed, or frozen), salt solutions (crystalloid), protein-containing fluids (colloid), or other osmotically active agents, such as dextran and starch. Whole blood is the fluid of choice despite some deficiencies of banked blood. Whole blood offers the advantage of the ability to transport as well as to on- and off-load oxygen and carbon dioxide, it contains most clotting factors in adequate supply, and it is a good buffer at physiologic pH. The disadvantages of banked blood include low storage temperature (4°C) with high thermal capacity; decreased clotting factors V and VIII; lack of functional platelets after 24 hours of storage; low pH; high potassium concentration (although it returns to normal with restoration of red cell sodium pump activity); decreased red cell survival; presence of citrate; risk of transmission of hepatitis, cytomegalic virus, and AIDS; decreased red cell 2,3-diphosphoglycerate (DPG) concentration, resulting in high hemoglobin affinity for oxygen; and presence of red cell membrane antigens, which requires typing and crossmatching of the patient's blood with the blood to be transfused. However, the US Army had highly favorable experience in Viet Nam using unmatched low anti-A, and anti-B titer group O, and the need for crossmatch for patients who have neither been pregnant nor received prior transfusion has been questioned.

Blood banks fractionate most whole blood into its component parts, separating plasma from red blood cells. Consequently, anesthetists may need to rely on packed red blood cells ordinarily spun to a hematocrit of approximately 70 percent.

To decrease viscosity and thus ease administration, packed cells should be reconstituted to an approximately normal hematocrit prior to transfusion. Sodium chloride, 0.9 percent, is the only fluid recommended by the American Association of Blood Banks for use for this purpose. However, we have reconstituted thousands of units of packed cells during the past 5 years, using a balanced salt solution containing magnesium instead of calcium, without a single instance of clot formation. Reconstitution with salt solutions containing calcium should always be avoided. Because packed cells contain little plasma, some of the advantages of whole blood are diminished. The quantity of clotting factors is decreased. Oxygen transport is not affected, however, and the CO_2 transport capability is only somewhat decreased, as is buffering capacity.

Although devices available for collecting, washing, and transfusing the patient's own shed blood can be successfully utilized in elective surgery, no such device is available which meets the specific needs of the situation surrounding intraoperative care of the major trauma victim. These devices require a significant degree of operator attention, take several minutes to process a unit of cells, and result in a product that contains *no* platelets or clotting factors. Calcium will be present only if it has been added to the suspension medium. Furthermore, many major trauma victims have intestinal injury, which, when present, precludes the transfusing of shed blood because of the risk of bacterial contamination. Therefore, we do not recommend the use of these devices in the initial operating room management of major trauma victims.

Despite considerable laboratory and clinical investigation, there is no firm evidence that the use of microfilters for blood administration is beneficial. The resistance of these greatly impedes rapid blood administration, and we therefore do not recommend their use in this setting.

Note that when extremely rapid infusion of viscous fluid is required, there are considerable differences in resistance to flow between various types of infusion equipment and blood warmers. Stopcocks offer high resistance because their internal diameter is smaller than that of intravenous tubing, and therefore they should not be used. Warming of banked blood not only is essential to prevent severe hypothermia (see below), but it greatly decreases blood viscosity and therefore allows for its more rapid administration.

Inevitably, until the trauma victim's blood is typed, fluids other than blood must be administered. Current evidence indicates that in this regard colloid is of no advantage over crystalloid and, in fact, may be detrimental. Given the expense of the former and the availability and ease of the administration of the latter, there seems to be little, if any, reason to administer colloid in the acute resuscitative period. We prefer a balanced salt solution which does not contain calcium, which we also use for reconstitution of packed cells (already discussed). Resuscitative fluids undergoing research and development include perfluorochemicals (fluorocarbons) and stromal-free hemoglobin, either in solution or encased in layers of lipid. The oxygen content of fluorocarbons is proportional to the partial pressure of oxygen in the fluid and reaches an acceptable level only at very high Po_2. Furthermore, fluorocarbons are extremely expensive, have extraordinarily long half-lives, are stored frozen, require at least 30 minutes for defrosting, must be mixed prior to use, are administered slowly, and have a significant incidence of allergic response. Relying on their use for resuscitation from major trauma is inappropriate.

Recently it has been possible to prepare hemoglobin with very little, if any, stromal elements, thus eliminating renal toxicity and offering the advantage of high oxygen content at normal Po_2. Furthermore, hemoglobin so prepared can be stored in its crystalline form at room temperature for prolonged periods of time, and since no red cell membranes and antigens are present, standard blood typing is unnecessary. Phosphorylation and cross-linking the molecules have extended the product's intravascular half-life to approximately 24 hours and increased its P_{50} to an approximately normal value. Stromal-free hemoglobin has been shown to be superior to albumin in supporting myocardial function. Should human testing demonstrate efficacy and safety, stromal-free hemoglobin may find its place in the earliest phases of resuscitation of the massively bleeding patient.

Persistent Hypotension Despite Apparently Adequate Fluid Administration

This situation is observed at some stage in the operating room management of many patients who have sustained extremely major injuries. The first checks should be of the accuracy of the monitoring system.

The zero setting and calibration of transducers should be checked. It is useful to have placed a blood pressure cuff on the limb that has been cannulated for the arterial pressure. The occlusion pressure can then be used to validate the measured intra-arterial pressure. Possible causes of the continuing hypotension must then be reviewed. These include undetected hemorrhage; hemothorax, pneumothorax, or pericardial tamponade; acidosis; hypothermia; or an error in administration of ventilation or anesthesia. Hypocalcemia may be present in extreme cases of hypoperfusion, hypothermia, and massive transfusion.

If correction of all other problems (to be discussed) is ineffective in restoring systemic pressure, we empirically administer calcium chloride, 1 g intravenously, since ionized calcium measurements are not readily available. However, frequent repeated doses of calcium are not recommended because of the danger of producing ventricular tachycardia or fibrillation, which may be refractory to all therapy. Calcium and other pressors including epinephrine, norepinephrine, dopamine, and dobutamine have diminished effectiveness during acidosis.

Myocardial failure in a previously healthy young trauma victim is distinctly uncommon unless the patient has had direct myocardial injury or prolonged myocardial hypoxia. However, if all other possible causes of persistent hypotension have been excluded or treated, additional fluids may be administered until the central venous pressure is 20 to 25 torr. If arterial pressure does not respond, as a *last resort,* pressor agents (dopamine or dobutamine, 3 to 12 μg/kg/minute IV initially) may be infused. It must be pointed out that *pressors must not be used in place of restoration of adequate circulating blood volume.* An unusual cause of myocardial failure following perforating chest injuries is coronary air embolism, which may be diagnosed by direct observation of the coronary arteries. The question of the existence of a "myocardial depressant factor" in hypovolemic shock is controversial. In addition to hemorrhage, metabolic acidosis and hypothermia are the two most common secondary aggravating factors in the massively bleeding traumatized patient.

Acid-Base Balance

Poor tissue perfusion results in decreased availability of oxygen at the end of the mitochondrial electron transport chain, which results in tissue accumulation of lactic acid. Hepatic uptake of lactate from blood is impaired during severe reductions of hepatic blood flow or during severe hypoxia. It is not clinically convenient to measure lactic acid concentrations. However, its appearance in the blood will result in an increase in base deficit. Base deficit may be rapidly estimated from measurements of arterial P_{CO_2} and pH, by use of Siggaard-Andersen's nomogram, Severinghaus's slide rule, or automated blood gas equipment using equations developed by the latter. Arterial blood gases and pH should be measured as soon as possible. The treatment of acidosis secondary to hypovolemia is volume replacement. If volume is restored and perfusion is satisfactory, the acidosis will be corrected as the liver extracts lactate from the blood and the tissues cease lactate production. Thus, treatment of acidosis per se will not be required. However, acidosis can result in persistent hypotension despite adequate restoration of circulating blood volume. Myocardial performance deteriorates at pH below 7.2. Ideally, the magnitude of the acidosis should be measured. If data are not yet available, it is safe to administer $NaHCO_3$ as a therapeutic test. It is unusual to observe clinically important cardiovascular effects of metabolic acidosis at base deficits less than 10 mEq per liter, and in this setting acidosis of considerably greater magnitude is common. Whole body base deficit is usually calculated from the formula 0.3 base excess (BE; mEq per liter) × body weight in kg. Thus, 200 or more mEq of $NaHCO_3$ may be required to correct a clinically important metabolic acidosis. Since cardiovascular instability is usually present when administration of $NaHCO_3$ is indicated, a calculated dose of bicarbonate will not provide exact correction. Frequent, repeated evaluation is necessary. P_{CO_2} and pH should be measured at 37°C and not corrected to the patient's temperature based on evidence that, over a wide temperature range, vertebrate plasma pH is closely related to the pH of water and the ionization of imidazole. In any event, over the clinical range, computation of base excess is very nearly independent of temperature.

It is not clear whether measured P_{O_2} should be corrected to the patient's temperature or reported at 37°C. However, temperature correction is necessary for computation of alveolar-arterial difference in oxygen tension $P(A-a)O_2$. Furthermore, in the hypothermic patient, if temperature correction results in error it is on the side of patient safety.

Hypothermia

Poor perfusion, opening of major body cavities, and administration of fluids of a temperature less than body temperature inevitably result in hypothermia. Hypothermia presents multiple dangers. Myocardial function decreases with temperature. Myocardial hypothermia is poorly tolerated in the clinical setting of decreased myocardial preload and prolonged poor myocardial perfusion. As myocardial temperature falls to approximately 30°C, arrhythmias become common. Refractory ventricular fibrillation frequently occurs when myocardial temperature falls an additional 1 to 3 centigrade degrees. Hypothermia adds to the coagulation defects (to be discussed) by causing sequestration of platelets. This phenomenon is reversible with rewarming. Additional problems of hypothermia include alteration of drug action and half-life, and confusion of interpretation of blood gas, pH, and acid-base data.

Temperature should be measured continuously by a thermistor or thermocouple placed in the esophagus, just behind the heart, or by use of the thermistor of a thermodilution pulmonary artery catheter, if one has been inserted. These sites are preferred to those that are more distal because of the life-threatening hazard of myocardial hypothermia. Rapid changes in myocardial and blood temperature will be reflected slowly at other sites, which are less central, such as the rectum.

Although it may not be possible to maintain normothermic conditions in the massively bleeding, traumatized patient, it is possible to prevent severe hypothermia. All administered intravenous fluids should be warmed. Some commercially available devices can warm blood effectively without adding important resistance to flow, thus allowing for high flow rates. A plugged-in connected circulating-water warming blanket should always be in place on the operating table. The device should be set at 40°C and switched on at first notice of a patient's likely transport to the operating room, since most of these devices require 10 to 20 minutes to reach operating temperature. Warming blankets, although useful, are of less than optimal value because of poor peripheral circulation during massive hypovolemia. Heated inspired humidity is of greater value in preventing serious hypothermia, since nearly all the right atrial output will be exposed as a thin layer to the inspired heat in the pulmonary circulation. If the foregoing measures fail, warm crystalloid solution should be placed in the chest or abdominal cavities. Since we have been routinely using heated inspired humidity and warming all administered blood and intravenous fluid for all major trauma victims, it has become unusual to require the filling of body cavities with warm saline.

Coagulation

A bleeding diathesis following massive blood loss and replacement is not uncommon. Causes are lesions of banked blood; hypothermia; consumption coagulopathy; and platelet dysfunction. The most frequent cause of a coagulopathy in the massively bleeding trauma patient is dilutional thrombocytopenia and/or platelet dysfunction. Platelet function is severely impaired within minutes of storage at 4°C, with survival limited to less than 48 hours. Many blood banks remove platelets from blood after its collection. Thus, nearly all blood transfused is free of functional platelets, creating a dilutional thrombocytopenia. Furthermore, hypothermia causes platelet sequestration.

The coagulopathy of massive transfusion occurs commonly when between one and two times the estimated blood volume has been administered. Treatment of the dilutional thrombocytopenia or platelet dysfunction is accomplished by administration of platelets. Ten units of platelet concentrates should be administered if further significant transfusion is anticipated or generalized bleeding is apparent. Most hospital blood banks do not stock platelets, thus they may need to be ordered well in advance. Additional units of platelets will be required if hemorrhage is not controlled. We administer an additional 5 units of platelets with each additional 5 units of whole blood or packed cells transfused. Since the plasma in which platelets are suspended contains quantities of coagulation factors similar to that of fresh frozen plasma (except for somewhat decreased but nevertheless hemostatic levels of factors V and VIII), administration of fresh frozen plasma may be unnecessary if platelets have been infused.

Development of a consumptive coagulopathy (possibly resulting from release of tissue thromboplastin) will further deplete the diluted platelets and already decreased clotting factors.

Coagulation factors V and VIII have storage half-lives of approximately one week. Fortunately, only 5 to 30 percent of normally present quantities of these factors are necessary for surgical hemostasis. Furthermore, the liver can rapidly produce large quantities of factor VIII once circulation has been restored. Fresh frozen plasma contains all coagulation factors, but no platelets. When decreased coagulation factors are diagnosed as a cause of the coagulopathy, 2 units of fresh frozen plasma should be administered.

Although precise diagnosis of a coagulation defect requires laboratory tests such as bleeding time, prothrombin time, activated partial thromboplastin time, and fibrin split product levels, logistics may preclude their use. The most convenient method for determining the etiology of a bleeding disorder in the victim of major trauma is to observe the coagulation time. Few if any intraoperative coagulopathies of trauma victims cannot be appropriately managed by this regimen. If a solid clot does not form in a glass tube within 15 minutes, decreased clotting factors are implicated. If the clot forms but does not retract, thrombocytopenia is the likely cause. If the clot lyses, fibrinolysis is likely.

Calcium is bound by citrate, the anticoagulant of banked blood. However, hypocalcemia has not been demonstrated as a cause of the bleeding diathesis of massive transfusion. We do not administer calcium routinely as prophylaxis against coagulation defects. However, we do administer calcium to treat the myocardial effects of hypocalcemia (already discussed).

We transfuse fresh whole blood (stored less than 24 hours) very rarely, only as a last resort, when all other modes of therapy for a coagulopathy of trauma and/or massive transfusion have failed.

The Patient with Multiple Injuries

Frequently, priorities must be allocated in order to determine not only which injuries require immediate intervention (e.g., correction of major hemorrhage, cardiac tamponade, subdural hematoma), but also whether to continue operating after the most life-threatening problems have been corrected. This latter decision frequently involves injuries such as facial and long bone fractures. Considerations include:

1. *Physiologic status.* When it is being decided whether to proceed with less urgent surgery, an assessment should be made of the patient's response to injury, anesthesia, and surgery. Factors to be considered include: (a) the magnitude of the proposed procedures, including probable duration and blood loss, (b) hemodynamic stability and acid-base status; (c) pulmonary gas exchange and mechanics; (d) blood volume replacement and coagulation status; and (e) temperature.

Prolonged major procedures involving substantial potential blood loss should not be contemplated in any patient who is not hemodynamically stable, who has impaired lung-thorax mechanics (e.g., from pulmonary edema or con-

tusion, distended abdomen, bronchospasm), or whose $P(A-a)O_2$ is greater than 250 to 300 mmHg when the FIO_2 is 0.99. If blood volume replacement has exceeded the patient's blood volume, proceeding with additional, prolonged surgery for injuries that are not life-threatening is relatively contraindicated. An obvious coagulopathy is an absolute contraindication to proceeding. Inability to maintain the patient's temperature at 33°C or greater is also a contraindication to proceeding.

2. *Prolonged anesthesia.* There is no generally applicable information relating outcome to length of anesthesia, independent of the magnitude of the surgical procedure. Therefore, of itself, this should not be a consideration.

3. *Evolving intracranial injury.* A conscious patient, with an obvious head injury, who has no lateralizing signs, may require urgent surgery for hemorrhage at site(s) other than the cranium. During anesthesia, it is not possible to detect an increase in intracranial pressure, except in the extreme, unless a cannula to monitor intracranial pressure has been inserted. Absence of pupillary changes is not a reliable index of satisfactory intracranial pressure. In such cases, the decision to proceed with less urgent surgery requires special consideration. In outline, there are four options: (a) proceed, based on neurosurgical opinion that the extent of the original head injury was trivial; (b) permit the patient to awaken from anesthesia in order to allow further neurosurgical assessment; (c) maintain anesthesia and proceed to CT scan; (d) insert a cannula to monitor ICP and determine whether to pursue further radiologic evaluation, carry out intracranial exploration, or proceed with other surgery.

4. *Sustaining anesthesia excellence.* Usually it is in the best interest of the patient for the same anesthesia personnel to remain with the patient from induction to emergence and, in many cases, for the subsequent postoperative period, especially if the patient is unstable. An exception is when, in prolonged operations, owing to tiredness, it is difficult to sustain vigilance and to make objectively based decisions. If multiple procedures involving various surgical teams are proposed, it may be appropriate to involve an anesthesia "team," members of which can take a break or, if necessary, be replaced. If this is deemed necessary, provision *must* be made for continuity, i.e., sufficient overlap to permit a clear understanding of the injuries, the surgical and anesthetic course, and the patient's responses.

Special Problems

Thoracic Injuries

Three problems may require special actions by the anesthesiologist.

Pulmonary Injuries. It is not uncommon for alveolar pressure to exceed pressures in adjoining perforated pulmonary vessels, resulting in systemic air embolism. Occasionally, a massive bronchial air leak may prevent effective mechanical ventilation. Placement of a double-lumen endotracheal tube provides maximal control of this problem and also prevents hemorrhage from one lung into the other. If it is not possible to place a double-lumen endotracheal tube, endobronchial intubation may be accomplished using a long endotracheal tube. This is more applicable for left-sided leaks, since the anatomy of the tracheal bifurcation renders right main bronchial intubation more probable. Since one-lung ventilation is likely to result in a degree of hypoxia, due to shunting of blood through the unventilated lung, these maneuvers are only short-term, emergent expedients. Inhaled agents should include only oxygen and anesthetic vapor until measurements of systemic arterial Po_2 are obtained.

Aortic Injuries. Prolonged suprarenal clamping of the aorta may increase myocardial afterload and cause renal and spinal cord ischemia. The higher the clamp, the greater the likelihood of resultant left ventricular failure from the great increase in afterload. These problems may be minimized by the placement of a shunt if control below the aortic injury is feasible. However, if distal control is not feasible and a shunt is not placed, an agent such as sodium nitroprusside may be required to decrease myocardial afterload and permit volume loading while the aortic clamp is in place. Arterial pressure monitoring should be from the right arm if there is possible injury to the arch of the aorta. If time permits, left ventricular filling pressure should be monitored.

Cardiac Injuries and Tamponade. Rapid surgical correction is essential. Needle aspiration of traumatic cardiac tamponade does not often alleviate the hemodynamic problem. Intravenous fluid should be administered to achieve and maintain high cardiac filling pressure. Although theoretically important, this is only a short-term, temporizing measure. There is no anesthetic agent that will allow for the maintenance of venous return and cardiac output in the presence of hemodynamically important cardiac tamponade. Anesthesia should not be induced until the patient is prepared and the surgeons are ready to initiate surgical measures to decompress the pericardium *immediately* upon induction of anesthesia.

Spinal Injuries

The approach to securing an airway has been discussed elsewhere in this chapter. Although use of succinylcholine is contraindicated several days after a denervation injury, there is no evidence of muscle membrane instability in the first few hours. Thus, if otherwise indicated, succinylcholine may be used. Patients in halo traction requiring anesthesia for other injuries should be intubated, while awake, under topical anesthesia, either orally or nasally. If necessary a fiberoptic bronchoscope should be used. "Spinal shock" may result from acute spinal cord injuries, especially those that are cervical or high thoracic. Large volumes of intravenous fluid may be required to maintain adequate cardiac filling and systemic arterial blood pressure. Central venous pressure should be monitored, and continuous infusion of an α-adrenergic agent (e.g., phenylephrine) may be used to compensate for the sympathetic denervation, provided cardiac filling and urine output are maintained.

Head Injuries

After securing the airway and providing required resuscitation, the goal is to achieve and maintain normal or low intracranial pressure, while maintaining acceptable systemic hemodynamics. This may be difficult. Intracranial pressure is decreased as much as possible by administration of mannitol or furosemide, induction of hypocapnia ($PaCO_2$ 25 torr), and maintenance of a low venous pressure. A mechanical ventilator waveform with rapid inspiratory flow rate may assist in minimizing intrathoracic pressure. Barbiturates and narcotics are used to minimize autonomic response to intubation and incision. They are probably preferable to the anesthetic vapors because of their less unfavorable effects on intracranial pressure. However, there is no strong evidence to support large-dose barbiturate therapy for brain protection in this setting. Marked hypotension immediately following intracranial decompression is common. Treatment is by administration of fluids and, if necessary, the judicious use of a pressor, such as ephedrine, to replace the sudden decrease of sympathetic activity. We routinely establish arterial and central venous pressure monitoring as soon as possible after induction of anesthesia. A coagulopathy is occasionally seen. The etiology of this disseminated intravascular coagulation-like picture is not clear, but fresh frozen plasma or fresh blood, or a combination of the two, is the therapy of choice. Neurogenic pulmonary edema following head injury may be seen in rare instances. Myocardial failure is not the etiology of this disorder, and therefore treatment with inotropic agents is not appropriate. Facilities must be available for intraoperative application of positive end-expiratory pressure.

The Open Globe

Facial injuries may include trauma to the globe of the eye. Loss of vitreous humor, iris, and lens may result in permanent blindness and require evisceration. To minimize this possibility, every effort is made to avoid raising intraocular pressure. Intraocular pressure and intracranial pressure are controlled by similar factors. Induction of anesthesia must be smooth, and there must be neither "squeeze" of eye muscles nor straining during surgery. The fasciculations that follow administration of succinylcholine cause a transient increase in intraocular pressure, but its clinical importance is uncertain. It is not known whether administration of a small dose of a nondepolarizing neuromuscular blocking agent prevents the increase in intraocular pressure caused by succinylcholine. Nevertheless, our preference includes the use of "precurarization," followed by a large dose of thiopental, and succinylcholine; or, if a smaller dose of thiopental would be safer, substituting a large dose of pancuronium (0.15 mg per kg) for the succinylcholine. Either way, the profound myoneural block is maintained and is monitored with a nerve stimulator. The ventilator is adjusted to maintain hypocapnia.

Immediate Postoperative Period

At the end of surgery, for all but the most massive trauma, when hypovolemia has been corrected and the hemodynamic status is stable, the temperature is greater than 34°C, and pulmonary gas exchange is satisfactory, it is usually appropriate to extubate the patient's trachea and to administer oxygen in the recovery room. Because of the danger of possible regurgitation and aspiration of gastric contents, the patient should not be extubated until awake with intact upper airway reflexes.

After major trauma, many patients remain unstable in a number of ways, including blood volume and hemodynamics, temperature, acid-base balance, and coagulation. In some instances, pulmonary edema is present as a result of pulmonary trauma or secondary to previous cardiac ischemia or massive fluid load. Intracranial pressure may require monitoring. Intensive care will be necessary, but the process of transfer is not simple. There will be a lapse of time before the patient is settled in the intensive care unit (ICU) with all monitoring systems functioning and the ICU staff conversant with the ongoing problems. There are various ways to meet this situation, but the guiding principles are as follows:

1. Establish and maintain as much monitored stability as is feasible in the operating room, that is, do not take a "blind leap" to the ICU with a hypovolemic, hypotensive patient whose blood gas levels and acid-base status are unknown. If necessary, stay in the operating room long enough to correct these defects.

2. Use portable electronic monitoring and mechanical ventilation equipment for the move to the ICU and ensure that these are functioning well before leaving the operating room. In patients with severely impaired cardiorespiratory status, a change to manual ventilation may result in a sufficient change in intrathoracic pressure to cause increased hypotension or intracranial pressure, or to permit a change in lung volume with resulting deterioration in oxygen exchange.

3. Forewarn the ICU to prepare the necessary ventilation and monitoring equipment and any other urgently required therapy, such as blood products, so that they are in place and ready upon arrival of the patient.

4. On arrival, establish continuity of ventilation and blood pressure monitoring ventilation as first priority. Stay with the patient until all monitoring and support systems are re-established and the ICU staff is familiarized with the patient's circumstances and orders.

WOUND MANAGEMENT

Juris Bunkis, M.D.
Robert L. Walton, M.D.

Most wounds resulting from trauma are relatively minor injuries and can be treated in an emergency room, with the patient returning home after treatment. The care of all wounds, however, is governed by the same biologic principles, and the essence of treatment in each case is proper wound care based on biologic principles—*not* on spinal reflexes, anecdotal empiricism, or handbook dogma.

The phenomenon of healing is manifested by various cellular and intercellular events including epithelization, wound contraction, and collagen synthesis. Wounds heal at their maximum rate only when allowed to do so. An understanding of the basic principles of wound healing and management is necessary to allow the surgeon to make the right decisions in order to obtain a superior result. The practical management of wounds should be based on knowledge of the nature of the injury, functional anatomy, and the reparative process.

WOUND ASSESSMENT

A pertinent history and physical examination are essential. As with any injury, priorities are given to life-threatening conditions. Regardless of wound appearance, attention must first be directed toward establishing adequacy of airway, ventilation, and circulation. The history should be obtained from the patient or, if unattainable, from a reliable witness. The mechanism of injury should be determined to shed light on the nature and extent of the injury. Is the injury due to an automobile accident, a fall, a stab, or a gunshot wound? Was a pen knife or machete employed? Is the wound due to a bullet from a small-caliber, low-velocity handgun or to a powerful, short-range shotgun blast? Did the patient fall from 3 or 30 feet? Is the injury due to a relatively clean plate-glass window or a barnyard pitchfork? How much time has elapsed since the injury? How much blood was lost at the scene? What symptoms—e.g., hemoptysis, dyspnea, hematuria, paresthesia—has the patient experienced?

Alterations in the body's capability to respond to injury may alter the healing process. Stress, diabetes mellitus, malnutrition, bleeding disorders, and immunotherapy or steroid therapy represent systemic factors that may impede wound healing. The presence of other local factors (e.g., peripheral vascular disease, prior radiation therapy, or cutaneous erruptions) that may affect the healing process should also be determined by the surgeon.

A thorough physical examination should be performed. Present comments will be limited to examination of the wound, but one must remember to begin the examination with an overall assessment of the patient's nutritional status, vital signs, and other aspects of his general condition.

The examining physician must first ascertain the location of the injury. A stab to the neck, thorax, or abdomen presents a different set of potential problems than a superficial laceration of the buttocks. Deep lacerations of the extremities also frequently involve important underlying structures. The evaluation and management of deep wounds of the head and neck, extremities, chest, and abdomen are discussed in separate chapters of this book.

The depth of injury—as determined by loss of function of the injured part as well as injury to underlying nerves, blood vessels, ducts, tendons, bones, and joints—should be noted. The location, extent, and cause of the wound will indicate which laboratory or radiologic studies are needed.

Gross contamination of the wound or the presence of foreign bodies should be noted, as should the viability of tissues and the possibility of tissue loss.

35

Careful examination of the wound is imperative for proper diagnosis and management. Such examination is possible only in an appropriate facility equipped with adequate lighting and instrumentation. Frequently, this will necessitate taking the patient to the operating room, but universal guidelines cannot be established owing to the variability of standards between different emergency departments. Except under conditions of significant vascular compromise, a tourniquet is helpful in providing a dry field for the controlled evaluation of extremity wounds. Needless to say, sterile technique and gentle handling of tissues are mandatory.

Definitive wound evaluation cannot be performed in an uncooperative patient. It may be necessary to consider restraints, sedation, general anesthesia, or even a delay of the evaluation until more favorable conditions (e.g., sobriety) can be obtained. If anesthesia is given for this purpose, a thorough functional (including neurologic) examination should be performed prior to administration of the anesthesia whenever possible.

WOUND CLASSIFICATION

Tissue injury is caused by mechanical forces. Shear, tensile, and compressive forces, alone or in combination, produce predictable patterns of tissue injury. Knowledge of the nature and magnitude of mechanical forces employed to produce the injury allows the surgeon to predict the extent of the tissue damage. The predictability of certain injury patterns has allowed classification of wounds into specific categories: abrasions, lacerations, contusions, avulsions, amputations, degloving, and bursting injuries.

Lacerations result from shear forces applied to the skin by sharp objects. Relatively little energy is required to produce such lacerations, and a minimal amount of tissue is injured. Consequently, the general demands for wound healing are easily satisfied and wound infections are relatively infrequent.

Tensile forces can tear soft tissue. When tensile force exceeds the elastic yield of tissue, stretching and eventually separation of the parts will occur. The extent of injury is greater than in simple lacerations because the amount of energy absorbed by the soft tissue is larger. Such injuries may produce intimal damage in surrounding blood vessels, with subsequent thrombosis and ischemia to the injured parts. The structural integrity of nerves, muscles, ligaments, and tendons may also be disrupted. Such an injury places a greater demand on the biologic process of repair, decreases wound defense mechanism, and enhances susceptibility to infection.

Soft tissue compression between two opposing forces results in the greatest amount of tissue damage. Hemorrhage occurs in the soft tissues, with subsequent ecchymosis and hematoma formation. Edema affects capillary blood flow and prolongs the inflammatory phase of wound healing. Intimal damage to blood vessels may result in thrombosis and tissue necrosis. If the forces of compression are of significant magnitude, actual separation of the skin and soft tissue can occur to produce a "bursting" or "degloving" injury. Such wounds are markedly impaired in their ability to heal.

Wounds can also be classified, according to the expected level of bacterial contamination, into the following categories: clean, potentially contaminated, or contaminated. A thyroidectomy incision produced under sterile operating room conditions represents an example of a clean wound. Potentially contaminated wounds include those in which a hollow viscus (e.g., gallbladder, trachea, ureter, appendix) has been entered, but gross spillage of infected contents has not occurred. Other examples of potentially contaminated wounds include stab wounds with a kitchen knife and lacerations with glass or other relatively clean objects. Contaminated wounds contain quantitative bacterial counts exceeding 10^5 bacteria per gram of tissue, and the high probability of wound infection exists if such wounds are closed primarily. A puncture wound with a dirty pitchfork, human bites, and wounds that have sustained gross spillage of infected secretions fall into this category.

For therapeutic purposes, superficial wounds can be classified as being either tidy or untidy. Tidy wounds are caused by sharp objects, result in minimal tissue injury and contamination, and can usually be closed under favorable circumstances. Untidy wounds, however, are manifested by extensive soft tissue injury or contamination and require major intervention to allow satisfactory wound healing. Management of untidy wounds may be influenced by the extent and location of the injury. A surgeon may be able to surgically convert an untidy wound to a tidy one, and thus permit immediate closure.

ANESTHESIA

Satisfactory anesthesia often must be provided to ensure the patient's comfort while the wound is being assessed and treated. The age and mental status of the patient, as well as the extent of the wound, dictate whether a local, regional, or general anesthetic is preferable. Local or regional anesthesia requires the cooperation of patient, surgeon, and, if present, anesthesiologist.

Frequently, a supplemental tranquilizing agent may be beneficial in an anxious patient. Diazepam (Valium) provides good sedative and amnesic effects, but minimal respiratory and circulatory effects, at the usual dose of 5 to 10 mg. In addition, diazapam increases the threshold to lidocaine-induced seizures. It can be given orally or intravenously. If given intravenously, the injection site should be flushed with normal saline to avoid tissue irritation from the diazepam. Intramuscular administration, which frequently results in erratic absorption, should be avoided.

A "pediatric cocktail" containing 2 mg/kg meperidine (Demerol), 1 mg/kg chloropromazine (Thorazine), and 1 mg/kg promethazine (Phenergan) is a useful supplement in the pediatric population during suturing of lacerations or other potentially painful procedures. Such a "cocktail," however, should not replace a gentle, personal approach to the patient.

Local anesthesia is recommended for most minor wounds. The anesthetic agent may be infiltrated directly into the wound to reduce the discomfort associated with injection. Infiltration directly into the wound risks spreading potential infection and should be avoided in heavily contaminated wounds. The pain associated with cutaneous injection is due in part to the stretching of sensory nerve endings in the dermis. This can be minimized by using smaller, more concentrated volumes of anesthetic and slower infiltration rates. The least amount of anesthetic that will provide adequate anesthesia should be employed to minimize distortion of important landmarks, particularly when dealing with facial lacerations. In certain critical situations (e.g., in approximating the vermilion border), the key anatomic structures may be approximated with a single 6–0 monofilament suture prior to instillation of any anesthetic solution. Alternatively, methylene blue tattoos can be placed at critical anatomic points prior to injection of the anesthetic agent to allow subsequent accurate alignment.

Hemostasis is frequently achieved following injury by vasospasm, platelet plugging, and fibrin clot formation. Lidocaine and similar anesthetic agents cause vasodilation, which may result in rebleeding. The addition of epinephrine to the local anesthetic solution will overcome this tendency. An epinephrine concentration of 1:80,000 provides as much vasoconstriction as a 1:200,000 solution, but more dilute solutions are virtually ineffective. A 1:200,000 solution is optimal, as it produces maximal vasoconstriction with minimal epinephrine-related side-effects.

Epinephrine-containing solutions can severely compromise the local wound defense mechanisms by their vasoconstricting effects, and therefore should not be used in heavily contaminated wounds. Their use is also contraindicated in areas such as fingers and toes, which are supplied by terminal, segmental blood vessels. Epinephrine should also be avoided in patients with heart and peripheral vascular disease.

Signs of toxicity, which are remarkably similar among the different local anesthetic solutions, are always dose related and include numbness, tingling, diplopia, mental confusion, and convulsions.

Allergy to the ester-linked local anesthetics (e.g., procaine, cocaine) is well documented, and cross-sensitivity exists between the ester-linked moieties. Allergy to the amide-linked local anesthetics (e.g., lidocaine, bupivacaine, mepivacaine) is virtually nonexistent, and most reported reactions are vasovagal in nature. No cross-sensitivity exists between the amide-linked and ester-linked local anesthetic agents.

Limiting the total dose of local anesthetic administered is the surest way to avoid systemic toxicity. The vasoconstrictive effect of epinephrine decreases the rate of anesthetic clearance from the wound, thus adding to the safety margin (Table 1). Should a toxic reaction occur, however, the surgeon must be prepared to hyperventilate the patient and administer intravenous diazepam to increase the seizure threshold to the local anesthetic, and place the patient in the Trendelenburg position to ensure adequate cortical blood flow.

Certain wounds are particularly adapted to regional anesthetic techniques. Such techniques allow wider exploration and manipulation of deeper tissues than possible with local blocks. Regional techniques also avoid distortion of local tissues and allow precise alignment of injured parts. Regional anesthesia is especially applicable in ex-

TABLE 1 Suggested Maximum Dosages of Local Anesthetics

Agent	mg/kg	Total Dose in Average 70 kg Patient
Lidocaine	with epinephrine	7	500 mg
	without epinephrine	4	300 mg
Procaine	with epinephrine	14	1,000 mg
	without epinephrine	8	
Cocaine		1	

tremity injuries (e.g., axillary block; isolated ulnar, median, or radial nerve blocks; digital nerve blocks; sciatic or femoral nerve blocks; spinal or epidural anesthesia; Bier blocks). Trigeminal nerve blocks are useful in providing segmental facial anesthesia. Details regarding specific anesthetic techniques are provided in the chapter on *Anesthetic Management*.

Lidocaine and most other local anesthetics do not provide satisfactory local anesthesia in areas of established infection. Biochemical and physical mechanisms have been postulated for this clinical finding. Local anesthetics, which are weak bases, are inactivated by the acidic environment (e.g., increased lactic acid production) found in areas of infection. In addition, diffusion of local anesthetic solution is hampered by loculations and other physical barriers present in infected wounds. If the wound cannot be adequately examined or treatment rendered with either local or regional nerve block techniques, general anesthesia may be indicated. After adequate anesthesia has been achieved, the wound may be examined and definitive management rendered.

WOUND PREPARATION

Hair Removal

Shaving the operative area with a clean disposable razor is frequently recommended. This may be particularly useful in dense hair-bearing areas. Clinical data suggest, however, that preoperative shaving is associated with increased wound infection rates. Depilatory use does not enhance the wound's susceptibility to infection. Although shaving may facilitate wound management, it may invite bacterial proliferation and wound infection if the infundibulum of the hair follicle is injured. This can be avoided by clipping the hair 1 or 2 mm above the skin, or by using depilatory agents. Care should be taken to remove all shaved hair from the wound, as any hair left behind in the closed wound will act as a foreign body, inviting infection and compromising the wound healing process.

Hair definitely should not be shaved if the laceration traverses the eyebrow or other hair-bearing area. The juncture between the hair-bearing and non-hair-bearing skin presents a critical landmark which will allow accurate alignment of wound edges, thereby avoiding a step-off deformity, particularly in the brow line.

Skin Degerming

Although it is possible to sterilize surgical instruments, one cannot completely sterilize the skin of either the surgeon or the patient without damaging or destroying it. Skin degerming techniques, however, have been developed to decrease bacterial counts on the surgeon's hands, within the wound, and on the surrounding skin. A distinction must be made between techniques employed to decrease the resident bacteria on intact skin and those designed to decrease the bacterial contamination of the open wound. One must avoid placing anything into the wound that may cause further tissue injury or impede wound defense mechanisms. In the final analysis, one should avoid placing anything into the wound that one would not place into the conjunctival sac of the eye.

Initial cleansing of the skin surrounding the wound should be carried out by the physician or a member of the operating team employing soap, a nonirritating solution, or a fat solvent. Ionic soap and detergents are satisfactory skin cleansers, but are extremely irritating to the open wound and, if allowed to bathe the wound, actually increases the potential for wound infection. After application to intact skin, the surgical scrub solutions should be removed by thorough rinsing with water. Such cleansing will remove transient microflora, gross contaminants, and coagulated blood from the skin surrounding the wound.

A degerming agent should next be applied to the intact skin surrounding the wound. Commonly used solutions include iodine and iodine compounds, hexacholorophine, and alcohol solutions. Povidone-iodine (Betadine), which is nonirritating to intact skin and has a rapid onset of action and a broad antimicrobial spectrum, is the most commonly used skin disinfectant. Such solutions reduce the number of resident and contaminating bacteria on the intact skin surface. The iodine in these compounds is bound to a nonsurfactant moiety (polyvinylpyrrolidine)—large molecules which, if absorbed through the wound, are retained by the body owing to the kidneys' inability to excrete them. In addition, if povidone-iodine gains access to an open wound, free iodine can be absorbed, leading to disturbingly high serum levels. When placed in an open wound, antiseptic solutions destroy not only bacteria, but also cells responsible for local defense and tissue repair. Therefore, such solutions should not be used in open wounds.

Necrotic tissue, exogenous debris, and bacteria promote the development of wound sepsis. A simple wash of the open wound with physiologic saline solution or a balanced salt solution may mechanically remove up to 90 percent of contaminating bacteria. Normal saline (pH 5.0), however, may be irritating to the wound, particularly to the intima of blood vessels; lactated Ringer's solution (pH 6.7) is preferable to saline. Antibiotics may be added to the irrigating solution for heavily contaminated wounds.

The efficacy of wound irrigation is related to irrigation pressure. In heavily contaminated wounds, simple irrigation with an Asepto syringe does not adequately reduce the bacterial concentration. Pulsatile pressure delivered at 7 to 10 p.s.i., however, effectively removes debris, including bacteria, from the wound without disseminating microorganisms into the tissues. Irrigation with a 35-ml syringe through a 19-gauge needle produces irrigation pressures of 7 p.s.i., a useful technique in an emergency room setting. Higher irrigation pressures are to be avoided, as tissue damage and increased potential for wound infection may result.

Mechanical cleansing of the wound by direct scrubbing techniques is effective for removal of particulate contamination and bacteria, but may further injure local tissues. If mechanical scrubbing is required, a highly porous sponge will minimize tissue trauma. Brushes and low-porosity sponges are apt to inflict further tissue injury in an open wound, but may be required to remove imbedded debris from abrasion tattoos. Soaps, detergents, and surgical scrub brushes should not be used in open wounds, as they inflict further tissue injury and decrease the wound's resistance to infection.

Surgical Debridement

Although conservative debridement is recommended for most wounds, it must be adequate. Necrotic wound edges must be debrided, regardless of the location or former importance of the devitalized tissue. Surgical debridement may also be required to remove severely contaminated tissues or wound edges that are so irregular as to make wound closure impractical. Closely parallel lacerations may be converted to a single wound by excising the intervening skin bridge.

The simplest method of debridement is total excision of the wound, creating a surgically clean one, but this should be limited to wounds that do not involve specialized structures. Complete excision of the wound is possible only in regions containing an abundance of soft tissues, such as the thigh or buttocks. Selective debridement of all grossly nonviable tissue is essential in wounds containing vital structures. Under special circumstances, tendons, fascia, or dura of questionable viability may be retained, but must be protected from further injury through desiccation. These structures may survive as free grafts if appropriate wound coverage is provided.

Guidelines for determining tissue viability must be based on careful examination of the wound and sound clinical judgment. A completely reliable test to predict tissue viability has not been perfected, although inspection of the wound with a Wood's lamp for fluorescence following an intravenous fluorescence injection does provide a reflection of tissue perfusion at that moment. Especially with burn, crush, and blast injuries, the exact extent of tissue damage may be difficult to determine during the initial evaluation. The diffuseness of the tissue damage makes precise initial surgical debridement impossible. In such circumstances, grossly devitalized tissue should be debrided, but tissue of questionable viability may be initially preserved. The demarcated necrotic tissue can be debrided at a "second look" procedure in 24 to 48 hours.

Avulsed or amputated tissue will become necrotic unless the part can be converted to a graft or the blood supply re-established. Unless cellular destruction has occurred, avulsed skin can frequently be debrided, defatted, and reapplied successfully as a free graft. Composite tissues rarely survive as free grafts, and microvascular revascularization should be considered if feasible.

Hemostasis

Thorough wound debridement and prevention of fluid collections are primary goals of good wound management. A blood clot acts as a foreign body and provides an excellent culture medium for bacteria within the wound. Hematoma is a common cause of skin graft loss, and its presence beneath a skin flap may compromise the flap's viability. Therefore, every effort must be made to obtain meticulous hemostasis before closing the wound. Even small clots within the deep recesses of a wound may lead to fibrosis and palpable thickening in the postoperative period.

Spontaneous hemostasis may occur in an acute wound owing to vasospasm, fibrin deposition, and platelet plugging. If a known vessel traverses the wounded area, it should be examined for injury, regardless of the presence or absence of bleeding at the time of exploration.

Hemostasis can be achieved by the application of pressure or biologic solutions (e.g., crystalline collagen, thrombin solution) to the wound or by direct manipulation of injured vessels. Vessels may be suture ligated, clipped, or electrocoagulated. Vessels larger than 2 mm in diameter should be precisely clamped with as little adjacent tissue as possible and clipped or tied with the finest appropriate ligature to avoid necrosis of a large mass of tissue distal to the tie. Metal and synthetic, absorbable (polydioxanone) ligature clips are commercially available. Sutures and clips, however, are foreign bodies and increase the wound's susceptibility to infection. Braided, nonabsorbable sutures have the highest propensity for infection in contaminated wounds and should be avoided. Quantitative bacterial studies have demonstrated that a single, buried silk suture will enhance the possibility of infection by a factor of 10,000 times. Monofilament synthetic sutures are least reactive, but their low friction coefficient makes them unsuitable as ligatures, except in the repair of large vessels. For these reasons, absorbable sutures (e.g., polyglycolic acid, polyglactin, catgut) are recommended for use as suture ligatures in acute wounds.

Smaller vessels may be electrocoagulated. Vessels must be precisely clamped and the minimal amount of electrical energy necessary to provide hemostasis employed. Indiscriminate electrocoagulation results in significant amounts of charred, necrotic tissue within the wound, which will increase the wound's susceptibility to infection.

Antibiotics

The reward for meticulous wound debridement and physiologic closure is timely healing without suppuration and rapid restoration of function. Fortunately, most civilian wounds are not heavily contaminated and contain less than 10^2 bacteria per gram of tissue at the time of presentation in the emergency room. Quantitative bacterial studies demonstrate that the critical factor in predicting wound sepsis is the number rather than the type of bacteria remaining in the wound at the time of closure. Infection will predictably occur if wounds containing more than 10^5 bacteria per gram of tissue are closed without adjunctive measures. The most important factor in preventing wound infection is adequate surgical debridement. If the likelihood of wound infection remains high, antibiotic prophylaxis is indicated.

Prophylactic antibiotics markedly decrease the risk of postoperative sepsis if the antibiotic can be delivered before the bacteria arrive in the tissues. Understandably, it is unlikely that the patient will have adequate antibiotic tissue levels at the time of acute injury, but, if indicated, antibiotics should be administered promptly in the emergency room following wound evaluation and after culture specimens have been obtained. The effectiveness of antibiotics in preventing subsequent wound infection is markedly reduced by any delay in starting therapy and by delaying wound closure. Prophylactic antibiotics have a negligible, if any, beneficial effect if initial administration is delayed four hours following injury and bacterial contamination. In elective situations, prophylactic antibiotics should be administered during induction of anesthesia.

It has already been mentioned that wound quantitative bacterial counts give an accurate prediction of subsequent potential for wound infection. Properly managed wounds containing less than 10^5 bacteria per gram of tissue at the time of closure will heal per primum without infection.

Insight into the magnitude of bacterial contamination is provided by knowledge of the mechanism of injury and by the clinical appearance of the wound, but a more definitive assessment of the degree of contamination can be obtained by quantitative microbiologic assays. The "rapid slide technique" can provide the surgeon with this crucial information within 20 minutes (Table 2).

Clean acute lacerations rarely present with bacterial counts greater than 10^5 bacteria per gram of tissue. Following proper irrigation and debridement, such wounds can usually be closed primarily without risk of infection and do not require prophylactic antibiotic therapy. Wounds resulting from crush or blast injuries, on the other hand, frequently contain large quantities of devitalized tissue, foreign debris, bacteria, and blood clots. The level of bacterial contamination should be determined following irrigation and debridement. If counts greater than 10^5 organisms per gram of tissue persist, but the extent of tissue injury does not contraindicate wound closure, prophylactic antibiotics may allow uncomplicated primary wound closure and healing. A Gram stain from the wound helps to determine the appropriate antibiotics. Antibiotics are only effective in preventing wound infection, however, if the bacterial levels are less than 10^9 organisms per gram of tissue. If closed, wounds containing greater than 10^9 bacteria per gram of tissue following debridement will suppurate regardless of the presence or absence of prophylactic antibiotics. Such grossly contaminated wounds (including those contaminated by feces, pus, or heterosaliva; puncture wounds) should not be closed primarily. In such circumstances, the wound should be debrided and topical antimicrobials (e.g., silver sulfadiazine) added to the wound management regimen until bacterial counts drop below 10^5 bacteria per gram of tissue to allow delayed primary closure.

Previous comments have been limited to the treatment of acute wounds. The same basic principles, however, apply to the management of chronic wounds. All chronic wounds (e.g., pressure sores, full-thickness burns, leg ulcers) contain granulation tissue—by definition, granulation tissue contains bacteria. Successful closure of chronic wounds is also predicated on the surgeon's ability to control the bacterial contamination. Regardless of the method employed for wound closure, suppuration will result if the final bacterial counts exceed 10^5 bacteria per gram of tissue and prophylactic antibiotics are withheld. Clinical

TABLE 2 The "Rapid Slide" Bacterial Quantitative Assay

1. Clean the surface of the wound biopsy area with 70 percent isopropyl alcohol.
2. Obtain the biopsy specimen with a 3- or 4-mm dermal punch or with a scalpel. No anesthesia is required for an open wound.
3. After the tissue is weighed, flamed, and diluted 1:10 with thioglycollate (1 ml/g), it is homogenized.
4. Spread exactly 0.02 ml of the suspension with a 20-lambda Sahli-pipette on a glass slide. The inoculum is confined to an area 15 mm in diameter.
5. Oven-dry the slide for 15 minutes at 75° C.
6. Stain the slide using either a Gram stain or the Brown and Brenn modification for tissue staining, to accentuate the gram-negative organisms.
7. Read the smear under 1.9 mm (magnification × 97) objective and examine all fields for the presence of bacteria.
8. The presence of even a single organism is evidence that the tissue contains a level of bacterial growth greater than 10^5 bacteria per gram of tissue.

evaluation of granulation tissue provides a notoriously inaccurate estimate of the degree of contamination; as in the management of acute wounds, the surgeon should validate his clinical impressions by obtaining a quantitative bacterial assay.

Intravenous antibiotics do not reach adequate levels in granulation tissue to have an effect on bacterial concentrations quantitatively, but may affect them qualitatively, leading to a more virulent, antibiotic-resistant organism. Intravenous antibiotics are not indicated in the treatment of chronic soft tissue wounds except to treat surrounding cellulitis. Reduction of excessive bacterial flora can be accomplished by meticulous attention to surgical techniques and by the judicious application of topical antimicrobials.

Any wound may provide the portal of entry for *Clostridium tetani*. Nail puncture wounds, splinter injuries, burns, and other traumatic wounds require tetanus prophylaxis (Table 3).

WOUND CLOSURE

Timing of Closure

Time elapsed since injury does not by itself represent a significant determinant for wound closure. The decision to close a wound is predicated upon many factors, the most important of which is the level of contamination. The primary goal is to reduce the bacterial inoculum below the critical

TABLE 3   Tetanus Prophylaxis

Type of Wound	Patient Not Immunized or Partially Immunized	Patient Completely Immunized Time Since Last Booster Dose	
		5 to 10 yrs.	10 yrs.†
Clean minor	Begin or complete immunization per schedule; tetanus toxoid 0.5 ml	None	Tetanus toxoid 0.5 ml
Tetanus prone	Human tetanus immune globulin, 250–500 units; tetanus toxoid, 0.5 ml, complete immunization per schedule; antibiotic therapy as indicated	Tetanus toxoid 0.5 ml; antibiotic therapy if indicated	Tetanus toxoid 0.5 ml; human tetanus immune globulin, 250–500 units; antibiotic therapy if indicated

N.B.: No prophylactic immunization is required if patient has had a booster within the previous five years.

level of 10^5 organisms per gram of tissue prior to wound closure. A laboratory test, however, must not replace sound clinical judgment. When faced with less than ideal circumstances (e.g., retained foreign body, necrotic tissue following debridement) or in light of diminished wound defense mechanism (associated with systemic illness, malnutrition, impaired local blood supply, and so on), primary wound closure may produce disastrous results, regardless of the initial quantitative bacterial counts.

The timing of wound closure represents a compromise between the likelihood of infection and the ability to provide favorable conditions for closure. If appropriate, primary wound closure is clearly advantageous over other methods. An open wound invites fibrous tissue proliferation and contraction, both of which will detract from final function and appearance. The wound should not be closed indiscriminately, as infection will defeat any possible gains from primary closure.

If left open, contaminated wounds gradually gain resistance to infection over a 4-day period. After initial debridement, the open wound may be dressed with sterile, fine-mesh gauze. A moist or greasy dressing will prevent wound desiccation. The presence of wound debris, drainage, or fever will dictate the frequency of dressing changes. On the fourth day, a quantitative bacterial assay helps to determine the appropriateness of wound closure. Following further debridement and antibiotic coverage as necessary, the wound may be closed using sterile technique. If the wound is not located in a critical area and if it is small, it may be preferable to allow healing by secondary intention.

The most aesthetically pleasing scars and the most satisfactory return of function usually result from healing by primary intention. Anything that interferes with primary healing may result in ad-ditional scarring and a less acceptable result. Proper wound debridement, closure, and postoperative management are prerequisites for satisfactory primary healing. Initial wound care has a significant influence on subsequent healing; surgical technique remains the most important determinant of successful wound closure. This includes gentle manipulation of injured tissues, precise sharp debridement, prudent use of electrocautery, avoidance of excessive or strangulating sutures, prevention of tissue desiccation, and diligent postoperative management.

Methods of Closure

Once the decision to close the wound has been made, the surgeon must choose an appropriate method. The decision requires an understanding of the objectives of repair as well as the materials implemented to effect such a repair. The ultimate goal of any closure is to achieve precise tensionless alignment of the injured parts without further injury to adjacent structures. This will allow prompt restoration of function and cosmetic appearance.

The choice of appropriate material for wound closure is based on its biologic and mechanical properties as well as characteristics of the tissues being approximated. Composition of the material, strength, knot efficiency, tissue response, and wound location should all be considered. The surgeon's armamentarium includes a variety of suture materials, stainless steel staples, and surgical tapes. To a degree, however, the choice of material for surgical closure is less important than the surgical technique. Each suture must be properly placed and tied without excessive tension to minimize ischemia of the wound edges. The least reactive and the smallest size and amount of suture material that will adequately effect tissue approximation, particularly in contaminated wounds, should be employed.

The necessity to close individual layers of the wound is based on knowledge of local wound stresses, presence of dead space, and the necessity for accurate approximation of tissues. Dense connective tissues (e.g., dermis, fascia, ligaments, tendons) represent the strength layers of any wound closure. These tissues heal slowly, however, and the suture material chosen to approximate them should be capable of maintaining its strength until satisfactory union has occurred. Ideally, such a suture should incite a minimal amount of local tissue reaction. Synthetic, monofilament, nonabsorbable sutures are best suited for this purpose.

Muscle and adipose tissues do not hold sutures well. Closure of these layers is occasionally necessary in order to obliterate dead space. In the laboratory model, dead space resulting from tissue loss has been shown to increase the likelihood of infection. Obliteration of dead space with sutures, however, enhances the possibility of infection because the sutures act as foreign bodies in the wound. Suturing of the dead space is particularly contraindicated in the closure of contaminated wounds. When necessary, the dead space should be obliterated with a minimal number of loosely tied absorbable sutures.

Skin closure may be performed in layers or by full-thickness percutaneous sutures. Surgical tapes or staples may also be considered. The choice of method depends on the location of the wound, its direction, and local stress factors. Wounds that are oriented in the direction of skin wrinkles are subjected to less tension during healing, and consequently produce a more favorable scar. Examples include transverse lacerations involving the forehead or neck. Wounds that cross the lines of maximal stress are subjected to increased tension during healing and have a propensity to widen and hypertrophy with time. Examples include lacerations over the deltoid region or the cheek. In most situations, the acute wound should be debrided and closed without any attempt at reorientation of the direction of the scar. The scar should be allowed to mature before considering scar revision.

The degree of wound gaping prior to epidermal reapproximation reflects the potential width of the scar. Particularly in areas of high skin tension, layered wound closure is indicated to minimize the final width of the scar. The dermis should be anatomically realigned with interrupted inverted sutures. A few well-placed 5–0 or 6–0 clear Nylon sutures will provide adequate reapproximation of the dermal layer until the wound has healed and the scar matured. Dermal Nylon sutures, however, may remain palpable or visible through the skin. Absorbable sutures are more frequently employed for dermal closure. Catgut sutures, which are made from animal protein (available either in the plain or chromic form), are frequently employed for dermal closure. Catgut sutures, however, display erratic behavior in loss of strength, absorption, and tissue reaction. For these reasons, many surgeons prefer to use synthetic absorbable sutures (e.g., polyglycolic acid, polyglactin) for dermal reapproximation. Even though these sutures do have longer holding power than catgut, they too lose their holding power before wound maturation is complete. Recent studies with polydioxanone monofilament absorbable sutures have demonstrated prolonged breaking strength retention, a reliable absorption profile, and minimal tissue reaction. Experience with polydioxanone is still limited, but perhaps this suture will prove to be the most appropriate material for dermal approximation. Following closure of the dermis, the strength layer of the wound, the epidermal layer can be adjusted with fine, nonabsorbable, monofilament sutures—chosen for their low tissue reactivity—or surgical tape. This method of wound closure is designed to provide the least noticeable scar and is most appropriate for facial lacerations.

Percutaneous sutures that incorporate both the epidermis and dermis and a small amount of underlying subcutaneous tissue are frequently employed to close wounds elsewhere in the body. Such sutures are usually removed 7 to 14 days later. Without dermal support during the subsequent maturation phase, the scar tends to widen and hypertrophy.

Factors in obtaining a satisfactory scar include eversion of the wound edges to effect precise epidermal coaptation and proper suture tension to minimize ischemia of the wound margins. In order to obtain everted wound edges, the sutures must be placed so that the depth of each bite exceeds its width. It has been clearly shown that the size of suture material employed is not so important as the tightness of the closure or the length of time that the sutures are left in situ. Sutures should be removed before the seventh day to avoid epithelization of the suture tracts with a resultant objectionable (railroad) appearance of the scar.

Monofilament, synthetic nonabsorbable sutures (e.g., nylon, polypropylene) are most frequently employed for percutaneous skin closure. Silk sutures, which are natural fibers, are significantly more reactive and have been shown to increase the incidence of wound infection. Silk should not be used in acute wounds, except occasionally for closure of intraoral mucosal laceration.

Stainless steel sutures, skin clips, and staples have been employed for years because of their presumed inertness. However, studies have suggested slightly increased infection rates, probably owing to the mechanical irritation because of their rigidity. This fact will be of little, if any, clinical significance if the staples are removed before the seventh postoperative day. A number of prepackaged skin staplers are now available. Most staplers are designed to produce an everted skin closure and can do so quickly. The main advantage of staplers is a significant reduction in wound closure time, particularly with extensive lacerations or in such specialized situations as securing multiple skin grafts.

Surgical tapes have the advantage of not requiring anesthesia or painful stimuli during wound closure. Such techniques are particularly attractive in the care of the pediatric population. Taped wounds also have the least propensity for infection. In certain situations, one may close the deeper layers of the wound (including the dermis) with sutures and coapt the epidermal layer with tape—thus avoiding the need to later remove skin sutures. Microporous, rayon reinforced wound tapes are widely used. Adherence is enhanced if all moisture is removed and the skin defatted with acetone prior to application to the skin. Tincture of benzoin may initially enhance tape adhesion, but it is quickly solubilized by skin oils and loses its adherence capabilities, thus contraindicating its use. Wound tapes do, however, have significant disadvantages. It is difficult to obtain precise anatomic approximation of the skin edges with surgical tapes, particularly with irregular lacerations. It is impossible to obtain an everted closure solely with tape. Moreover, tape only approximates the superficial portion of the wound and leaves deeper layers vulnerable to biomechanical stresses, which may result in widening and a more prominent scar.

Wound Drains

Justification for drains has been stated to include obliteration of dead space and to allow egress of material foreign or harmful to a particular location. Drains are rarely, if ever, indicated in the closure of acute superficial wounds. Percutaneous drains constitute foreign bodies, enhance tissue necrosis, and serve as conduits for bacterial contamination. Contrary to popular opinion, drains do not prevent the formation of hematomas or seromas. If good surgical technique has been employed, it will be unnecessary to drain most superficial wounds in the acute situation. If bleeding cannot be controlled at the time of operation, delayed primary wound closure should be considered. Drains may, however, be an important adjunctive measure in the treatment of superficial abscesses. The specific indications for drainage of body cavities and organs are discussed in separate chapters.

POSTOPERATIVE WOUND CARE

The surgeon's responsibilities do not end with wound closure. The surgeon must provide maximal support of the patient and a suitable environment for satisfactory wound healing, and he must direct the patient's rehabilitation.

Although wound healing may be considered a local phenomenon, the ideal milieu for the wound can only be provided by total patient care. Attention must be paid to associated injuries. In addition, nutrition, blood volume, and oxygenation must be maintained. A social worker may provide valuable assistance to a patient with a physically disabling injury. Likewise, a psychiatrist may help a patient to cope with an altered body image following a disfiguring injury.

The sutured wound should be protected from the environment with a dressing impervious to exogenous microbial contamination. Experimental studies have demonstrated that closed wounds can be infected by surface bacterial contamination within the first 2 or 3 days. Following this period, sutured wounds gain considerable resistance to infection, and dressings no longer serve a protective role. Taped wounds demonstrated superior resistance to infection, becoming resistant to surface contamination within 2 hours following wound closure.

A dressing may serve a number of functions that may contribute to healing. Ideally, a dressing should provide an atmosphere conducive to satisfactory wound healing. The dressing should keep the wound surface free of excess fluids to minimize maceration and bacterial proliferation while, at the same time, avoiding desiccation. The main functions of a dressing may be listed as follows: protection, immobilization, compression, absorption, debridement, medication, and cosmesis. As the wound heals, its needs may change and necessitate a different type of dressing.

Most dressings consist of a contact layer, an absorptive layer, and an outer wrap. Plastic-coated dressings (e.g., Telfa) or gauze impregnated with bismuth ointment (e.g., Xeroform) or petrolatum provides a satisfactory contact layer. A bulky intermediate layer should be applied to absorb wound exudate. A plaster or aluminum splint may be added to the dressing to enhance immobilization.

Dry gauze is frequently applied to a freshly closed wound. Such a dressing will adhere to the epithelium and vascular tissue of the wound and may result in interference with wound healing during dressing changes. Preferably, the contact layer should consist of nonadherent plastic-coated material or gauze impregnated with a bland ointment. This contact layer should be applied as a single sheet to allow continued egress of wound fluid through the contact layer. Fluffed gauze sponges, mechanics' waste, and bulk cotton may be added as an absorptive layer, to allow the dressing to conform to a desired shape, and to provide immobilization of the wounded part. Nonstretchable, firm, roller gauze bandage and adhesive tape complete the typical occlusive dressing, thus providing a compact and stable immobilizing influence.

Occlusive tapes limit vapor transmission, promoting tissue maceration and bacterial growth. Porous paper tapes are preferable as they allow moisture to be transmitted through the interstices of the tape, with resultant dry skin beneath the tape, which inhibits bacterial proliferation.

Immobilization may avert further tissue damage. Immobilization of the site of injury is essential in the managment of contaminated wounds because lymphatic flow is thus reduced in the immobilized part, thereby minimizing the spread of wound microflora. Immobilization places the wound at rest, thus decreasing pain and metabolic demands of the tissues. In addition, immobilization may protect the newly formed capillaries from disruption, thus avoiding small clots and allowing the wound to heal more expeditiously. When combined with elevation and pressure, the transudation of fluid is minimized. Immobilization may be aided by bulky dressings, skin tapes, or splints. The length of immobilization varies according to the demands of local tissues and the status of the

wound. Prolonged immobilization, however, may defeat its possible advantages.

One cannot overemphasize the advantage of elevating the injured part to minimize edema with its resultant deleterious effects. This is particularly applicable to extremity injuries. Edema, which has been stated to be "the mother of scar," slows down the machinery of repair and increases fibrous tissue proliferation. Elevation of the wounded part above the level of the heart is the simplest method of limiting the amount of edema. In certain situations, compression of the wound with bulky dressings may subserve the benefits of elevation. However, one must not apply tourniquet-like constriction to proximal parts or distal venous and lymphatic congestion could result. In extremity injuries, compression dressings should extend from the most distal point proximally, but access to the toes or fingertips should be maintained to allow assessment of the neurovascular status. Maximal wound edema occurs within the first 48 hours and gradually resolves over the next week. It may be necessary to adjust an extremity dressing during periods of fluctuating tissue edema.

A clean wound should have very little drainage and require few dressing changes. Unless clinical signs dictate otherwise, the initial dressing should be left intact over most sutured wounds for the first 48 hours. As mentioned previously, sealed wounds will be highly resistant to surface bacterial contamination by this time, and further dressings may be unnecessary. In most clinical situations, the patient with a well-healing wound may shower by the third day. Wounds that continue to drain serous fluid, however, require continued protection with an appropriate dressing.

Certain wounds are not amenable to the satisfactory application of a dressing. It is frequently difficult to apply a conforming dressing to sutured facial lacerations. Meticulous suture line care may provide a reasonable alternative. This involves frequent cleansing with saline or dilute hydrogen peroxide solution to remove adherent coagulum, thus decreasing the likelihood of stitch abscess formation. Following cleansing, a thin layer of antibiotic ointment should be applied to the suture line.

Dressings may also be used to debride an open wound. The traditional wet-to-dry method utilizes avulsion of adherent tissues to provide the debridement. This method is effective if performed properly, but one must remember that the dressing does not discriminate between viable and nonviable tissues and tissue injury results with each dressing change. Moistening the dressing prior to removal defeats the purpose of such a dressing. A wet-to-dry dressing should not be employed in wounds containing viable periosteum, perichondrium, paratenon, or perineurium because such tissues desiccate during the "dry" phase, resulting in further tissue damage.

Enzymatic debridement provides an alternative to the wet-to-dry dressing. An enzyme produced by *B subtilis* (Travase) is effective in removing particulate necrotic debris and coagulum without producing significant injury to viable tissues.

Medicated dressings are occasionally indicated. Topical antimicrobial agents, particularly silver sulfadiazine (Silvadene) and mafenide (Sulfamylon) are frequently employed to control surface contaminants in chronic granulating wounds. These agents are also useful in the management of partial-thickness injuries or wounds containing marginally viable tissues to decrease the potential for bacterial invasion with subsequent conversion to a full-thickness injury and necrosis. Topical agents, however, retard wound epithelization and should be discontinued as soon as their objectives have been reached (mainly bacterial counts less than 10^5 organisms per gram of tissue).

A surgeon should not discount the importance of a neat dressing. To the patient or casual observer, the sight of a wound may be abhorent and incite fear or anxiety. A carefully applied dressing reassures the patient that the best possible wound care has been provided.

Rehabilitation may require the assistance of a physical or occupational therapist. The surgeon's responsibility to the patient does not end until the scar has matured and the patient has returned to the mainstream of life.

NEUROLOGIC INJURY

Henry M. Bartkowski, M.D., Ph.D.
Lawrence H. Pitts, M.D.

HEAD INJURY

Head injuries account for approximately half of trauma fatalities and result in more than five million days of hospitalization and 30 million days of work lost annually in the United States. While prevention of head injury ultimately will reduce morbidity and mortality most effectively, we currently must direct our attention toward aggressive management of craniocerebral trauma after impact. Primary mechanical brain damage that occurs at the moment of injury cannot be repaired by therapeutic intervention; thus management of head injury attempts to prevent secondary insults to the traumatized brain.

During initial treatment of head injury, restoration of normal cardiopulmonary function is of paramount importance. Resuscitation must be accomplished promptly in the emergency room. Unconscious patients should be intubated immediately for airway protection as aspiration can cause sudden pulmonary compromise leading to hypoxia and hypercapnia, which cause additional insult to the brain. Even without evidence of aspiration, between 30 and 50 percent of patients with traumatic coma are hypoxic when first treated, and endotracheal intubation allows mechanical ventilation with increased arterial P_{O_2} and decreased P_{CO_2}. Head injury alone does not produce shock except in the terminal phases of brain death, when medullary failure leads to cessation of respiration and to agonal hypotension. The significance of shock cannot be overemphasized. Patients presenting with severe head injury and hypotension suffer a 90 percent mortality, whereas patients with a similar degree of head injury who are not in shock have a 50 percent mortality. Hypotension must be assumed to be due to hypovolemia and its cause sought from bleeding into the chest, abdomen, or extremities.

In order to reverse possible hypoglycemia or narcotic overdose, which may contribute to neurologic depression, we routinely administer 50 ml of 50 percent dextrose and 0.4 mg of naloxone to comatose patients after obtaining blood and urine specimens for routine and toxicologic studies.

Physical Examination

The initial physical examination must include sufficient observations to determine an accurate baseline evaluation, recorded in a manner that will allow clinical changes to be readily appreciated by subsequent examiners. Vital signs are, of course, essential. Abnormalities of pulse and blood pressure may reflect a primary cardiac event as the etiology of the patient's disorder. On the other hand, it is well established that hypertension with bradycardia, the Cushing reflex, is a sign of increased intracranial pressure and signifies an intracranial mass lesion until proved otherwise. Associated injuries must be identified and therapy instituted because such injuries may lead to airway compromise, blood gas abnormalities, or shock, all of which will compound neurologic damage (Table 1). A cervical spine injury should be assumed to exist, and the head and neck kept in a neutral position until a lateral film of the cervical spine excludes spine instability.

The scalp must be inspected carefully for lacerations or puncture wounds. Small puncture wounds may be the only outward sign of penetrating injuries. They may occur anywhere on the scalp and commonly may be missed by the examiner if located in the dependent occipital area. Depressed fractures may or may not be identified by digital palpation of the scalp or exploration of a laceration. As in the case of puncture wounds, depressed fractures may involve any portion of the calvarium. In the case of an open brain injury, no

47

TABLE 1   Multisystem Injuries Associated with Major Head Injury

Head injury and facial injury	14%
Head injury and chest injury	16%
Head injury and extremity injury	20%
Head injury and abdominal injury	21%
Head injury and at least one other injury	39%

further inspection is warranted; these wounds must be debrided and closed in the operating room.

Basilar skull fractures are diagnosed on the basis of physical findings. Circumscribed unilateral or bilateral periorbital ecchymoses or "raccoon eyes" are indications of intraorbital bleeding from fractures of the floor of the frontal fossa. Blood in the external canal indicates a basilar fracture through the lateral portion of the temporal bone. A temporal bone fracture medial to the tympanic membrane results in a hemotympanum. Ecchymosis overlying the mastoid, Battle's sign, represents blood dissecting to the skin from a mastoid fracture; it usually is delayed for 12 to 24 hours after initial injury. Leakage of cerebrospinal fluid via the nose (rhinorrhea) or the ear (otorrhea) is a manifestation of meningeal disruption at the site of a basilar fracture and carries the risk of meningitis. Damage to the seventh or eighth cranial nerve may accompany temporal bone fractures. Facial palsy of immediate onset represents direct facial nerve inury at the site of temporal bone fracture and requires early diagnostic evaluation and possible early surgical repair. Delayed onset facial palsies usually resolve spontaneously without surgical intervention. Tearing and stretching injuries to the auditory and vestibular nerves severely disrupt hearing and balance and are irreparable by any currently available surgical or medical treatment.

Emergency Neurologic Examination

The initial neurologic examination must be rapid and complete; immediate therapeutic and diagnostic actions hinge on the findings. The examination must determine the level of consciousness, brainstem or spinal cord dysfunction, and the presence of any peripheral nerve injury. Level of consciousness has been described poorly by a variety of imprecise words such as lethargy, stupor, or obtundation, which imprecisely describe changes in neurologic function in different patients or in the same patient at different times. An alter-

native to these terms has been the Glasgow Coma Scale (Table 2). This system records the patient's response to verbal and painful stimuli and has been widely adopted at trauma centers. It is a valuable tool for following a patient's improvement or deterioration, is highly reliable, and is accompanied by remarkably little variation among examiners.

The integrity of midbrain, pontine, and medullary function is determined by cranial nerve examination. The pupillary light reflex allows evaluation of the optic and oculomotor nerves. A pupil that is dilated and unresponsive after injury indicates ipsilateral transtentorial herniation from an expanding mass lesion. The oculocephalic reflex (doll's eyes maneuver) consists of conjugate eye deviation contralateral to the direction of head rotation. The reflex evaluates connections between the vestibular apparatus, pontine gaze centers, and sixth and third nerve nuclei in the pons and midbrain. The head should be turned to elicit the response *only* if a cervical fracture has been excluded by appropriate cervical spine x-ray studies. In the event of a cervical fracture, the pontine gaze center and its connection to the third and sixth cranial nerves can be evaluated by the oculovestibular reflex (caloric testing). The expected response to cold water irrigation of the auditory canal in a comatose patient is conjugate deviation of the eyes toward the irrigated ear. Supraorbital pressure can be used to elicit a facial grimace to test seventh nerve function in a comatose patient. Cough and gag reflex can be used to evaluate lower cranial nerve and medullary function.

Diagnostic Procedures

In the emergency room, when a comatose patient is being initially evaluated, a chest roentgenogram and a lateral cervical spine film should be taken immediately, the former to rule out pneumothorax, hemothorax, or other pulmonary lesions that may lead to hypoxia or hypercapnia and the latter to rule out a cervical spine fracture. Skull films should be obtained for any penetrating injury if a fracture is suspected on physical examination, or if injury produced loss of consciousness for several minutes or more. If a patient is neurologically intact following head injury, without headache, nausea or vomiting, lethargy or focal deficit, radiographs of the skull are not warranted. Computerized tomographic (CT) scanning has largely replaced arteriography and ventriculography in the

TABLE 2   Glasgow Coma Scale

Eye Opening	Best Motor Response	Best Verbal Response
4 Spontaneously	6 Follows commands	5 Oriented
3 To voice	5 Localized painful stimulus	4 Confused
2 To pain	4 Complex arm movement	3 Inappropriate words
1 None	3 Reflex flexor posturing	2 Incomprehensible sounds
	3 Reflex extensor posturing	1 None
	1 Flaccid	

diagnosis of traumatic intracranial lesions. Radioisotope scanning has no role in the early phases of head trauma.

Classification

Head injured patients can be placed into four groups, depending on the severity of injury.

Brainstem Dysfunction

Patients with signs of brainstem dysfunction require immediate aggressive investigation and treatment. Transtentorial herniation is accompanied by the triad of ipsilateral sluggish pupillary constriction to light, depressed consciousness, and contralateral or ipsilateral hemiparesis. This complex requires immediate treatment consisting of:

1. Emergency endotracheal intubation to optimize arterial oxygenation, allow hyperventilation, and protect the airway against obstruction from blood, vomitus, or pharyngeal soft tissue.

2. Maintenance of normal blood pressure by intravenous fluid resuscitation and placement of the patient in Trendelenberg position, since lowering of systemic pressure in the face of elevated intracranial pressure (ICP) can cause inadequate cerebral perfusion and cerebral ischemia.

3. Use of hyperosmotic agents such as mannitol (1.5 g/kg infused rapidly intravenously).

4. Immediate transport to the operating room for placement of an emergency temporal burr hole on the side of the dilated pupil. If an extracerebral hematoma is found, a craniotomy is performed to evacuate the clot. If a hematoma is not found by burr hole exploration, the patient is taken for an immediate CT scan (if available, otherwise cerebral angiography) to diagnose intraparenchymal lesions including hemorrhage and focal edema. It is essential to relieve brain stem compression as quickly as possible to prevent irreversible ischemic damage.

5. Based upon a clinical trial in our institu-

tion, corticosteroids are ineffective in improving outcome from severe head injury. The efficacy of barbiturates in improving outcome has not been adequately established, and their use is accompanied by substantial cardiovascular side-effects; thus they cannot be recommended for widespread use until appropriate trials are completed.

Focal Neurologic Deficit

Patients with focal neurologic deficits (e.g., hemiparesis, dysphasia) in the absence of brain stem compression (e.g., pupillary dilatation, abnormal eye movements) should be evaluated by CT scanning if available, or by cerebral angiography. If the patient has a decreasing level of consciousness while the study is being performed, mannitol should be given (1.5 g/kg infused rapidly intravenously), followed by surgery if indicated by the diagnostic study. If CT scanning reveals a mass lesion, immediate decompression is performed via craniotomy. Speed is the most important factor in treating a mass lesion; the sooner the brain is decompressed the better the outcome.

Depressed Consciousness: No Focal Deficit

In patients with a depressed level of consciousness but no focal deficit, careful serial observation may be employed to determine whether the patient will improve neurologically without specific intervention. If the patient fails to display neurologic improvement within a few hours or shows any deterioration, a CT scan or cerebral angiogram should be performed. If a mass lesion, infarct, or edema is not found, a thorough metabolic work-up should be done to determine the cause of altered consciousness.

No Apparent Neurologic Deficit

Patients who are neurologically intact following head injury are unlikely to develop delayed complications. Even patients with classic "lucid intervals" before deterioration usually have significant headache or some degree of lethargy when seen after injury. Short periods of retrograde or anterograde amnesia are of no prognostic importance; however, prolonged amnesia manifest by continuing confusion and inability to answer simple questions is a significant neurologic deficit and requires close observation. Nausea and vomiting are common after head injury in children and generally of no prognostic value. However, severe vomiting may necessitate hospitalization for treatment of dehydration. The child is intravenously hydrated at two-thirds maintenance intake so as to avoid overhydration and worsening of any brain edema that may be present.

Patients who have skull fractures and in whom there was a loss of consciousness for greater than several minutes should be hospitalized for close observation for a 24-hour period, since the patient initially may be lucid, but then deteriorate as with an epidural hematoma. If the circumstances surrounding the head injury are unclear, and problems such as seizures or syncopal episodes may have precipitated the injury, admission should be considered to evaluate these possibilities. If the patient can be observed by reliable and intelligent family members or friends, he or she may be observed at home with careful instructions given for recognition of signs of possible deterioration and for obtaining additional medical consultation or care if necessary.

Compound depressed fractures require immediate operation to prevent development of late intracranial infection. These fractures are debrided, and the bone fragments are washed in an antibiotic solution (such as bacitracin, 50,000 units in 500 ml of normal saline) and reserved for immediate replacement. Dural and brain lacerations are debrided and the dura repaired either primarily or by the use of pericranial or fascia lata grafts. Large dural lacerations overlying basilar fractures may be repaired by onlay grafts of temporalis fascia, fascia lata, or pericranium.

Intracranial pressure is monitored in all postoperative and comatose nonoperative patients via a catheter placed into the lateral ventricle, if possible, or in the subdural space. Alternatively, a threaded bolt can be placed through a small drill hole in the skull, under which the dura has been opened. An intraventricular catheter gives the most accurate readings and can be used as a therapeutic measure by the withdrawal of intraventricular fluid to reduce intracranial pressure.

The catheter system is filled with an antibiotic solution, such as tobramycin or gentamycin, 10 mg in 20 ml of normal saline. This same solution is used to fill the transducer. Epidural fiberoptic intracranial pressure monitors are being used more widely and offer a satisfactory alternative to the fluid-filled systems. They do not permit withdrawal of cerebrospinal fluid for control of intracranial pressure, which is possible with intraventricular catheters. Intracranial pressures up to 20 mmHg are considered to be within normal limits; above that level the pressure is considered to be abnormal and appropriate treatment is indicated to reduce the pressure.

Postoperative Care

Supportive care following the initial resuscitation and/or surgical intervention is a critical phase in the management of head injury and is optimally provided in an intensive care unit. The skills of the anesthesiologists and medical and surgical subspecialists can be added to those of intensive care nurses and respiratory therapists to keep the patient as stable as possible during the posttraumatic period.

When it occurs, intracranial hypertension is most pronounced in the first 2 or 3 days after trauma. Exceptions to this rule include such patients as those with diffuse cerebral swelling in whom the ICP may remain elevated for 10 to 14 days. Patients with ICP above 20 torr show a significantly higher morbidity and mortality than those whose ICP can be controlled below this level. Death almost uniformly results with uncontrolled intracranial hypertension above 40 torr. It is imperative to obtain adequate control of intracranial hypertension using a combination of the following:

1. *Surgical decompression.* Removal of even relatively small quantities of hematoma or necrotic brain may markedly lower ICP and prevent herniation.

2. *Head elevation.* This measure enhances venous drainage and lowers venous pressure.

3. *Ventricular fluid drainage.* This can immediately lower ICP. In the case of diffuse cerebral swelling, it is of limited value, for little cerebrospinal fluid (CSF) is available for removal.

4. *Hyperventilation*. Cerebral vessels constrict in response to hypocapnia. It is best used for short periods, being allowed to return to mildly hypocarbic levels (Pco_2 28 to 32 torr) as other methods of controlling hypertension are employed.

5. *Hyperosmotic therapy*. Mannitol may be administered in doses of 0.5 g/kg every 3 hours. Its use is best guided by actual ICP monitoring. Mannitol should not be used when serum osmolality exceeds 340 milliosmoles, since osmotic levels above this level can cause cerebral dysfunction.

6. *Diuretics*. Furosemide (Lasix) may decrease elevated ICP both by dehydration secondary to diuresis and by inhibiting production of CSF by the choroid plexus. Diuretics may be used alone or in conjunction with hyperosmotic therapy. A common dose is 0.5 to 1 mg/kg every 4 to 6 hours.

7. *Maintain normothermia or moderate hypothermia (35 to 37 degrees centigrade.)* This lowers cerebral metabolism and may reduce elevated ICP. Attempts to lower body temperature may be accompanied by generalized shivering, and this increased muscular activity can elevate ICP by thoracic contraction and elevation of central venous pressures.

8. *Barbiturate coma*. Its efficacy in head injury has not been clearly established and requires further evaluation.

Anticonvulsants are routinely used in patients with coma-producing head injuries. The presence of intracranial hematomas, depressed fractures, or post-traumatic amnesia lasting longer than 24 hours increases the likelihood of early seizures. Relatively few seizures occur after the first year following injury, and these late seizures are not diminished in frequency by the early use of anticonvulsant therapy. Diphenylhydantoin or phenobarbital should be used during the first 12 months after head injury and then gradually discontinued over several months if the patient has remained seizure-free. We recommend 300 mg of Dilantin daily or 30 to 45 mg of phenobarbital t.i.d. as maintenance dosage. Anticonvulsant therapy can be restarted in the small population of patients who develop late seizures.

Late sequelae of head injury include the post-concussion syndrome and cerebrospinal fluid leaks. The former, which consists of headache, dizziness, and memory deficits, has no specific therapy, but usually resolves within weeks to months. Late CSF leaks may occur following basilar skull fracture. These usually do not subside spontaneously and generally require surgical repair.

SPINAL CORD INJURY

The primary responsibility of emergency personnel is to identify spinal cord injury and prevent further cord damage. Careful physical examination is crucial in the assessment of an injured patient's spine and spinal cord function. Spinal cord injury evaluation requires determination of the level of damage and a differentiation between complete or incomplete spinal cord injury.

Immediately after a spinal cord injury, there occurs a transient period of disordered function called "spinal shock." During this time no reflex or voluntary activity can be elicited distal to the level of injury, as determined by a careful motor and sensory examination. Once some reflex activity has returned, and if there is no distal sensation or voluntary motor control, the cord lesion can be deemed complete and without chance of functional recovery. The bulbocavernosus reflex is the earliest to recover from spinal shock; it involves the contraction of the anal sphincter in response to glans penis or clitoris compression or by gentle traction on an indwelling urinary catheter.

It is important to differentiate between nerve root injuries and damage to the cord itself by a detailed neurologic examination and careful radiologic work-up. Roots just proximal to a cord injury often are contused and may not function initially, but may recover over several days, weeks, or months. Injuries of the thoracolumbar junction may involve the conus medullaris. This injury carries a poorer prognosis than a cauda equina injury, since the former involves anterior horn cell distribution and the latter may only reflect a peripheral nerve injury, which has a much better chance of recovery. Most incomplete cord injuries improve; obvious deterioration is uncommon, and if it should occur, emergency diagnostic studies and possibly surgical decompression are warranted.

X-ray studies of the cervical spine must be obtained before moving the neck of an unconscious or obtunded trauma patient, and in any alert individual who complains of neck pain. Neurologic examination identifies the presence and extent of cord injury; however, radiographs better indicate the severity of damage to the vertebral column and the risk of further injury to the cord.

Anterior prevertebral soft tissue swelling or slight malalignment of vertebrae might be the only suggestion of gross ligamentous instability. One should be aware that injuries may involve multiple spinal levels. Flexion and extension views are not indicated in an emergency setting and should only be performed under the direct supervision of a neurosurgeon. CT scanning has added a new dimension to the radiology of spine trauma and may demonstrate more clearly than plain roentgenograms the anatomy of the spine injury and possible spinal canal compromise. Radiologic assessment of dural compression with a myelogram or CT-metrizamide scan has been proposed as a guide for planning early treatment of spinal cord injuries; however, the significance of a myelographic block remains controversial. If angulation, dislocation, or fragment retropulsion compromises the spinal canal, it should be corrected as rapidly as possible, starting with traction, but employing open surgical reduction of dislocations as necessary.

Spinal cord injury patients may require treatment for hypotension, respiratory failure, paralytic ileus and urinary retention. Insensitive skin must be protected from pressure by careful turning of the patient at least every 2 hours and bridging high pressure areas such as heels, sacrum, and occiput. The efficacy of corticosteroids in spinal cord injury is uncertain; a multicenter clinical trial is in progress to evaluate the use of steroids. In the absence of neurologic deterioration, there is no convincing evidence that surgical treatment for decompression or stabilization promotes neurologic recovery.

PERIPHERAL NERVE AND BRACHIAL PLEXUS INJURY

There are many causes of peripheral nerve and brachial plexus injury, and in 60 percent of cases gross continuity of the nerve is preserved. Proper management and eventual recovery depend on various pathophysiologic factors. These factors are assessed on the basis of a thorough history of the circumstances and mechanics of injury, serial clinical examinations, and electrodiagnostic studies of the lesion. Decisions regarding whether to operate, when to operate, and what to do once the lesion is surgically exposed should be based on an intimate understanding of neural regeneration as well as a respect for the practical limitations of functional recovery.

When it is likely that a peripheral nerve has been transected, management is relatively straightforward. A sharply divided nerve, particularly at the brachial plexus level or for the sciatic nerve at the buttock level, is an indication for immediate primary suture. If there is associated blunt trauma to the nerve, repair should be delayed two or three weeks to allow demarcation of the injury of the proximal and distal stumps of the divided nerve. When acute wound exploration is necessitated by vascular injury and it reveals divided and contused nerves, the surgeon should identify proximal and distal stumps and affix them to muscle or fascia to minimize stump retraction until definitive nerve repair is done 2 or 3 weeks later. The in-continuity nerve lesion challenges the clinician to determine accurately the need for resection and suture. If there is neither clinical nor electrodiagnostic evidence of regeneration within 8 weeks of injury, the lesion should be explored and nerve action potentials should be evaluated intraoperatively. If intraoperative nerve stimulation does not transmit an action potential across the lesion, resection and suture are indicated. If electrical conduction through the lesion can be shown at the time of nerve exploration, significant function will return in 95 percent of cases and nerve resection is contraindicated.

Functional recovery from peripheral nerve injury depends on the patient's age, the type of injury, the particular nerve involved, the level of injury, and the length of delay until repair. Prognosis is better for the sharply transected nerve, if repaired immediately, than for stretch injuries or nerve contusion that require major resection with or without graft. Distal injuries generally have better recoveries than proximal ones because the regeneration distance to end-organs is shorter and because regeneration pathways are more direct with fewer interfascicular connections and fewer misdirected regenerated fibers. The longer the delay between injury and treatment, the poorer the recovery. A surgical delay of more than 6 months usually is incompatible with functional recovery, except with distal lesions in favorable nerves or with children. Regeneration is very poor in elderly patients. Poor rehabilitative efforts adversely affect the quality of the distal field the regenerating axons must reinnervate. The patient must be started in a rehabilitative program as soon as is possible if maximum functional recovery is to be achieved.

MAXILLOFACIAL TRAUMA

Robert L. Walton, M.D.
Juris Bunkis, M.D.
Judith J. Petry, M.D.

Injuries of the maxillofacial region are common, particularly in urban areas, where victims of automobile collisions and physical assaults constitute a large proportion of the emergency room traffic. The severity of injury is not often reflected in initial appearances. Copious bleeding, early swelling, and associated neurologic disturbances frequently make accurate clinical assessment difficult, if not impossible. Early management, therefore, is often limited to control of life-threatening emergencies and other time-dependent problems such as compromised vision.

This chapter constitutes a summary of the techniques we have found useful in the management of acute injuries of the maxillofacial complex. Although this chapter focuses primarily on the management of facial fractures, we have included special sections addressing facial nerve, parotid, and laryngeal injuries.

GENERAL CONSIDERATIONS

The timing of therapy depends on numerous variables of which age, associated injuries, and antecedent medical problems play a pivotal role in the decision-making process. Obviously, each patient must be individualized. Our philosophy has been to effect wound closure and fracture reduction as early as possible. From a wound healing point of view, this approach makes good sense, yet the factors governing this act defy generalization. In the heat of the resuscitation/stabilization battle, there is little chance or sense in pursuing a precise, comprehensive therapeutic assault. For facial fractures, a "grace period" of about 10 days (except for mandibular fractures) allows time for an organized "team" assessment and operative plan. Massive soft tissue swelling is perhaps a relative contraindication to early operative reduction

of facial fractures. If surgery is delayed, every effort to hasten the dissolution of swelling should be implemented. This includes debridement and simple closure of open wounds, elevation of the head, and immobilization of the fracture. The latter may require the simple implementation of a liquid diet (usually through a straw), a Barton bandage, or gross wire fixation of the dentition. Contamination of mandibular fractures through the oral cavity usually is not a major consideration unless operative reduction is delayed beyond 2 to 3 days or there is a significant amount of periodontal disease or dental caries. In these situations, we prefer to irrigate the oral cavity with a Cleocin solution, 300 mg/100 cc water, every 6 hours. This method has significantly decreased the incidence of infections in our patients.

In patients with severe midfacial and/or mandibular trauma, presenting with acute upper airway obstruction, a cricothyroidotomy is preferred over direct oral or nasotracheal intubation because it is quick, carries minimal risk, and avoids unnecessary manipulation of the injured parts. Furthermore, it is difficult to perform a precise midfacial fracture reduction encumbered by the tether of a nasotracheal tube. In the same context, oral tracheal tubes are not employed in fractures of the mandible or maxilla. Moreover, both of the latter techniques are quite uncomfortable for the patient. The cricothyroidotomy is left in place until after the operative management of the facial fractures, when the patient has recovered sufficiently to maintain an adequate airway. The airway can be maintained safely via the cricothyroidotomy. Rarely is it necessary to convert a cricothyroidotomy to a tracheostomy if the injury has been confined to the maxillofacial region. A primary tracheostomy is performed in the operating room for those maxillofacial injuries associated with laryngeal or hypopharyngeal obstruction, intracranial injury, chest or high spinal cord injury, or anticipation of prolonged postoperative airway problems. If the airway is not acutely compromised, nasal or oral tracheal intubation is preferable prior to tracheostomy, provided this can be accomplished by direct visualization of the hypopharyngeal structures; otherwise a cricothyroidotomy is performed first.

A thorough physical examination is performed prior to any diagnostic studies. Evaluation of the cervical spine is a first-line priority which precedes any detailed facial study. Most facial fractures can be diagnosed easily with a minimum of radiographs. A stereo Water's roentgenogram is perhaps the single most informative view in the standard "facial series." Specialized views of the mandible (posterior-anterior, lateral oblique, or Panorex) are often necessary in evaluating fractures of the subcondylar regions or assessment of dentition in the fracture line. If available, the computerized axial tomogram (CAT) is an extremely accurate tool in the radiologic examination of the facial skeleton. This method exposes the patient to less radiation than does standard tomography and allows visualization of areas that cannot easily be examined by conventional techniques. Over the past 2 years, we have exclusively employed the CAT examination for all complex upper and mid-facial fractures.

SOFT TISSUE INJURIES

The basic precepts of wound management will be dealt with in another chapter. Suffice it to state that the maxillofacial region constitutes a complex anatomy with specialized structures that serve innumerable important functions. For this reason, extensive debridement of the facial wound should be avoided. The rich vascular supply to this region allows salvage of tissues that otherwise might be discarded. In heavily contaminated wounds, minimal debridement and delayed closure are perhaps the most appropriate therapy. Specialized injuries of the face, such as those involving the facial nerve, the parotid gland and its duct, and the larynx, will be addressed.

Facial Nerve Injuries

Any wound that lies in the anatomic distribution of the facial nerve must be carefully assessed for injury to the nerve. In the conscious, cooperative patient, a thorough motor test is appropriate. Because of the extensive interneural communication of the buccal and zygomatic branches of the facial nerve, a simple laceration of one or several branches may not produce any significant loss of motor function. Nerve lacerations medial to the pupil are not repaired because it is at this level that the nerve arborizes extensively and enters the facial musculature. In the unconscious patient or the uncooperative patient, all wounds suspect for facial nerve injury are explored in the operating suite. If major life-threatening injuries are present, the facial wound is simply closed with skin tapes or monofilament suture and explored at a later date. Early exploration and repair is mandatory for an optimum result. In all cases, the operating microscope is employed utilizing magnifications of 16 to 25 power. A nerve stimulator is used to help identify the cut distal end of the nerve—this is only effective during the first 4 days following nerve injury owing to the loss of conductivity of the distal nerve end, which accompanies neuronal degeneration, another key consideration for early primary repair. To the inexperienced surgeon, locating the divided ends of the facial nerve is no easy task. Here, a keen familiarity with local anatomy is paramount to success.

First the wound is gently irrigated to remove all clots and debris. Next, the superficial myoaponeurotic system (SMAS) is identified. This lies just below the superficial fat as a fine fibrous layer which is continuous with the platysma inferiorly and the superficial temporal fascia superiorly. Just beneath this layer lies the plane of the facial nerve. Utilizing ocular loupes ($2.5\times$ to $4.0\times$ magnification), the wound is then explored to identify the nerves. Not all nerves are of the motor type—many sensory nerves lie in this area as well. The nerve stimulator (set at 0.5 mv) will help to identify the motor branches. After a distal branch is identified, it is tagged with a 6–0 monofilament suture, and its corresponding proximal counterpart is located. In this fashion, the entire wound is explored. After all the nerves have been identified and tagged, the deeper layers of the wound are closed. Next, using the operative microscope and microsurgical technique, the cut nerve ends are coapted with two 10–0 sutures placed through the epineurium. If a clean division of the nerve is present, simple cleaning of the fibrous tissue 1 to 2 mm from the nerve end is all that is necessary.

Irregular or jagged lacerations are prepared by sharp amputation with a broken razor blade. Care is taken to avoid any unnecessary manipulation of the cut nerve end. Extremely small branches or branches which lie together easily, without tension, are repaired with a single epineural suture. Lacerations involving the main trunk of the facial nerve are repaired with fine epineural suture after precise fascicular alignment of the proximal and distal ends.

If segments of the nerve (greater than 1 cm) are missing, primary nerve grafts are employed if the condition of the wound, as well as the patient, permit. The greater auricular nerve is an excellent source of autogenous tissue for grafting the facial nerve and its branches. Other cutaneous sensory nerves, such as the antebrachial cutaneous and sural nerves, are also employed, but are less desirable because of their size discrepancy and distant donor site location. If for some reason a primary neurorrhaphy or graft cannot be performed, the proximal and distal nerve ends are tagged with 6–0 monofilament suture. The suture is placed through the entire thickness of the nerve end and 5 mm long tails are left for later identification. Reexploration of these wounds has shown that, even with tagging, the nerve ends are extremely difficult to identify owing to their diminished size and local scarring.

After the nerve repair has been completed, the skin is closed in layers and reinforced with skin tapes. Skin tapes placed directly over the wound closure site help to splint the area of nerve repair and minimize vascular oozing and possible disruption of the repair. This splinting is maintained for three weeks.

Even in the best of circumstances, the amount of recovery from a total facial nerve laceration is less than 50 percent of the original function. Dyskinesis (mass action) is a frequent complication of facial nerve repair, particularly if the level of injury is at a major division or of the nerve trunk itself. Lacerations of the marginal mandibular branches are notorious for poor recovery.

Parotid Injuries

The majority of parotid injuries are characterized by a penetrating wound that lacerates the capsule and separates the parenchyma or parotid ducts. Because of the intimate association of the parotid gland and Stenson's duct with the buccal branch of the facial nerve, injury to one structure should be suspect for injury to the other.

Simple lacerations of the parotid capsule are managed by closure with an absorbable suture. Division of some of the minor collecting ducts from the parenchyma requires no specific therapeutic intervention except for the usual wound debridement and closure. Salivary leakage from these severed ducts is contained by the wound and usually ceases as the wound heals. Occasionally, a sialocele forms and is resolved by serial aspirations.

Transection of Stenson's duct requires surgical intervention; otherwise, a salivary fistula may result. The wound is explored and enlarged if additional exposure is needed. The distal duct is located by passing a Silastic catheter through its mucosal orifice. The injecting of methylene blue or other dye through this duct for purposes of localization is to be avoided because it is rarely necessary and the dye causes staining of the surrounding tissues, which further complicates the anatomy. The proximal duct end is more difficult to find. It is helpful to dry the wound with a sponge blotter and then gently compress the parotid parenchyma. The proximal duct is usually found at the site of salivary pooling. Once identified, the duct is cannulated in-continuity and the two segments are repaired. A single-layered repair is employed, avoiding the ductal mucosa. Direct repair of the epithelial mucosa of this duct is complicated by the formation of an obstructing intraluminal mass—the result of a retained nidus of suture material.

The Silastic cannula is secured to the buccal mucosa with a nonabsorbable suture and then removed after 7 to 10 days. It is not necessary to drain these wounds.

Injuries that result in loss of the anterior portion of the parotid duct and its orifice are managed by rerouting the proximal duct through the buccinator muscle and suturing the duct end to the edges of a buccal mucosal slit. The duct is kept cannulated for 10 to 14 days to allow maturation of the new orifice.

Complete loss of the extraparenchymal portion of Stenson's duct represents a major therapeutic challenge. In most cases, primary reconstruction is impractical and carries the risk of further soft tissue injury. In these cases, it is perhaps wise to accept a controlled parotid fistula. This is easily created by cannulating the remnant parenchymal portion of the duct and directing the salivary flow to the oral cavity. Delayed reconstruction is then performed weeks or months later.

Ligation of the parotid duct has been advocated as an alternative method of management, but carries a substantial risk for the production of a parotid fistula. If significant parenchymal and/or ductal injury precludes salvage or reconstruction, it is probably best to excise the entire gland. Radiation therapy will eliminate salivary secretion by destroying the glandular components of the parotid. This method, while effective, results in extensive soft tissue fibrosis, pigmentation of the skin, and unknown potential future sequelae. It should be reserved for those isolated cases that cannot easily be managed by surgical excision.

Blunt trauma to the parotid will cause parenchymal injury, hematoma, or both. The parotid will be massively swollen, quite tender, and susceptible to infection. In most cases, bleeding within the parotid capsule is diffuse and subsequently resorbed by the parenchyma. For these cases, supportive measures such as iced compresses, broad-spectrum antibiotic prophylaxis, analgesics, and a bland diet will result in rapid resolution of the problem. Massive hematomas should be drained immediately. Needle aspiration is rarely effective and thus a direct incision and evacuation of the clot is preferred. These wounds are then drained to allow egress of the necrotic glandular debris. Salivary fistulas occasionally result from this procedure, but rarely are permanent unless the major ductal system has been injured.

Parotid abscesses can complicate blunt trauma to the gland. These are managed by simple drainage and antibiotic therapy. Care must be exercised, however, to avoid injury to the facial nerve branches.

Laryngeal Trauma

Blunt or penetrating trauma of the larynx requires immediate attention to the airway. Blind or hastily placed endotracheal tubes carry the risk of extending the injury, and attempts at their placement may be unsuccessful. If the airway is acutely compromised, an emergent tracheostomy is performed. This should be conducted with expedience under good illumination and adequate instrumentation. Gaping wounds of the larynx can be intubated directly until the patient is stabilized and can be transported to the operating theater for formal tracheotomy. Blunt injuries to the larynx must be

observed carefully if minimal or no airway obstruction is encountered at the initial examination. Edema or hemorrhage into the neck over the ensuing 48 hours may subsequently obstruct the traumatized air passage, necessitating tracheostomy. Similarly, progressive subcutaneous emphysema requires direct management.

Contusions of the anterior neck may not result in fracture of the cartilaginous skeleton of the larynx or acute compromise of the airway. These patients are placed at bedrest with the neck stabilized and the head of the bed elevated at least 30°. Humidified oxygen by facemask keeps the traumatized airway moist and reduces the patient's tidal volume. Swallowing will be quite painful and is often accompanied by pharyngeal spasm and/or aspiration. For this reason, no oral feedings are instituted for at least 48 hours. The patient is supported with intravenous fluids and, ideally, hyperalimentation. Antibiotic therapy is instituted as a prophylaxis and continued for approximately 72 hours. Analgesics and sedatives are kept to a minimum to avoid depression of the respiration and possible precipitation of an airway obstruction. These patients generally do well with conservative therapy, though some may experience lingering voice changes or difficulties with swallowing.

Blunt trauma causing acute airway obstruction signifies fracture and collapse of the laryngeal skeleton. As such, the larynx must be explored and repaired to establish a functional organ. After tracheostomy, the larynx is explored through a transverse anterior neck incision, exposing the anatomy from the hyoid bone to the trachea. The strap muscles are separated in the midline and retracted laterally. These can be detached from the hyoid superiorly for greater exposure. The larynx is next examined, and specific consideration is given to the anatomic relationships between the hyoid and cricoid cartilages and the stability of each. Fracture, collapse, or separation of either is an indication to perform a laryngotomy. Simple, relatively stable fractures of the thyroid cartilage are repaired with fine monofilament or wire sutures placed through small drill holes on each side. One should avoid placing these sutures through the laryngeal mucosa—a possible advantage in preventing suture granulomas.

The laryngotomy is performed through a midline incision, which first divides the thyroid cartilage. An oscillating saw or knife is used to make a vertical incision, which extends down to, but not through, the laryngeal mucosa. Occasionally, the thyroid cartilage is vertically fractured, making this incision unnecessary. In any event, the mucosa behind the thyroid cartilage is carefully dissected for approximately 5 mm on each side of the midline. Next, a vertical incision is made through the cricothyroid membrane in the midline and is carried up to the anterior commissure of the glottis. The anterior commissure is divided exactly at its apex, and the incision is then directed laterally just below the epiglottic cartilage. Care must be exercised to avoid injury to the internal branch of the superior laryngeal nerve during this dissection. Illumination of the operating field is facilitated by a fiberoptic headlight or a disposable, goose-neck light placed from above into the larynx.

The lumen of the larynx is then carefully explored. The mucosa may be hemorrhagic and edematous, and there may be lacerations. The articulations of the cricoid, thyroid, and arytenoid cartilages are examined. Any dislocations should be manually repositioned and secured by simple sutures through the appropriate ligaments. It is particularly important to repair the avulsed ligaments with fine absorbable sutures (5–0 or 6–0), incorporating just enough tissue to allow stability. A major problem lies in the post-traumatic fibrosis of the cricoarytenoid joint, which severely impairs vocalization. This can be minimized by fine surgical technique.

Mucosal lacerations are trimmed and carefully closed with absorbable sutures. In these types of injury, mucosal loss is rare. However, if any defects remain they can be closed by local mucosal advancement or the placement of a mucosal graft (preferably from the cheek). It is not desirable to create flaps from the adjacent laryngeal mucosa because these tend to distort the laryngeal lumen, and their viability may be compromised as a consequence of the original trauma. Split-thickness mucosal grafts are excellent for this purpose. The graft is tailored to match the mucosal defect and then secured to the bed and adjacent mucosa with fine catgut. We have not found it necessary to stent these grafts, unless a particularly large area is being resurfaced. Stents are foreign bodies, quite irritating, and can themselves contribute to laryngeal fibrosis. If a stent is used, it is secured to the anterior larynx with pull-out sutures, so that the larynx and stent move in unison.

The laryngotomy is closed in layers, using fine interrupted catgut sutures for the mucosa. The cricothyroid ligament and extramucosal soft tissues are repaired with synthetic absorbable suture

material. The thyroid cartilage is then reapproximated with 5–0 stainless steel wire. Horizontal mattress sutures placed through small drill holes across the isthmus of the thyroid cartilage work well in securing the two halves. Care must be taken to avoid twisting the wires too tightly because they can cut through the cartilage. The remaining cartilage fractures are then repaired.

The avulsed or detached laryngeal muscles and ligaments are then repositioned and secured to the laryngeal framework with absorbable sutures. If severe disruption of the laryngeal anatomy has occurred, the repaired larynx can be suspended from the hyoid bone to help stabilize the parts and to remove tension from the repair. Two absorbable sutures are anchored laterally to the hyoid and then affixed to either the cricoid cartilage or the first tracheal ring. The tension is set firmly, causing the larynx to "rest" in the neck untethered.

The skin is closed over drains placed alongside the larynx. The tracheostomy is kept in place for 7 to 10 days or until it can be plugged and removed without compromising the airway.

Penetrating trauma of the larynx is managed in the same way as described for severe blunt trauma, except that the laryngotomy may have to be modified somewhat to suit the anatomy of the laryngeal wound. In addition, these wounds should be suspect for nerve, vascular, or esophageal injury. Division of the superior laryngeal or recurrent laryngeal nerves should be managed by precise repair utilizing microsurgical technique and magnification. With these injuries, careful postoperative care must be administered to prevent aspiration and/or airway obstruction.

In the extreme case, despite diligent care, laryngeal function rarely returns to normal. At minimum, permanent voice changes will be encountered. The sequelae of fibrosis, joint immobility, airway compromise, and skeletal distortion will give cause for further attempts at reconstruction.

FACIAL FRACTURES

Nasal Fractures

Nasal bone fractures are the most frequently encountered fractures of the facial skeleton. Bleeding from the nose is the most common presenting sign and, in some patients, may be copious (particularly in hypertensives). The thin membrane bones of the nose shatter in unpredictable fashion when broken. Most fractures, however, are minimally displaced and thus represent a minor therapeutic problem. Roentgenograms of nasal fractures are not particularly useful from a therapeutic point of view and so are not generally obtained. The key points in assessing these injuries are the alignment of the nasal pyramid and septum, the symmetry of the nasal profile, and the presence of a septal hematoma.

If the condition of the patient permits, the head is elevated and ice packs are placed over the root of the nose. The patient is sedated with diazepam (5 to 10 mg IM) and generally given an analgesic/antiemetic (Demerol, Thorazine) parenterally. If massive swelling is present, a simple intranasal examination is all that is performed initially, allowing 3 to 4 days for the swelling to subside before instituting definitive therapy. A thorough intranasal examination is performed at the time of reduction. This requires excellent lighting—preferably a head lamp or reflector. Instrument requirements are minimal and consist of a rubber-shod elevator, a long-bladed nasal speculum, alligator forceps, Asch nasal forceps, a needle-point cautery, and suction. Topical and local infiltration anesthesia is most commonly employed. Cocaine hydrochloride is an excellent topical anesthetic for use intranasally. Its vasoconstrictive effects are indispensable in shrinking the edematous nasal/septal mucosa. Prior to administering this drug, a careful history should be obtained regarding possible allergies or sensitivities. The surgeon should also be familiar with the systemic effects of cocaine and the signs of toxicity (headache, anxiety, chills, tachycardia, irregular respirations, nausea, numbness or tingling of the extremities). Overdoses of this drug should be rapidly treated by discontinuance of the drug followed by intravenous administration of a short-acting barbiturate. Instrumentation for artificial respiration should also be available should respiratory arrest occur.

With regard to dosage, 5 to 10 cc of a 5 percent solution of cocaine hydrochloride is enough to moisten six small cotton pledgets, which are placed intranasally. This dosage rarely causes toxic reactions in an adult patient. Into each naris, one cotton pledget is introduced and the septum and lateral nasal walls are swabbed throughout. One pledget is then directed posteriorly along the nasal floor below the inferior turbinate to a depth of 4 to 6 cm. A second pledget is introduced and the swabbing repeated. This pledget is directed posterosuperiorly below the middle turbinate until resistance is encountered (site of sphenopalatine ganglion). A third pledget is impacted high in the nasal vault at the root of the nose. The pledgets are left in position for 10 to 15 minutes. During this time, one can perform local and regional percutaneous infiltration of Xylocaine (2 percent) with epinephrine (1:200,000) solution. A total of 6 to 10 cc is sufficient for blocks of the infraorbital and infratrochlear nerves, as well as local infiltration along the nasal-malar groove, dorsum, tip, and nasal spine. The anesthetic is used sparingly to avoid soft tissue distortion.

The nasal vaults and septum are examined with a speculum. Septal hematomas are evacuated through a vertical mucosal incision and the cavity is examined for bleeding points, which are cauterized. It usually is not necessary to suture these incisions. Septal fractures and dislocations are then reduced with an elevator or the Asche forceps and held in this position with bilateral nasal packs. Comminuted fractures of the nasal septum, if unstable, require stent fixation. For these purposes, sterilized x-ray celluloid is excellent stent material. A stent is simply tailored with scissors to conform to the septal anatomy. Greasy medicated gauze is applied over each side of the reduced nasal septum and is backed with the celluloid stent material. The stent-septum-stent sandwich is then fixed with through-and-through sutures of 3–0 Prolene. Care must be taken to avoid excessive tension in the sutures to prevent septal necrosis or ulceration. The stents are left in place for 2 weeks and removed.

In most instances, displaced fractures of the nasal bones can be reduced by direct intranasal manipulation with an elevator or by simple external molding with the thumb and forefinger. A dislocated nasal septum is often reduced by these maneuvers as well. After reduction, the intranasal structures are re-examined. Any small irregularities are then reduced and molded with the Asche forceps. The end point for reduction is primarily visual—a straight nose, symmetry of the nasal walls, and a midline septum.

Some greenstick fractures of the nose are quite stable on reduction and require no additional support. Comminuted, unstable fractures of the bony, cartilaginous nasal pyramid are best managed by intranasal packing and external splinting. We prefer a petrolatum-impregnated intranasal pack placed according to the method described by Kazanjian and Converse (layered gauze strips carefully packed into the nasal cavity). It is often helpful to first insert a small rubber or Silastic tube along the nasal floor to serve as an airway as well as a pressure equalizer in the nasopharynx. These tubes make the patient more comfortable by preventing the "plugged-ear" sensation that accompanies swallowing.

The nasal packs are left in place for 4 to 5 days, which is usually enough time for the fractures to become "sticky" enough to not require support. The presence of an intranasal pack causes mucosal irritation and copious rhinorrhea. This nuisance can be reduced by administering a decongestant such as pseudoephedrine.

There are different types of external nasal splints, all of which have their particular advantages and disadvantages. We prefer the following method: after reduction of the nasal fracture and intranasal packing, the nasal dorsum is cleaned with an alcohol solution. Microporous ½-inch tape is applied in overlapping, transversely oriented strips from the nasal root to the tip. This is backed in similar fashion with ½-inch cloth adhesive tape. Next, plaster strips are cut and applied over the taped area in "sloppy-wet" fashion until a 3- or 4-ply thickness is achieved. The plaster is then smoothed gently with the finger, congealing all the layers, and the excess water is blotted with a dry sponge. Care is taken to avoid getting any of the plaster into the eyes. After the custom splint is dry, it is secured by cross-taping to the cheeks. A small 2 × 2 gauze nasal drip pad is placed and held into position with a rubber band. This pad is changed when soiled by nasal discharge. The external nasal splint is removed in 5 to 7 days.

Nasal Fractures in Children

Nasal and septal fractures in children are at risk for producing growth disturbances and thus require special consideration. Any injury causing nasal bleeding in a child should be interpreted as a possible nasal/septal fracture. Examination and therapy are best performed under general anesthesia. Cocaine nasal packs are employed to shrink the edematous mucosa. Particular attention is directed to injuries of the nasal septum. Septal hematomas are quite devastating in this age group and require immediate drainage. If associated with a septal fracture, the hematoma may be bilateral. In these cases, a small portion of the cartilage should be removed, and the opposite hematoma evacuated through the same mucosal incision.

Naso-Orbital Fractures

Severe blows to the nasal bridge may result in a communition of the supporting bony structure of the intercanthal region. These injuries are complex and represent the most difficult to manage of the maxillofacial region. There is often associated neurologic trauma resulting from telescoping of the nasal pyramid posteriorly and superiorly through the cribriform plate. Neurosurgical intervention may be indicated if signs of frontal lobe injury, intracranial bleeding, or extensive dural lacerations are present. CSF rhinorrhea is a common finding and, in the absence of neurologic signs, is not a contraindication for surgical reduction of the fractures. There is no evidence that a broad spectrum antibiotic is effective as a prophylaxis against meningitis. CAT scan imagery of the upper midface is the best noninvasive diagnostic tool for evaluation of these injuries. If a neurosurgical emergency exists upon presentation a definitive, combined intracranial and extracranial approach is effected. Otherwise, the patient is stabilized and the surgical repair is performed at a convenient time when the swelling has subsided (see Table).

Goals of Therapy

The goals of management lie in restoration of the anatomic continuity of the fractured parts, drainage of the affected paranasal sinuses and lacrimal apparatus, and soft tissue repair. The thin, eggshell bones of the medial orbital wall, the honeycomb ethmoidal labyrinth, and the floor of the frontal sinus shatter unpredictably as the nasal root is imploded by the point of impact. A precise anatomic reduction of these fragments is neither possible nor practical. The key here is to re-establish correct relationships of the nasal pyramid to the frontal root and base of the skull and to realign the major pillars of the orbital-nasal complex (e.g., supraorbital rims to frontal bone and its nasal process, nasal bone to frontal bone and frontal process of maxilla, frontal process of maxilla to maxilla and zygoma). The position of the medial canthal tendon is altered in these injuries, producing a traumatic telecanthus deformity (pseudohypertelorism). Usually, the tendon attachment to a fragment of the medial orbital wall is preserved. This allows for repositioning of the fragment back into its normal anatomic position, where it is secured to the stable nasal pillar and maxillary process as

TABLE 1 Facial Fractures: Composite of Clinical and Radiographic Findings, Surgical Approaches, and Complications for Specific Facial Fractures

Fracture	Clinical Presentation	Radiographic	Surgical Approach	Complications
Naso-orbital	Symptoms: pain, visual abnormalities. Signs: massive periorbital and upper facial edema and ecchymosis, epistaxis, traumatic telecanthus, foreshortening of nose with telescoping. Associated intracranial injuries.	Views: CAT Scan. Findings: disruption of interorbital space and comminution of nasal pyramid. Frontal, zygomatic, orbital, maxillary fractures common.	ORIF via coronal "Meisterschmitt" approach or direct "open sky" approach through wound. Severe comminution may require outrigger suspension to head frame. Frontal sinus repair/drainage. Canthal tendon alignment and fixation.	Residual upper mid-face deformity ("dish face"). Telecanthus. Frontal sinus/nasolacrimal system pathology with mucocele, mucopyocele, dacryocystitis.
Zygoma Arch	Symptoms: pain lateral cheek, inability to close jaw. Signs: swelling, crepitus over arch, obvious asymmetry.	Views: Water's submentovertex. Findings: depression of arch, comminution.	"Greenstick fractures": closed reduction via brow or temporal approach. Comminuted: reduction and stabilization by circumosseus wiring to external rigid stent. Unstable: ORIF by direct coronal approach.	Contour irregularities of arch area, flattening of arch.
Body "Tripod Fracture"	Symptoms: pain, trismus, diplopia, numb upper lip, lower lid bilateral nasal area. Signs: swelling, ecchymosis of malar and periorbital areas. Palpable infraorbital rim "step-off". Entrapment of extraocular muscles with disconjugate gaze. Scleral ecchymosis, displacement lateral canthal ligament.	Views: Water's submentovertex, CAT scan. Findings: clouding, air/fluid level maxillary sinus, separation of zygomaticomaxillary, zygomaticofrontal and zygomaticotemporal sutures lines.	Non- or minimally displaced: conservative. Displaced/comminuted: ORIF via brow and infraciliary approach. Entrapment: orbital floor exploration and reconstruction via infraciliary approach. Caldwell-Luc with sinus stent. Complex comminuted: outrigger suspension.	Residual malar deformity, enophthalmos, diplopia, infraorbital nerve anesthesia, chronic maxillary sinusitis.
Orbital floor	Symptoms: diplopia, orbital pain. Signs: periorbital edema, ecchymosis, enophthalmos, extraocular muscle entrapment, disconjugate gaze. Hyphema, subluxation of lens, retinal detachment, rupture of globe with direct eye trauma.	Views: Water's, CAT scan, tomograms. Findings: air/fluid level maxillary sinus, herniated adnexae and/or orbital floor fragments in maxillary sinus.	No entrapment, enophthalmos, or adnexal herniation: conservative therapy. Entrapments, enophthalmos or herniated adnexae: orbital floor exploration via infraciliary approach, reconstruction (cartilage, bone or alloplastic material). Antrostomy with sinus stent.	Enophthalmos, diplopia. Recurrent orbital cellulitis with implant (alloplastic) extrusion.
Mandible Condyle	Symptoms: pain at fracture site, referred pain to ear.	Views: AP, oblique, Water's, Panorex.	Non- or minimal diplacement: IMF.	Ankylosis of TMJ. Chronic TMJ symptoms.

Site	Signs/Symptoms	Views/Findings	Treatment	Complications
	Signs: crepitus, excessive salivation, swelling in condylar region, deviation of jaw toward fracture, cross-bite or open-bite deformity.	Findings: nondisplaced, or displaced anteriorly and medially.	Displaced: ORIF via submandibular or transoral route.	Non-union, malunion osteomyelitis.
Angle	Symptoms: pain at fracture site, inability to close mouth. Signs: swelling at angle of jaw, ecchymosis, crepitus, malocclusion.	Views: Panorex, mandibular series. Findings: nondisplaced (favorable) or posterior fragment displaced upward and medially (nonfavorable).	Favorable: IMF Nonfavorable: ORIF via intraoral or submandibular route.	
Body	Symptoms: pain at fracture site, limitation of movement. Signs: swelling, ecchymosis, crepitus, malocclusion.	Views: Panorex, mandibular series. Findings: nondisplaced (favorable), or post. fragment displaced upward and medially, anterior fragments rotated lingually (nonfavorable).	Favorable: IMF. Nonfavorable: ORIF, via extraoral approach. IMF with lingual splints.	Osteomyelitis. Infection (tooth in fracture line.)
Symphysis	Symptoms: pain. Signs: malocclusion, frequent association with soft tissue wounds of lower lip, tongue.	Views: mandibular series, submentovertex. Findings: nondisplaced or lingual rotation of anterior fragments, may be associated with angle or condyle fractures.	ORIF via submental incision. IMF with lingual splints.	Residual malocclusion, loss of chin projection, asymmetry. Osteomyelitis.
Maxilla LeFort I (transverse)	Symptoms: pain upper jaw, numb upper teeth. Signs: midfacial edema and ecchymosis, epistaxis, malocclusion, mobility of maxillary dentition.	Views: Water's, Panorex, CAT scan. Findings: opaque maxillary sinus, displacement of fragments of alveolus if comminuted. Fracture through maxillary sinus and pterygoid plates.	Disimpaction, IMF with skull cap or internal fixation to pyriform margin.	Loss of teeth, infection, malocclusion.
LeFort II (pyramidal)	Symptoms: pain midface, numb upper lip, lower lid, lateral nasal area. Signs: midfacial edema and ecchymosis, epistaxis, malocclusion, mobility of midface, nasal flattening, anesthesia infraorbital nerve territory.	Views: Water's, CAT scan. Findings: opaque maxillary sinuses, separation through frontal process, lacrimal bones, floor of orbits, zygomaticomaxillary suture line, lateral wall of maxillary sinus and pterygoid plates.	Disimpaction, IMF with suspension to internal wire fixation to solid structure above fracture (infraorbital rim, frontal bone). Direct transosseus wiring via infraciliary approach.	Nonunion, malunion, lacrimal system obstruction, infraorbital nerve anesthesia, diplopia, malocclusion.
LeFort III (craniofacial dysjunction)	Symptoms: pain face, difficulty breathing. Signs: "donkey-face" deformity, malocclusion, mobile face, marked facial edema and ecchymosis, epistaxis, CSF rhinorrhea.	Views: Water's, CAT scan. Findings: separation of mid-third of face at zygomaticofrontal, zygomaticotemporal, and nasofrontal sutures, and across orbital floors. Opaque maxillary sinuses.	IMF and cranial suspension to wire fixation at frontal bones. Direct wiring via brow incisions, naso-orbital incisions.	Nonunion, malunion, malocclusion, lengthening of midface, lacrimal system obstruction.

well as to the opposite tendon by a through-and-through wire. The positioning of these tendons correctly is quite difficult and prone to considerable error, which is not apparent at the time of reduction unless a wide exposure is achieved.

Surgical Exposures

Some surgeons prefer a direct approach through the nasal root via an "open-sky" technique. We occasionally use this approach if there is an open wound here which provides access or can be enlarged satisfactorily without producing an objectionable scar. The retraction of the soft tissue causes distortion of important landmarks, which are particularly important in gauging bone to soft tissue relationships. We prefer the Meisterschmitt or degloving exposure for these injuries. A coronal scalp incision is made from ear to ear, and the scalp is dissected forward below the galea to the supraorbital rims. The periosteum is incised high above the orbital rims, and a subperiosteal dissection is continued over the supraorbital rims and laterally below the temporalis muscle. The superior orbital neurovascular bundle may be dissected from its foramen with a fine osteotome to provide greater exposure. Centrally, a subperiosteal dissection is continued over the nasal bones to the upper lateral nasal cartilages. The medial orbital wall is exposed, and the lacrimal sac is dissected from its fossa, leaving the nasolacrimal duct intact. The anterior ethmoidal vessels are identified here and divided. The subperiosteal dissection is continued inferiorly, exposing the infraorbital rim and frontal process of the maxillary bone. If greater exposure of the maxilla and infraorbital rim is needed, a subciliary incision is made along the lower eyelid medially to the lacrimal punctum. The orbicularis muscle is divided, and the dissection is continued behind the muscle to the orbital rim.

This exposure gives excellent visualization of the entire naso-orbital complex. Reconstructive efforts can then be based upon the full "birds-eye" view of normal and abnormal anatomy.

Surgical Repair

First priorities are given to reconstruction of the stabilizing pillars of the naso-orbital region. Preoperative radiographic assessment will determine if this can be safely done without a craniotomy. Occasionally, neurosurgical exploration with exposure of the anterior cranial fossa is the most conservative and safest approach. This can easily be performed through a frontal craniotomy via a Meisterschmitt exposure. The nasal pyramid is disimpacted with an Asche forceps and is brought forward. The nasal bones are then secured to the stable frontal root with stainless steel wires (26-gauge). The nasal processes of the maxillary bone are wired to the maxilla and the nasal bones. If severe comminution of these bones is present, each piece is carefully positioned anatomically and wired at two points to neighboring pieces with No. 30 stainless steel wire. In this fashion, the puzzle is reconstructed, but no attempt is made to wire together the thin, delicate flakes of the lamina papyracea, lacrimal, or ethmoid bones. These pieces are usually attached to periosteum or mucosa, and upon reduction and fixation of the naso-orbital pillar, they generally lie in satisfactory position. If severe comminution is present with marked lateral displacement of the ethmoidal bones, reduction can be accomplished by direct gentle molding with an Asche or Walsham forceps. This "pinching" together of the nasal bridge is quite effective in maintaining the anterior projection of the fractured segments.

Medial Canthal Tendons

The medial canthal tendons are usually repositioned in the reconstruction of the naso-orbital pillar. This reduction can be reinforced internally or externally to maintain the projection of the nasal bridge and the security of the canthal fixation. Internal reinforcement is preferred when the lateral walls of the pyramid are not comminuted and, when reduced, maintain their anatomic position. In these cases, a No. 26 stainless wire is passed through two drill holes that traverse the nasal bridge just above the attachment of the canthal tendons. When tightened, this wire maintains a rigid fixation of the central structures.

Medial Orbital Walls

If the medial orbital walls are comminuted, a simple internal wire fixation is insufficient for support, but allows collapse of the surrounding fragments. These fractures are best stabilized by external splint fixation. After the nasal bridge, canthal tendons, and medial orbital wall fragments have been positioned and wired, through-and-through wires are placed across the nasal bridge just superior to the canthal tendon attachments. These wires are then brought through the nasal skin on each side and attached to contour pledgets fashioned from Alumifoam splints (foam side toward the skin). The splints aid in molding the fractured bridge framework as well as in maintaining the requisite anterior projection of the nasal pyramid. If the medial canthal tendons have been avulsed from their bony attachments, they are reattached by fixation to the reconstructed nasal bridge. It is important to delineate the exact point of fixation here to avoid postoperative discrepancies in palpebral orientation. A helpful solution is to gauge the fixation points of the *lateral* canthal tendons. A line (wire) connecting these two points will fall across the bridge at the correct point of fixation for the medial tendons. A small hole is drilled through the nasal bridge at this level. It is important to position this hole anterior to the lacrimal fossa or its remnant to ensure proper positioning of the canthal tendon. (The canthal tendon normally splits and attaches to the anterior and posterior rims of the fossa.) Next, the medial canthal tendons are wired to each other through the hole. A No. 30 stainless steel wire is excellent for these purposes.

Occasionally, severe comminution of the naso-orbital complex precludes adequate internal or splint stabilization. In these cases, outrigger fixation via a plaster head cap or cranial "halo" device is necessary. We prefer the halo device, which is fixed to the cranium. This is more precise and allows visualization of the scalp and frontal region, a feature that is particularly advantageous following craniotomy. Plaster head caps become loose with time and are a source of constant complaint. A wire is secured to a stable fragment or passed through the canthal block and attached to the outrigger device. The vector of traction is determined by the direction of collapse. If satisfactory reduction can be maintained by simple traction, the wire is secured to the outrigger appliance at the proper point. This is maintained for 2 weeks or until bony fixation is adequate. Combinations of internal wiring, external splint, or outrigger fixation may be necessary to achieve and maintain the desired reduction.

The Nose

After reduction and stabilization of the naso-orbital pillar and medial canthal tendon attachments, the nose is examined. Disruption of the bony-cartilaginous juncture of the nasal dorsum can cause severe deformities of the nasal profile and is also a harbinger of possible septal fractures or dislocation. A careful intranasal examination is performed, with topical cocaine hydrochloride used to shrink the edematous mucosa. Any septal fractures or dislocations are reduced (see *Nasal Fractures*). Septal hematomas are evacuated. The nose should not be packed in the presence of CSF rhinorrhea. If a combined intracranial, extracranial approach is used, and the dural defect repaired, a light nasal packing is inserted and removed in 3 to 4 days. The dorsal nasal cartilage is fixed to the nasal bones with fine wire sutures placed in horizontal mattress fashion through small drill holes. Absorbable sutures are insufficient to maintain reduction here and should not be used.

Sinuses

The next consideration is given to the drainage of the ethmoidal, sphenoidal, and frontal sinuses. If an adequate reduction is achieved, these sinuses will drain satisfactorily. In severe impaction-type injuries, the ostia of the frontal sinus may lose its continuity with the ethmoid. This may result in the formation of a frontal sinus mucocele or mucopyocele. The cause is obstruction of the nasofrontal duct. In these cases, drainage of the frontal sinus must be effected. Access to the frontal sinus can often be achieved through a fracture of its floor or anterior wall or through craniotomy; otherwise a 5-mm sinusotomy is performed anteriorly and a drainage tract is established by probe exploration through the nasofrontal duct. The probe is directed to beneath the anterior portion of the middle turbinate. This tract is maintained by stenting with a No. 12 F Silastic catheter, which is brought out through the naris and sutured to the nasal floor. The tube is left in this position for 3 to 4 weeks. It is irrigated daily with a sterile saline solution. Both frontal sinuses should be drained. In some cases in which wide exposure of one sinus is present through a fracture segment, the intersinus septum can be burred away, creating a common sinus for unilateral drainage.

Lacrimal Apparatus

The lacrimal apparatus must be inspected for injury. Common sites of disruption occur in the lacrimal sac and the nasolacrimal duct. Canalicular injuries should be suspected if the medial canthal tendon has been avulsed from its bony attachments. If no injuries are detected by gross visualization, it is helpful to cannulate the lacrimal punctum on the upper or lower eyelid and inject 2 to 3 cc of saline solution into the lacrimal system. If saline returns via the noncannulated punctum and into the nose beneath the inferior turbinate, this is good evidence that the lacrimal system is patent and all components communicate with each other. If the saline leaks into the wound, careful inspection of the canaliculi and lacrimal sac is necessary to determine the site of injury. We repair lacerated canaliculi with fine 9–0 monofilament nonabsorbable sutures over a Silastic stent using operative magnification. Lacrimal sac injuries are first probed to determine patency of the nasolacrimal duct. If resistance to probing is encountered, adjacent fracture segments in line with the nasolacrimal duct are manipulated until the probe can be easily passed into the nose below the inferior turbinate. The duct is stented with a Silastic catheter gauged to fit snugly, but not tightly. The catheter is sutured to the nasal floor and left in place for 3 weeks. The lacrimal sac is then closed in one layer with fine interrupted 8–0 monofilament sutures.

In severe crushing or avulsion type midfacial injuries, the lacrimal collecting system may be so traumatized that repair is impossible. In these cases, it is best to close the wound and perform a dacryocystorhinostomy or other drainage procedure at a later time. In some cases, a primary dacryocystorhinostomy is performed if the nasal wall has not been comminuted and is stable.

Primary Bone Grafting

Injuries resulting in the loss of bony support of the medial orbital wall, nasal bridge, orbital rim, or floor are treated by primary reconstruction using bone grafts. This technique is preferred over a staged reconstruction because it achieves the desired goal in one operation and is unencumbered by the formation of difficult scar tissue. A cortical-cancellous bone graft is harvested from the iliac crest and tailored according to the demands for reconstruction. Onlay grafts are generally employed for isolated reconstruction of an orbital wall, floor, or rim. In massive injuries with loss of the entire nasal root and medial orbital walls, a "butterfly" graft is employed with the body serving as the nasal root and dorsum, and the folded wings as the medial orbital walls. In these cases, remnants of the ethmoid sinus are removed with a rongeur. The frontal sinuses are drained, and a nasal lining is constructed using septal and lateral mucosal flaps. The grafts are fixed to the adjacent stable bony structures with interosseous wire. These wounds are not usually drained, although every effort is made to obtain absolute hemostasis prior to closure. Broad-spectrum antibiotics are administered preoperatively, intraoperatively, and postoperatively for 48 hours unless CSF rhinorrhea persists, in which case they are continued until the problem is resolved.

The coronal scalp incision is closed in layers and an occlusive bulky head dressing is applied. Postoperatively, the patient is kept at bedrest with the head elevated 30°. Dressings over the face, and particularly the eyes, are avoided. Vision and neurologic status checks are performed at intervals of 4 to 6 hours. Swelling, which is usually quite extensive, begins receding by the third day. Most patients tolerate liquids without difficulty by the second postoperative day. The diet is advanced as conditions permit. Analgesics are given parenterally in frequent small doses (morphine is preferred). Severe postoperative pain is uncommon and, if persistent, signals a potential complication.

Frontal Sinus Fractures

A blow of significant magnitude is required to fracture the frontal bone, especially the supraorbital rims. These injuries are frequently associated with intracranial injury and are often managed at the time of craniotomy. Simple, nondisplaced fractures of the frontal sinus require no intervention. Broad-spectrum prophylactic antibiotic therapy is occasionally instituted.

Comminuted outer table frontal sinus fractures are explored through the adjoining forehead laceration or via a coronal scalp exposure. The sinus cavity is examined and the nasofrontal duct is probed to ensure patency. The fracture fragments are carefully reduced and secured with interosseous wires if the reduction is unstable. Even in severely comminuted fractures, the anterior wall can be reconstructed safely provided sinus drainage is ensured and a rigid interosseous fixation achieved. It is not necessary to "obliterate" the frontal sinus in these injuries; there is no biologic basis for filling the sinus cavity with devascularized fat or muscle.

Inner table fractures of the frontal sinus are associated with dural and brain injuries and frequently require craniotomy. The bone of the inner table is relatively thin and shatters upon impact, at times making reconstruction impossible. If the fragments can be reduced to reconstruct a continuous inner table, this method is preferred. At times, a painstaking effort must be made to precisely fit the individual fracture pieces into their proper position. Fine No. 28 stainless steel wire is employed for these purposes. When the inner table is fractured beyond repair, the segments are completely removed and the edges of the sinus cavity are smoothed of any irregularities. The sinus is stripped of its mucosa to the nasofrontal duct. Careful submucosal dissection of the orifice of the duct is performed so that a sleeve of duct mucosa is mobilized. This is doubly ligated with fine (5–0) synthetic absorbable suture and trimmed of any excess mucosa. The stump is then cauterized. Any remnants of suspected mucosa in the sinus cavity are likewise cauterized. A plug of cortical/cancellous bone harvested from the craniotomy site or outer table is tapped into the orifice of the nasofrontal duct after the edges of the duct have been freshened with a burr. The outer table is reconstructed as previously outlined. The sinus cavity will fill with serum, CSF, and clot initially, but will gradually become occupied by the frontal portion of the brain. If both walls of the sinus have been destroyed, the preferred procedure is "cranialization" combined with a primary bone graft reconstruction of the outer table.

Supraorbital rim fractures occasionally involve the frontal sinus. The key here is assurance of patency of the nasofrontal duct by stenting or a "window" procedure through the intersinus septum for drainage through the opposite side. Bony defects are reconstructed primarily with cortical/cancellous iliac crest or split rib bone grafts. Alloplastic materials such as Methylmethacrylate, Silastic, and Teflon have been utilized for reconstruction of the frontal region in acute trauma. Their advantage lies in ease of reconstruction, avoidance of a donor site, and availability. We prefer autogenous material if the patient's general condition permits and if no penetrating intra-abdominal injury is present. Autogenous bone is better tolerated by the patient, is permanent, and when healed is a less susceptible nidus for bacterial infection.

Fractures of the Zygoma and Orbit

Lateral or oblique blows to the midface are absorbed by the malar region. Although the zygoma itself is uncommonly fractured, its attachments to the maxilla, frontal, and temporal bones are vulnerable to disruption. If the zygoma is displaced, disruption of the orbital floor and lateral wall is encountered. Direct forward blows to the orbit are absorbed by the orbital rims. The eye and ocular adenexa are compressed in the orbital vault, causing the weakest part, the floor, to fracture. There is probably a component of both mechanisms in a large percentage of malar complex fractures. In assessing these injuries, primary attention is given to the eye and its function. The maxillary sinus, which is involved in all fractures of this sort, is considered not only as a route of operative access, but also as a source of complication if inappropriately managed (see Table).

Indications for Surgery

Surgical management of these fractures is performed as early as possible, particularly when entrapment of the extraocular muscles or massive disruption of the orbital floor is present. Delay of surgical intervention in these cases not only continues the inevitable inflammatory process, but also invites progressive ischemia of fat and muscle leading to fibrosis, diminished extraocular muscle function, and enophthalmos. Undisplaced fractures do not require surgical treatment. Our indications for surgery are as follows: (1) clinical or radiographic displacement of the zygoma or orbital floor, (2) documented enophthalmos, and (3) early diplopia with a positive forced duction test.

The goals of surgical therapy are basically twofold: restoration of normal function and appearance. Release of entrapped or herniated orbital contents, precise reduction of displaced fractures, primary reconstruction of bony and soft tissue defects, and sinus drainage procedures constitute the therapeutic sequences employed to achieve these goals.

Isolated Zygomatic Arch Fractures

Isolated zygomatic arch fractures are usually of the "greenstick" variety and are easily managed via the Gillies' approach through a temporal incision. Local anesthesia with general standby may be employed for the majority of these cases. Occasionally, muscle relaxation may be required for reduction of the fracture. A vertical incision is made within the hairbearing scalp directly over the temporalis muscle. A blunt elevator is slipped below the temporalis fascia to the undersurface of the zygomatic arch. The depression of the arch is palpated and slight counterpressure is applied here to "control" the reduction. The fracture is then elevated, using the forefinger as a fulcrum for the elevator. These fractures can be heard or felt to "click" back into normal position. After reduction the fracture is palpated for stability; if it is stable, a protective splint fashioned from a finger splint is molded to arch over the fracture site. It is taped to the forehead and mandibular angle and left in place for 10 days. A soft diet is recommended during this time as it is possible, with forceful chewing, to dislodge the fracture segments.

Unstable or Comminuted Zygomatic Arch Fractures

Unstable or comminuted zygomatic arch fractures require internal or external fixation. Numerous adjunctive techniques have been employed based on the temporal fossa "packing" principle. Balloon catheters, vaginal gauze, and rubber drains have all been employed as packs placed beneath the zygomatic arch to maintain an anatomic reduction. This technique is not favored because it is imprecise, creates an "open fracture" situation with the risk of infection, and is quite bothersome for the patient. Open reduction of the unstable arch is a more direct approach and can be accomplished through a coronal incision or an incision placed over the arch in a wrinkle line. Both approaches require general anesthesia, expose the patient to the risk of injury to the facial nerve, and are time consuming. We have occasionally performed an open reduction of a comminuted zygomatic arch in conjunction with another procedure involving fractures of the frontal/orbital complex. The coronal "degloving" approach gives a wide exposure of the entire arch, making open reduction quite easy. A simple method of external fixation is achieved by placing a percutaneous wire suture around the depressed arch and securing this to a stable arch splint (contoured finger splint), which is taped to the forehead and cheek or mastoid eminence. In severe comminution, two or more wires can be used to obtain and maintain an accurate reduction. Postreduction radiographs are taken to check the fracture alignment; adjustments of the wire tension can be made if any displacement is encountered. The splint is left in position for 10 to 12 days and then removed.

"Tripod" Fractures of the Zygoma

Classic "tripod" fractures of the zygoma are managed by open reduction when displaced. If there is clinical or radiographic evidence of orbital content herniation into the maxillary sinus, entrapment of the extraocular muscles, or marked disruption of the orbital floor, exploration of the orbital floor is performed. For minimally displaced fractures, a brow incision is made to expose the zygomaticofrontal suture line and this access is used to reduce the fracture with a blunt elevator through the temporal fossa. Careful palpation of the arch and infraorbital rim during this reduction will determine its end point. If the fracture remains stable, the brow incision is simply closed. The Gillies' temporal incision is not a good approach for these fractures because the unstable fracture will require a brow incision anyway.

Unstable and Severely Displaced Fractures

If the fracture is unstable or if severe displacement or comminution is present, a brow and lower eyelid exposure is performed. The zygomaticofrontal suture line is cleaned of its periosteum and a figure-of-8 No. 26 interosseous wire is placed either anteriorly or posteriorly through fine drill holes. The wire is not twisted. Next, the orbital rim and floor are exposed via an infraciliary transmuscular incision. The line of incision on the lower eyelid is marked as it is for a blepharoplasty—2 to 3 mm below the lash line, extending laterally in a wrinkle crease, but not beyond the orbital margin (scar becomes apparent here). The skin and subcutaneous tissues are infiltrated with a solution of 1 percent Xylocaine with epinephrine (1:200,000), and 7 to 10 minutes are allowed for the full vasoconstrictive effect. The incision is begun laterally and is extended medially to the lateral lash margin. Next, the underlying orbicularis muscle is divided and precise hemostasis effected with the electrocautery. Using blunt-tipped tissue-cutting scissors, a tunnel is dissected behind the orbicularis to the lacrimal punctum. The scissors are used to cut the skin and muscle along the inscribed line. Two fine sutures are placed through the upper cut edge of the lid incision and connected to clamps for upward retraction of the eyelid; this protects the cornea and tenses the tissues to allow easier dissection. The composite skin-muscle flap of the lower eyelid is dissected to the orbital rim. Care is taken to keep the dissection just behind the muscle in the fine fibroareolar tissue in front of the orbital septum. This plane is relatively bloodless, though small bleeders will be encountered medially and laterally. Precise hemostasis is obtained at all times with a fine needle-point electrocautery. Alternative exposures to this region include the transconjunctival and the infraorbital rim approaches. The transconjunctival approach carries the risk of corneal abrasion and does not provide adequate exposure if interosseous wire fixation is required. Its benefits lie in ease of dissection and a concealed surgical scar. The infraorbital rim approach is relatively bloody, carries the risk of injury to the infraorbital nerve, and creates a conspicuous scar on the face. Its advantages lie in its direct approach to the inferior orbital rim and floor and the avoidance of ectropion formation in the lower eyelid. The infraciliary lower eyelid approach is believed to represent a compromise between these two approaches and incorporates some of the advantages inherent in each. Ectropion of the lower eyelid has occurred with this approach, but in most cases is a temporary phenomenon that resolves by gentle massaging of the eyelid. For the most part, ectropion can be avoided by employing fine surgical technique and obtaining absolute hemostasis prior to wound closure.

The inferior orbital rim is exposed medially beyond the zygomaticomaxillary suture line (fracture line) and laterally to the point of ascendancy of the lateral orbital rim. If the medial portion of the inferior orbital rim is fractured, the dissection is continued along the rim until a stable buttress is encountered. Occasionally, a counter-incision placed anterior to the lacrimal fossa in the nasomalar crease facilitates this exposure. After the entire orbital rim defect has been exposed, a periosteal incision is made along the lower margin, and a subperiosteal dissection of the rim and lateral orbital floor is performed. Usually, the lateral orbital floor or a portion of it is intact, allowing the dissection to commence in "known" territory. The subperiosteal dissection is continued posteriorly to the inferior orbital fissure and medially to the rim of the fracture. At the zygomaticomaxillary juncture, the infraorbital nerve and artery will be encountered. Care is exercised here to avoid injury to these structures. The dissection is continued medially to expose the stable components of the orbital rim and medial orbital floor. After the medial and lateral dissections are complete, there is usually encountered a tether or actual herniation of the periorbital soft tissues through the fracture line in the orbital floor. It is important *not* to forcefully attempt to retract this tissue from its impingement for fear of causing permanent nerve, muscle, or fat injury. In these cases, distraction of the fractured zygoma will allow atraumatic manipulation and reduction of these tissues. For these purposes, it has been found advantageous to secure a traction wire on the zygomatic portion of the orbital rim (through a small drill hole) and to use this anchor to help distract the zygoma while manipulating its reduction via the brow approach. The wire anchor helps in directing the reduction to the appropriate position after the orbital contents have been freed.

When extracting the herniated or entrapped tissues, it is important to employ a gentle technique and to make every attempt to visualize the anatomy clearly. Usually, the contents are easily freed by distraction. Occasionally, in delayed cases, swelling, inflammation, and early fibrosis will be encountered. The herniated tissues must then be gently dissected or "teased" from their abnormal position. After the soft tissues have been freed, the zygoma is reduced and secured by interosseous wiring of the zygomaticomaxillary suture line and tightening of the previously placed zygomaticofrontal wire. A two-point stabilization is adequate for most fractures of this type.

After the zygoma has been reduced, the orbital floor is carefully examined. In most cases, there will be adequate bony support to prevent herniation. If the orbital floor is comminuted and the fractures are unstable or a defect is present which allows collapse of the orbital soft tissues, a reconstruction is performed. First, all of the loose fragments are removed and foreign body fragments are extracted from the maxillary sinus as these may provide a nidus for infection. The resultant orbital floor defect is closed with a bone graft harvested from the anterior wall of the maxillary sinus, the vomer, with nasal septal cartilage, or with an auricular cartilage graft. We prefer autogenous material for reconstruction of the orbital floor because it is better tolerated by the patient and has been associated with fewer complications. Certainly, a good number of antral bone grafts placed in the orbital floor are resorbed and replaced by fibrous tissue, but this is of very little clinical significance because the remnant fibrous sling is quite stable and provides excellent support of the orbital contents. It is difficult to rationalize the biologic sense of placing an alloplastic material (Silicone, Teflon) in a potentially contaminated site comprising the roof of a paranasal sinus cavity. The orbital floor graft is placed over the defect or wedged between the adjoining sides of the floor remnants. The rim periosteum is closed to help stabilize the graft. Prior to wound closure, the operative site is carefully explored for bleeding points and these are cauterized. The brow and lower eyelid incisions are closed in layered fashion.

Postoperatively, the zygoma is protected by an external splint or cup. Careful assessment of the vision is performed in the recovery room. The head is elevated to reduce swelling, and the patient is advised to avoid bending over or blowing the nose for 6 weeks following operation. Prophylactic antibiotics are administered in the perioperative period if a graft was employed and discontinued 48 hours after surgery. These patients frequently experience photophobia and require sunglasses for as long as 6 weeks following discharge from the hospital.

Comminuted Fractures of the Zygoma

Comminuted orbital rim and zygomatic body fractures are managed by piecemeal reduction and interosseous wire fixation of all the fragments. Periosteal attachments are preserved if they do not interfere with the drilling and wiring of the fragments. Care must be exercised when dissecting laterally over the zygomatic body to avoid injury to the zygomaticofacial sensory nerve, which exits the main body 1 to 2 cm inferior and lateral to the orbital margin. Injury to this nerve can be a source of annoying pain and discomfort to the patient.

After the rim and zygomatic body have been reconstructed and fixed to the rigid medial and lateral components, the complex often is unstable and prone to collapse—a common cause of postoperative malar deformity. In these cases, outrigger stabilization becomes necessary. One or two points along the orbital rim and/or zygoma are chosen for support. Stainless steel wires (No. 30) are passed through small drill holes at these points and brought out through the lower eyelid flap. At the completion of the procedure, the wires are connected to an outrigger appliance (preferably a skeletal head frame). Postoperative radiographs are used to gauge the external reduction. We do not use elastics for traction in these cases because there is a tendency for overcorrection leading to an exaggerated projection of the malar eminence or orbital rim, which is quite difficult to correct once the bones become rigid.

Primary Bone Grafting in Zygomatic Fractures

Primary bone grafting is employed for acute fractures of the zygoma and orbit when there is severe comminution and/or loss of bone. Prerequisites include a stable patient and adequate soft tissue coverage. The inferior orbital rim and floor are reconstructed with contoured iliac crest bone grafts. Split-rib grafts are an alternative source of graft material; they work well in children but have a high resorption rate in the adult. Interestingly, grafts placed in children enlarge with the normal growth of the surrounding facial skeleton. In some, however, graft enlargement is not proportional, and a hypoplastic skeletal deformity may develop; the factors governing these phenomena are not completely understood. Alloplastic materials are occasionally employed as an alternative. As stated previously, they are not considered equivalent substitutes for autogenous material, particularly when utilized around the paranasal sinuses. Here, deficiencies in soft tissue coverage give rise to implant migration and sinus tract formation. We do not use alloplastic materials in children. Contour defects of the malar eminence, zygomatic arch, or orbital rim in adults, however, are ideally suited for these grafts.

Orbital Blow-out Fractures

Blow-out fractures of the orbital floor are managed in the same way as those associated with zygomatic fractures. The key exception here is the lack of distraction capability in the zygomatic fragment. If the herniated/entrapped contents cannot be easily reduced without injury, the floor fracture is widened, bit by bit, by shaving the fracture edges with a No. 15 scalpel blade until the mass is easily delivered. The orbital floor defect can be repaired with a bone or cartilage graft, as previously described. A Caldwell-Luc antrostomy is occasionally employed to facilitate the reduction of difficult trap-door fractures or large comminuted fractures of the orbital floor. A 4- to 6-cm incision is made just below the apex of the labial gingival sulcus, and a subperiosteal dissection of the anterior wall of the maxilla is performed. A large antral window is made with a fine diamond-tipped burr, and the sinus cavity is entered. (The antral bone graft thus harvested is saved and used for reconstruction of the orbital floor.) After the old blood and mucus are evacuated, the sinus cavity is explored. All loose fragments and sharp spicules of attached bony floor are removed to exclude possible foreign bodies in the sinus and prevent any potential injury to the adnexal structures during reduction. An elevator is used to gently elevate the bone and soft tissues back into the orbital cavity. Care is taken to avoid stabbing the herniated adnexa with the instrument. Usually, a piece of attached orbital floor can be found which will serve as a platform for the elevator as the reduction progresses. After reduction of the fracture has been accomplished by this method, the floor is rarely stable unless a single large piece remains intact and can be wedged into position. If there is no significant bony defect in the orbital floor, the reduced fragments can be supported from below with a maxillary sinus pack. Numerous materials have been employed for this purpose and all have their advantages and disadvantages. Nonadherent inert materials work best. Gauze packings are quite malodorous and adhere to the bony fragments. Balloon catheters are easy to insert, but often do not elevate the orbital floor at the correct point. They may also cause pressure necrosis of the sinus mucosa. Custom low-pressure balloon catheters work well, but are expensive and frequently unavailable. We prefer a long half-inch Penrose drain. The drain is easily inserted and removed. It is nonadherent, maintains a good reduction of the orbital floor, and is well tolerated by the patient.

A medial wall antrostomy is made below the inferior turbinate, and the drain is passed from the maxillary sinus window into the nose and secured to the membranous septum with a silk suture. The sinus is then carefully packed in layers until the orbital floor fractures are in good position and stable. Excess drain is cut off, and the remaining end is notched with a "V" to ensure completeness of removal. The vestibular incision is closed in layers with absorbable sutures. The antral pack is left in this position for 10 to 14 days and then removed.

Antral packing is occasionally used for severely comminuted fractures of the zygoma and maxilla. We do not employ this technique, preferring direct wiring instead. When used, however, a balloon catheter, placed through a medial wall maxillary sinus antrostomy, has the requisite rigidity to immobilize the surrounding fragments. Unfortunately, this method remains somewhat imprecise.

Fractures of the Mandible

The mandible is unique among facial features owing to its functional detachment from the facial skeleton. Strong muscular forces applied to the mandible influence the direction and severity of displacement of its fractures. Unlike fractures of other facial bones, the mandibular fracture must be held in reduction by stronger methods of fixation and for longer periods of time. This key observation determines the ultimate mode of management. Timing of therapy is dependent on the relative severity of associated injuries and their importance in the overall status of the patient. Early therapy is preferred, especially in children, in whom fracture consolidation occurs rapidly (7 to 10 days). All mandibular fractures involving the teeth are considered open fractures because of the nature of the periodontal attachment, even if a laceration is not evident. Antibiotic prophylaxis is considered wise practice in such cases. If fracture management is delayed beyond 48 hours, we generally prescribe clindamycin (300 mg/100 cc saline every ten hours) mouthwashes as an additional measure, particularly when significant periodontal disease or dental caries are present. The bathing of the fracture site with saliva and oral cavity bacteria causes massive contamination, which, if allowed to persist, can lead to nonunion or osteomyelitis of the fracture site.

The mainstay of mandibular fracture management is based on the concept of intermaxillary fixation. In general, this represents the most conservative treatment that will effectively reduce and stabilize the fracture. Other methods of mandibular fixation include interarch dental fixation, interosseous fixation, and external fixation. These methods may be employed in addition to intermaxillary fixation for specific fractures.

In managing these injuries, attention must be directed to the presence or absence of serviceable teeth on either side of the fracture. Fractures of the mandible may be favorable or unfavorable, depending on their direction or bevel and the influence of the muscles of mastication on specific parts. A keen understanding of these relationships is necessary before embarking on any therapeutic plan. Inasmuch as the goal of therapy is the reestablishment of normal or pre-injury mandibular function, the teeth serve as both the diagnostic and therapeutic means to this end (see Table).

Intermaxillary Fixation

A metal brace affixed to the dental arch with circumdental wires is the most common method of intermaxillary fixation in both closed and open procedures. These are applied to the upper and lower teeth, and the jaws are brought into occlusion. Elastics placed between the arch bars guide and hold the fragments in position with the maxillary dentition. The elastics are initially employed to effect a "gradual" reduction over several days. This is an excellent means of overcoming muscle spasm, which might be present initially. Once reduction is achieved, the elastics are replaced by wires. To be successful, intermaxillary fixation requires a reasonable complement of teeth. Large gaps of dentition, particularly around the fracture site(s), must be compensated by additional support (special splints or direct wiring). Arch bars alone do not afford sufficient stabilization for fractures of the mandibular body or symphyseal region or those fractures classified as "unfavorable." In addition, circumdental wiring tends to cause extrusion of the teeth—a point to consider in children or in adults with significant periodontal disease. A distinct advantage of arch bar intermaxillary fixation is that it can be done under local anesthesia with a minimum of instrumentation.

Lingual splints are useful adjuncts to arch bar fixation. They provide rigid stabilization, which checks unwanted rotational forces, and they also aid in preventing extrusion of the teeth. These are fashioned from dental models preoperatively or in situ at the time of operative reduction. The former method is preferable because it is more precise and saves operating time.

Other appliances used for intermaxillary fixation include interdental wiring (e.g., Stout, Risdon, Ivy loops), orthodontic bands, and acid-etch composite dental resins. Interdental wiring is occasionally useful as a temporizing measure to stabilize the fractured parts until the time is appropriate for a more definitive procedure. Although once used routinely in the management of mandibular fractures, this method has generally been replaced by direct arch bar fixation. It remains, however, an excellent method of stabilization in the cooperative patient with a full complement of teeth. Orthodontic bands are quite effective in stabilizing the dentition. They are particularly useful in children because they do not cause extrusion of the dentition—a major problem when wiring primary teeth. Their application, however, is time consuming and extremely expensive. Acid-etch composite dental resins represent a new generation of fixation devices. When applied properly, they provide excellent stabilization, do not cause extrusion of the teeth, and are not obstructive to the maintenance of daily oral hygiene. Their disadvantages lie primarily in their variable adhesiveness to the teeth—they are prone to fracture. These and similar appliances may soon supplant the standard circumdental wire.

Interosseous Fixation

Direct wiring of the fracture segments is indicated when intermaxillary fixation alone is insufficient in maintaining a proper alignment, as in cases of:

1. Fractures of the edentulous mandible
2. Displaced fractures in which one or more fragments do not contain teeth
3. Displaced fractures in children having deciduous dentition
4. Fractures of both mandibular arches with a "floating" inter-arch segment.

The advantages of interosseous wire fixation of mandibular fractures are numerous. As with other fractures, direct exposure and wiring provide for a more precise, controlled means of reduction and stabilization. With internal support, the mandible can be released from intermaxillary fixation earlier (4 vs. 6 weeks). The fixation provided is quite strong and is less susceptible to the forces of muscle pull. Disadvantages of this technique include the potential for operative injury to the facial or mandibular nerve, the creation of a facial scar, and possible infection. For the most part, these disadvantages can be minimized by careful operative technique and placement of incisions in the lines of minimum skin tension (wrinkle lines).

The placement of the interosseous wire should be planned so that the point of fixation is advantageous regarding the direction of muscle pull on the fragments. For example, an unfavorable fracture of the mandibular angle may open superiorly if a single wire is placed along the inferior border. In this case, a figure-of-8 wire or two wires may be necessary to effect a rigid stabilization.

When placing the drill holes, one must avoid injury to the dental roots and the mandibular nerve. If a high fixation is needed in the tooth-bearing position, wire fixation of the outer cortex will prevent injury to the cancellous components. In most cases, however, arch bar or lingual splint stabilization precludes the use of interosseous wiring in this area.

For most fractures of the mandible stabilized by interosseous wiring, we use a No. 24 or No. 26 stainless steel wire. It is important not to strip the periosteum extensively for fear of devascularizing the fracture segments. The fracture is reduced and held in reduction manually or with a bone clamp. Drill holes are made with a fine high-speed drill, and the site is constantly irrigated with saline solution to avoid "burning" the bone. The wire is introduced, and both ends are pulled to engage the fragments. The ends are then twisted while maintaining moderate tension on the pull. The end point of twisting is based primarily on experience—we stop when the wire loop feels snug and elicits no play with movement. The wire will break just after it loses its sheen at the apex of the twist. After the wire is secured, it is cut off about 10 to 15 cm from the apex and bent (while twisting) into one of the drill holes. When bringing the wire around the inferior border of the mandible, it is often helpful to notch the border with a burr and use this to seat the wire. This technique is helpful in preventing migration of the wire ligature and in preventing the palpable and sometimes painful wire lumps that can be felt through the skin. Every attempt must be made to close the periosteum over these repairs as well as to close the oral mucosa. These are contaminated wounds that contain a foreign body (wire). Synthetic absorbable sutures are preferred for the periosteal and/or fascial closures because of their decreased reactivity. Chromic gut (3-0) is used for the oral mucosa because it dissolves rapidly as the mucosa heals. (Synthetic absorbable sutures are not readily degraded in the oral cavity and often require removal.) We do not generally drain these wounds.

In most cases, the interosseous wire is left in position permanently; infection or irritation of the soft tissues is an indication for removal.

Other methods of interosseous fixation of the mandibular fracture include osteosynthesis compression plating, stapling, and K-wire fixation.

Compression plating of the mandibular fracture is a recent development borrowed from the orthopedic experience. The method involves applying a special plate across the fracture site and securing the plate with screws into the outer cortex. This provides a rigid fixation of the fracture segments and requires less dissection than interosseous wiring. The technique is accurate and rather simple, though some experience is required to avoid errors in placement and drilling. Specially designed plates and screws constructed from stainless steel/molybdenum alloy are applied with a custom tool pack designed especially for this purpose. The hardware is quite expensive and this remains the greatest disadvantage of this technique. In early cases, using the osteosynthesis plating, it was recommended that the hardware be removed 6 weeks following surgery. As more experience has been gained with the materials and technique, and as the plates have been magnified, these appliances may now be left in permanently.

Large metallic staples have been employed for stabilizing fractured mandibles. The custom staples are tapped into small drill holes on each side of the fracture. These are sometimes used for the fixation of fractures of the edentulous mandible, particularly when there is a high degree of alveolar resorption and a rather fragile, thin mandibular remnant. The many problems associated with the use of these appliances include migration, breaking, splintering of the mandibular fragment during introduction, and extrusion. Their advantage lies in simplicity of application.

K-wire stabilization of mandibular fractures is occasionally employed either as a primary or a secondary means of fixation. It can also be used in temporary splinting of the fractured segments. Minimal periosteal dissection is required in the insertion of the K-wires—a potential advantage when treating comminuted fractures. K-wires are also helpful in maintaining correct spatial relationships of the fractured parts and are particularly useful when there are missing parts (i.e., as in blast injuries). They are best inserted with a power tool because of the density of the cortical bone of the mandible. Slower manually operated drills cause warping of the wire during insertion, with the production of large bone holes and a tendency for aberrant migration. Threaded K-wires are not recommended if the wire crosses through soft tissue (floor of the mouth) because the threads tend to grab the tissue and avulse resistant parts, such as nerves and blood vessels. A square "C-wire" is advantageous in some instances because it impacts the bone snugly and has less tendency for loosening and migration.

The disadvantages of K-wire insertion in the mandible are primarily that of infection, the potential for loosening and migration, and avulsion injury to soft tissue parts. Infection is related to the looseness of the K-wire and its proximity to the oral cavity. Loose wires should be removed. As a general rule, we avoid entering the oral cavity. In some instances, however, this is not practical. If the K-wire is rigid, bone infection is rare. In placing the K-wire, care should be taken to avoid major nerves and blood vessels. It is helpful to make a small incision (if the fracture has not been exposed) through the skin at the proposed entrance site and dissect bluntly to the bone, thus avoiding the soft tissue contacts with the wire as it engages and minimizing possible nerve or vessel injury.

External Fixation

Biphasic external fixation devices are excellent adjuncts to managing comminuted mandibular fractures, fractures complicated by missing parts, or fractures of the edentulous mandible. There are numerous methods for constructing a biphasic appliance. We prefer a simple but reliable technique, utilizing an endotracheal tube and threaded K-wires. The fracture segments are first reduced and brought into occlusion with the maxillary dentition. Arch bars, acrylic splints, dentures, or combinations of these are used to re-establish a correct dental alignment. Two K-wires, which pass through both cortical layers approximately one centimeter from the inferior margin are inserted into each mandibular fragment. In placing these wires, it is important to make adequate soft tissue incisions to avoid engagement of the surrounding soft tissues. The wires should also be oriented in a congruent horizontal plane. Next, an endotracheal tube is cut to match the appropriate arch span incorporating the protruding wires. The wires are cut approximately 4 cm above the skin level, and the shortened tube is impaled on the ends of the wires through small incisions placed on its facing surface. The positioned tube is filled with acrylic polymer injected through one end from a large truncated-tipped syringe. The polymer hardens after 10 minutes, creating a rigid external fixation device.

Biphasic appliances can be used in this fashion as an adjunct to interosseous fixation of the severely comminuted mandibular fracture or as an external "spacer" device for fractures complicated by missing parts. When properly secured, they can be employed for monomandibular fixation. Their disadvantages lie in the potential for infection, soft tissue injury during insertion and removal, and a rather imprecise means of fragment stabilization.

These devices are not recommended in children because of possible injury to the unerupted tooth buds.

Craniomandibular fixation with a head frame or skull cap is not usually employed for isolated mandibular fractures. These methods are occasionally used in conjunction with other fractures of the facial skeleton and particularly those associated with subcondylar fractures of the mandible.

Teeth in the Line of Fracture

One is often confronted with the question whether to remove or retain a tooth in the line of fracture. There are many arguments for both sides of this controversy. Certainly, vital, firm, functional teeth in the line of fracture should not be removed. Conversely, one could not object strongly to the extraction of teeth with fractured roots, nonrestorable teeth, extremely loose teeth, or teeth with periapical or periodontal disease that are in the line of fracture. In many instances, teeth in the line of fracture aid in stabilization. Our philosophy in these cases is to remove all teeth in the line of fracture that might contribute to the development of infection. We do not consider any benefit gained from stabilization to outweigh the potential sequelae of infection.

Similar controversy exists regarding removal of impacted or partially erupted mandibular third molar teeth associated with the line of fracture. In these cases, we prefer to extract the tooth and secure the fragments with an interosseous wire through the buccal cortical plate. This approach has not, in our experience, caused any complication and indeed removes a lingering problem.

Treatment of Mandibular Fractures

The treatment of mandibular fractures can be divided into four major categories based on the anatomic region involved: (1) condylar fractures, (2) angle, ramus, and coronoid fractures, (3) body and alveolar ridge fractures, and (4) anterior fractures. There are numerous other classifications, but this method simplifies an otherwise complex arrangement. The following treatment plans take into account an understanding of the influence of the various muscle groups as they act on the fracture segments.

Condylar Fractures

Undisplaced or minimally displaced fractures of the condylar neck are treated conservatively by closed reduction and intermaxillary fixation for 3 weeks. In bilateral condylar fractures treated by closed reduction, intermaxillary fixation is continued for 4 weeks because of the tendency to develop an open-bite deformity.

Displaced condylar fractures are best managed by open reduction and internal fixation in conjunction with intermaxillary fixation. Absolute indications for this approach include (1) displacement of the condyle into the middle cranial fossa, (2) lateral displacement of the condyle, (3) the presence of foreign body (e.g., bullet, shrapnel), (4) displaced condylar fractures in children, and (5) the inability to obtain proper occlusion by closed reduction. Open reduction and internal fixation should also be considered for displaced condylar fractures in patients having a social or medical problem that would preclude intermaxillary fixation (e.g., alcoholism, seizure disorder, neurologic problem).

The type of surgical approach used for these fractures depends primarily on the location of the fracture and the type of internal fixation to be employed. Two basic exposures are used: (1) the submandibular approach, and (2) the periauricular approach. The submandibular approach is most commonly used and gives adequate exposure for most condylar fractures except the very high neck fractures. An incision is made approximately 2 cm below the mandibular angle in a convenient neck crease. Care must be exercised to avoid injury to the marginal branch of the facial nerve, which is encountered just deep to the platysma anterior to the angle. Variations in the course of this nerve must be anticipated. In most cases, the inferior course of the nerve is not beyond 1.5 cm of the lower mandibular margin. The identified nerve is reflected superiorly and protected. At the level of the mandibular angle, the muscle insertions are divided, and a subperiosteal dissection of the lateral surface of the ascending ramus is performed to the fracture site. The distal fragment is retracted inferiorly to facilitate the exposure. The condylar fragment is usually displaced medially. Occasionally, it is helpful to bluntly dissect upward along the lingual surface of the ramus to engage the condylar fragment and guide it into position with digital manipulation. Muscle relaxation is a helpful adjunct during this part of the procedure.

After the condylar fragments have been reduced, the fracture is stabilized with an interosseous wire, a wire loop, or by intramedullary pinning. We prefer the intramedullary pin technique because it is simple and temporary, and provides excellent stabilization during healing. A small burr hole is drilled on the lingual surface of the angle until cancellous bone is encountered. A square "C-wire" is inserted through the skin and drilled up the medullary canal of the ramus into the condylar fragment, stopping in the head of the condyle. Intraoperative radiographs are taken to check the pin and fragment positions. Retrograde pinning of the fracture is occasionally employed if aberrant pin migration is encountered with the antegrade method. The fracture site is exposed, and a percutaneous pin is directed through the open end of the distal fragment and captured as it exits the angle. The fracture is reduced and the pin drilled into the proximal fragment.

The pin is cut 2 to 3 cm from the skin surface and capped with a cork. It is removed after 3 weeks. Intermaxillary fixation is continued for 2 weeks and then a soft diet is begun.

Very high displaced neck fractures of the condyle cannot easily be reduced by the angle approach and are best managed by direct exposure and interosseous wiring. This may be accomplished through a postauricular incision, which divides the ear canal. The facial nerve and parotid gland are reflected to expose the lateral and posterior surfaces of the temporomandibular joint. Care must be exercised to preserve, as much as possible, the soft tissue attachments to the condylar fragment; otherwise, aseptic necrosis of this structure will occur.

Bilateral subcondylar fractures are notorious for producing severe open-bite deformities if displaced and are managed according to the guidelines stated previously. Subcondylar fractures in children carry the risk of growth arrest leading to abnormalities in jaw development and ankylosis of the temporomandibular joint. Most of these fractures are managed conservatively without intermaxillary fixation. A soft diet allows early mobilization of the condyle—a possible prophylaxis against ankylosis. In the same context, a displaced condylar fracture should be managed by open reduction, with special care to avoid unnecessary periosteal stripping. Jaw motion is begun at 2 weeks because these fractures heal quite rapidly.

Dislocation of the Temporomandibular Joint. In the absence of fracture, the condylar head is displaced anteriorly out of its fossa, tearing its capsule. The jaw becomes locked in an open-bite position, and there is considerable pain associated with muscle spasm.

Most of the dislocations will spontaneously reduce by the simple injection of lidocaine solution (1 percent) into the joint capsule. If this is unsuccessful, a manipulative reduction is required. The patient must be cooperative. Sedation is often helpful though not mandatory. The operator's thumbs are placed in the patient's mouth over the molar dentition with the fingers grasping the mandibular bodies. Gradual firm pressure is exerted to push the posterior mandible downward while pulling the anterior mandible upward. The jaw will "click" into position, and the patient notices immediate relief. A general anesthetic may be required to overcome the muscle spasm in some cases.

Angle, Ramus, and Coronoid Fractures

By definition, these fractures do not contain tooth-bearing segments. Consequently, their stabilization depends on the indirect influence of intermaxillary fixation. Favorable fractures whose line of obliquity lies against the masticatory muscle pull are best managed by intermaxillary fixation if adequate upper and lower dentition is present. In the edentulous patient, dentures can be used to effect this stabilization. The dentures are secured to the mandible by circum-mandibular wiring and to the maxilla by suspension wires from the piriform aperture, nasal spine, infraorbital rim, or zygoma. Intermaxillary fixation is generally concluded by the fourth week and followed by graded physiotherapy to improve opening and closing.

Open reduction of these fractures supplemented with intermaxillary fixation is reserved for those characterized by displacement, an unfavorably oriented fracture line, or bilateral fractures. The preferred surgical approach is through a submandibular or angle incision.

Fractures of the coronoid process generally do not require open reduction and can be managed adequately by intermaxillary fixation.

Body and Alveolar Ridge Fractures

These fractures are characterized by the inclusion of tooth-bearing segments. If stable teeth are present on both sides of the fracture and a complement of occluding maxillary dentition is present, intermaxillary fixation is the procedure of choice. Open reduction of these fractures is indicated if (1) teeth are present on only one side of the fracture and the fracture angle is unfavorable, (2) there are no stable occluding maxillary teeth in the presence of an unfavorable fracture, or if (3) the mandible is edentulous.

For body fractures, a submandibular approach gives the best exposure. One or two interosseous wires are affixed and the jaws are secured by intermaxillary arch bars or denture appliances. In children, open reduction and internal fixation of these fractures carries the hazard of injury to the unerupted tooth buds. In these cases, one must make every effort to place the wires very low along the inferior mandibular margin. Osteosynthesis plates may also be employed to stabilize the reduced fracture fragments—their use may eliminate the need for intermaxillary fixation.

Alveolar ridge fractures do not generally require open reduction unless they are "flail" and attached to a substantial piece of bone. Loose nonviable teeth are removed along with the small detached remnants of the alveolar ridge. The remaining teeth and attached alveolus are reduced to the dental arch and secured to an arch bar. In these cases, we do not like to use circumdental wiring because it tends to extrude the teeth. Dental bands or acid-etched adhesive appliances are best employed for this purpose. Occasionally, special acrylic lingual or occlusal splints are used when the adjoining dentition is absent or there are associated anterior or body fractures of the mandible.

Avulsed Teeth. Successful replantation of avulsed teeth is dependent on the conditions under which the tooth has been stored and the time interval between injury and replantation. The tooth should be kept moist if replantation cannot be performed immediately. The best storage medium is the saliva of the oral cavity. The replanted tooth is kept splinted by dental banding or an acid-etched adhesive appliance for a minimum of one week to allow repair of the periodontal ligament.

Anterior Fractures

Symphyseal or parasymphyseal fractures require special attention because they cannot be maintained in adequate reduction by simple arch bar stabilization. The pull of the attached muscle groups causes the fragments to gape at their inferior margins, and the obliquity of the fracture line allows overriding of the fragments, producing a lingual tilt of one side. Rare midline fractures of the symphysis may not demonstrate these tendencies and are amenable to closed reduction.

Open reduction and intermaxillary fixation is the procedure of choice for the majority of these fractures. In the case of a symphyseal fracture associated with an angle or body fracture, a lingual splint is necessary to provide additional support for the intervening mandibular segment.

Open reduction is performed by one of two approaches: the intraoral approach or the submental approach. We prefer the submental approach for comminuted fractures because minimal periosteal dissection is employed, thereby diminishing the chances of devascularizing a fracture segment. A 4 to 5-cm curvilinear incision is made under the chin, just inferior to the submental skin crease. The dissection is extended through the platysma to the fascia of the digastric muscles and then anteriorly to the inferior border of the mandible. At the fracture site(s), the periosteum is incised and elevated anteriorly and posteriorly just enough to allow placement of the drill holes along the inferior margin. The fracture is cleaned of debris and granulation tissue. If the fracture courses obliquely from anterior to posterior, a single hole is drilled through the overlapping segments and a wire is passed through the hole and secured tightly around the inferior margin. Perpendicular fractures are best stabilized by wiring through two adjoining holes or placement of a figure-of-8 ligature. The use of osteosynthesis plates as an alternative means of internal fixation has greatly simplified stabilization in these fractures. The periosteum is repaired with fine synthetic absorbable sutures, and the wound is closed in layered fashion. The gingival mucosa is usually disrupted in these cases, and this tissue should be debrided and closed when it is practical to do so. After the internal fixation is performed, the teeth are stabilized in proper occlusion by intermaxillary fixation. The additional support provided by a lingual splint is quite helpful in controlling the comminuted fracture and does not contribute to the extrusion of the incisor teeth (which in these cases may be loose, particularly those bordering the fracture). The advantages inherent to lingual splint stabilization have led us to use them more frequently for these fractures.

The intraoral approach is employed for simple fractures of the anterior mandible and fractures of the edentulous mandible. An incision is made in the labial gingival mucosa above the sulcus and a subperiosteal dissection is performed over the alveolar ridge of the mandible at the level of the fracture. A wire is placed through paired drill holes

along the upper border and secured. This placement has the advantage of providing a fulcrum against the surrounding muscle pull, which tends to gape the fragments when the wire is placed along the lower border. Care must be taken to "seat" the wire or other appliance away from the alveolar crest to avoid denture erosion.

The intraoral "degloving" technique provides a very wide exposure of the anterior mandible, but necessitates rather extensive dissection. It is occasionally used for simple anterior fractures of the dentulous mandible or for comminuted fractures if osteosynthesis plating is to be employed. (This does not require a posterior periosteal dissection.) Using this approach, we prefer a supraperiosteal dissection to the inferior border, where a 2 to 3-cm flap of periosteum is elevated, exposing the fracture site. The advantages of this technique lie in the wide exposure obtained and the avoidance of an external scar.

K-wires are occasionally employed for stabilization of these fractures. They are particularly useful in comminuted fractures when open reduction might jeopardize fragment viability. The fragments are manipulated into reduction and the K-wire is inserted percutaneously to engage the mandibular fragments and fix them to their stable counterparts. We avoid entering the oral cavity to minimize contamination. Although this method is rather imprecise, and for the most part has been supplanted by other techniques, it remains useful as a temporary means of stabilizing the anterior mandible.

Primary Bone Grafting

In the treatment of mandibular fractures characterized by loss of bone (in severely comminuted fractures with extensive devascularization or injuries resulting in direct loss of bone) consideration is given to (1) stabilization of the remnant mandibular segments according to their normal anatomic relationships, (2) reconstruction of the mandibular defect, and (3) provision of adequate soft tissue coverage.

All nonviable bone and soft tissue are debrided. If there are teeth on both sides of the defect, these can be used to help position the fragments in relationship to the maxillary dentition. Acrylic occlusal splints are extremely valuable for this purpose. Internal or external stabilization can be used to secure the fragments. We prefer a biphasic external appliance because it avoids a lot of cumbersome and rather irritating intraoral hardware. Also, this appliance can be maintained during subsequent jaw reconstruction with bone grafts.

The question of placing a bone graft into an acute mandibular defect should be reserved for those rare instances in which (1) there has been minimal soft tissue trauma, (2) there is adequate soft tissue coverage, and (3) a modicum of contamination is present.

Blast injuries to the jaw represent an absolute contraindication to primary bone grafting. The ideal situation exists in the comminuted mandibular fracture or those defects resulting from "clean blows" (e.g., machete, hatchet). For small defects, a cortico-cancellous bone graft from the iliac crest is excellent donor material. Some surgeons prefer a metallic mesh tray, which cups around the defect and is filled with cancellous bone chips. Both methods have their proponents as both work well. We prefer the former method because it contains minimal foreign body and does not require a secondary operation for tray removal. Absorbable synthetic trays, which do not require subsequent removal, are now available as well.

Large mandibular defects represent a major reconstructive problem and should probably be delegated to the management of post-traumatic sequelae. The recent techniques gained from our microsurgical experience, however, allow the transfer of vascularized bone with the additional benefit of soft tissue for a composite reconstruction. The clinical application of this technique for acute traumatic defects remains limited to date.

Maxillary Fractures

Although the standard categorization of the maxillary fractures is represented by the Le Fort classification, it is infrequent that any patient presents with a "pure" form of the classic pathology. More commonly, a mixed type of injury is encountered with variable degrees of comminution of the involved structures. A characteristic not often associated with other facial fractures is the frequent occurrence of severe hemorrhage from the nose and nasopharynx. In most cases, bleeding usually stops with elevation of the head and the application of iced compresses. Occasionally, posterior and anterior nasal packs are necessary to control the hemorrhage. In the unusual circumstance, direct ligation or embolization of the internal maxillary artery or other branches of the external carotid system may be indicated.

Standard radiographs and CT assessment, while important, do not supersede the information gained from a detailed physical examination. The occlusion is particularly important as this represents a key in the operative management. Therapy is directed toward the restoration of functional dental occlusion. Some believe that equal emphasis should be given to esthetics, and we agree. Severely comminuted midfacial fractures can give rise to dishface deformities and elongation or shortening of the central facial height.

Direct wiring of the maxillary bone fragments and skeletal suspension have become the standard form of therapy, replacing older techniques such as chin straps, complicated head caps, and outrigger appliances. A stable mandible and a full complement of teeth simplify the management of these fractures. Broken or avulsed teeth, an edentulous jaw, and a fractured mandible are given first consideration. In these cases, the mandible is stabilized and custom acrylic occlusal splints, bite splints, spacers, or dentures are employed to guide the disharmonious segments into the proper position. The maxilla is "floated" into a functional occlusion with the mandible, and the two structures are thus immobilized by intermaxillary fixation. In this fashion, the maxilla is passively aligned to the mandible and then fixed to the stable facial skeleton by direct interosseous wiring or skeletal suspension. Care must be taken to ensure that the mandibular condyles are resting in their centric position at the completion of the reduction to avoid later temporomandibular joint problems (see Table 1).

Alveolar Fractures

Simple segmental fractures of the alveolus are manipulated into reduction and stabilized by direct ligature or arch bar fixation to the adjacent dentition. An acrylic palatal-alveolar splint constructed from a plaster dental model is an ideal method for stabilizing comminuted tooth-bearing segments of the alveolus as well as palatal fractures. Occasionally, a distracted fragment may be recalcitrant to the manipulative reduction and alignment to the remaining dental arch. In these cases, we prefer a direct open reduction and interosseous wire fixation through the vestibular mucosa. Precise dental alignment is completed by the employment of a single arch bar. The alternative method of applying upper and lower arch bars and elastic traction to guide the dental bearing fragment into position is often complicated by incomplete reduction, rotation of the fragment, or labial eversion. In addition, this method requires a class I type of occlusion to be successful.

Le Fort I Fractures

Transverse fractures of the maxilla can be managed by a variety of techniques, yet the prerequisite common denominator is primary establishment of correct occlusal relationships. This is accomplished by intermaxillary fixation. Arch bars are applied to the upper and lower dentition. The tooth-bearing maxillary fragment is disimpacted with Walsham forceps and brought into proper occlusion with the mandible. Elastics are applied, bringing the two components together. We like to orient the elastics forward from the maxilla to the mandible so as to overcome the tendency to an open-bite deformity. The maxillary fragment is reduced to its normal position with the facial skeleton. By placing a finger in the external meatus of the ear one can palpate the mandibular condyle to check its position in the fossa. It is important not to leave the condyle distracted after maxillary reduction, for reasons already explained.

In isolated Le Fort I fractures, reduction and intermaxillary fixation alone may provide sufficient stabilization. Some argue that it is necessary to fix the maxillary fragment to the stable facial skeleton in order to prevent a long-face deformity. Comprehensive study of this concept, however, has not borne out this statement, but it is probably safest to stabilize these fractures with suspension wiring. A variety of methods are available, and all employ the attachment of stainless steel wires to a stable part of the facial skeleton (infraorbital rim, lateral orbital rim, zygomatic arch), and then to the maxillary arch at a point of suspension. We prefer stabilization to the lateral orbital rim just above the zygomaticofrontal suture line. This approach is simple and places the suspension point more central and posterior to the others; it has the advantage of preventing the common posterior collapse of the maxillary dentition—a major cause of open-bite deformities in these fractures.

After the maxillary fracture has been reduced and stabilized to the mandible by intermaxillary arch bar fixation, the lateral supraorbital rims are exposed through bilateral brow incisions. A No. 26 wire is connected to a pull-out wire and passed through a small drill hole in the supraorbital rim. The two ends of the wire loop are passed through the temporal fossa attached to a long curved wire passer. The wires are delivered into the mouth at

the level of the upper first molar on each side. After the maxillary reduction and the position of the mandibular condyles are checked, the wires are fastened to the maxillary arch bar and twisted until snug. The pull-out wire is brought out through the skin above the brow and attached loosely to a button.

Elastics securing the intermaxillary fixation are replaced with wires after 48 hours or when the teeth look and "feel" like they are in good occlusion. The teeth are left in intermaxillary fixation for approximately 4 weeks. During this time, a rigorous course of oral hygiene is implemented. Frequent mouthwashes and brushing are extremely important in preventing gum and dental disease. Dietary counseling is often necessary as intermaxillary fixation necessitates a liquid diet with attendant restriction of food intake and the disturbance of normal eating habits. The arch bars are left in place for 1 or 2 weeks after intermaxillary fixation is terminated. The diet is advanced to solid foods during this time. Careful frequent checks of the occlusion are made with special consideration given to the development of an open bite. Any shift of the dentition is treated by resumption of the intermaxillary fixation (with elastics, then wire) for an additional 2 weeks.

Le Fort II Fractures

These pyramidal fractures of the midface are best managed by direct interosseous wiring of the infraorbital rims and nasofrontal process followed by suspension wiring from the zygomatic process of the frontal bone. An intact mandible and correct occlusal alignment are prerequisite to fixation of the maxilla. Frequently, there will be associated zygomatic and orbital fractures, which should be reduced and stabilized to the facial skeleton prior to management of the maxilla.

Injuries to the lacrimal sac and canaliculi should be suspected in all Le Fort II fractures. Function is usually maintained with proper fracture reduction. In severely comminuted fractures, exploration of the medial orbital wall and drainage of the lacrimal apparatus may be indicated (see *Naso-Orbital Fractures*).

Comminuted Maxillary Fractures

Severely comminuted fractures of the maxilla are reconstructed by piecemeal interosseous wiring through an intraoral approach. It is important to remove all bone fragments and foreign bodies (teeth) from the maxillary sinus to prevent possible infection. If the anterior maxillary wall is unstable, the sinus is packed with a rubber drain to provide additional support. The maxillary sinus pack is removed after 7 days, when the fracture segments have consolidated.

Panfacial Fractures

Combined fractures of the facial skeleton are the result of high-velocity impact usually sustained in automobile or motorcycle accidents. The tremendous force absorbed by the head in these injuries is frequently manifested by intracranial and cervical spine sequelae. The patients may not demonstrate any airway difficulties initially, but may soon succumb to the effects of massive hemorrhage and inevitable swelling. A cricothyroidotomy should be performed as a part of the initial trauma management.

The surgical philosophy employed in these injuries is reduction of the fractures into their anatomic positions, fixation to a stable support (usually the skull or a craniofacial outrigger appliance), and soft tissue repair.

In the acute situation, therapeutic priorities are given to the control of hemorrhage, ophthalmologic emergencies, and frontal bone or other fractures communicating with the cranial cavity. If massive swelling is present, definitive management of the remaining fractures is delayed for approximately 5 days, and supportive measures are employed (e.g., temporary stabilization of the fractures, wound closure, oral lavage).

Mandibular fractures are repaired first, followed by sequential reduction and stabilization of the zygomas, nasoethmoid region, orbital floors, and maxilla. Comminuted fractures are treated by direct interosseous wiring of the fracture segments with stabilization of the repaired "bloc" to a rigid support, such as an adjacent facial bone, the orbital rims, frontal bone, zygomatic arch, or an outrigger appliance. Considerable improvisation is required as these fractures rarely follow any stereotyped pattern. Intermaxillary fixation, with the reconstruction of a normal or "preinjury occlusion," correct projection of the facial parts, and facial symmetry, are key end points of therapy.

Blast Injuries to the Face

The devastating effects of a high-velocity projectile, as from a gun or a bomb, represent the most complex of facial injuries. Such injuries may produce extensive destruction of soft tissue, comminuted fragmentation of bone, loss of composite facial parts, and widespread impregnation of foreign bodies. These wounds are difficult to assess at the outset. Initial care is directed to the establishment of an airway and restoration of blood volume. Arteriography should be performed if there is suspicion of vascular injury. CAT scan assessment is, at times, quite valuable, but may be clouded because of the deflections caused by metallic foreign bodies.

Operative management of these injuries is staged and consists of initial cleansing, minimal debridement, and hemostasis. Antibiotic and tetanus prophylaxis is instituted at the outset. Broad-spectrum therapy (penicillin, erythromycin, cephalosporin) is recommended.

As a rule, we do not close these wounds primarily because of the high propensity to infection and the indeterminability of tissue viability. Repeat wound exploration is performed in 24 to 48 hours, and further debridement of the devitalized bone and soft tissue is effected. Wound closure is planned as a secondary procedure, incorporating a multidisciplinary approach. First considerations are given to the re-establishment of bony relationships and appropriate drainage of the paranasal sinuses. Direct interosseous wiring, craniofacial appliances, acrylic splints, and intermaxillary fixation constitute the primary means of fixation for this purpose. Bone grafting is reserved for the reconstruction of the orbital walls, rims, and floor, and the major facial buttresses, provided adequate soft tissue coverage is available. Nasal, septal, palatal, and mandibular reconstructions are performed as delayed procedures after the initial wounds have healed.

After the facial skeleton has been repaired, the soft tissues are closed. Despite the impressive defects encountered, many of these wounds can be closed by approximation. Others may require the introduction of skin grafts, local or regional flaps, or simple skin-to-mucosa closure. Because of the nature of the injury, fibrosis of the soft tissues is a common sequela and can pose significant problems in later facial reconstruction. For this reason, it is advantageous for bony defects that are not reconstructed primarily to be supported with temporary obturator devices to check the tissue contraction. This is particularly applicable in the region of the anterior mandible, the maxilla, and the palate.

TRAUMA PRINCIPLES AND PENETRATING NECK TRAUMA
Donald D. Trunkey, M.D.

WOUND BALLISTICS

Stab wounds are relatively benign injuries unless a major blood vessel has been lacerated or unless a particularly vital structure has been injured. Rarely do these result in much morbidity. Gunshot wounds, on the other hand, may cause devastating injury, particularly if they are from high-velocity weapons or close-range shotguns. Table 1 lists common handguns and weapons with their respective muzzle velocities.

Terminal ballistics, the amount of energy imparted to tissues by the missile, largely determines the injury and killing power. The most widely accepted terminal ballistic theory is the kinetic energy theory, which states that kinetic energy released to tissues equals mass times velocity squared, divided by two times the gravitational constant. This is thought to provide the best estimate of wounding capacity, and it thus follows that modest increases in velocity will result in tremendous increases in the kinetic energy of the missile and resultant killing and wounding power. Simple calculation, using this formula, demonstrates that a .22 Magnum is capable of eight times the energy release of a .38 revolver. Generally, weapons capable of generating a missile velocity in excess of 2,000 ft/sec are said to be high-velocity weapons.

The amount of energy imparted to the tissue is estimated to be kinetic energy on impact minus kinetic energy on exit. Thus, bullet design becomes important, and to inflict the greatest possible tissue damage, a bullet should dissipate all of its energy to the tissue with no residual exit energy. This has led to the development of missiles that disintegrate on impact, such as soft-point and hollow-nose bullets. Increased muzzle velocity and disintegrating missiles cause extensive tissue damage. Some missiles, for example, can create a temporary cavity 30 times the size of the entering bullet, the size of this cavity being dependent on ballistics, type of bullet, and the tissue that is transgressed. The damage produced can be worsened by secondary missiles or fragments of disintegrating bone and other tissue. Recent studies show that missile yaw within tissue is very destructive, particularly when the velocity is greater than 2,800 ft/sec. The same studies, and others, also show that it is not necessary to do radical debridements with high-velocity wounds, as was once believed. Debridement of obviously dead tissue and delayed primary closure of the skin are the hallmarks of wound management.

Close-range shotgun blasts undoubtedly cause the most devastating injuries of any weapon to which civilians are normally exposed. Sherman and Parrish have classified shotgun wounds into three categories: type I shotgun injuries, sustained at long range (greater than 7 yards); type II shotgun injuries, sustained at close range (3 to 7 yards); and type III shotgun injuries, sustained at very close range (less than 3 yards). Type I injuries usually present as scatter types and may not even penetrate visceral cavities from distances greater than 40 yards. At 20 yards, penetration is increased, and yet expectant management may sometimes be warranted. Type II injuries usually involve damage to deep structures and require more aggressive management. Type III wounds produce massive tissue injury and carry a very high mortality rate (85 to 90 percent).

BLUNT TRAUMA

Blunt injury can be caused by direct impact, deceleration, rotary forces, and shear forces. Direct impact may cause significant injury, and the severity can be estimated by knowing the force and duration of impact as well as the mass of the patient contact area. Table 2 demonstrates the most common sites of injury from motor vehicle accidents; ejection, steering assembly impact, windshield impact, instrument panel impact, and rear collision account for the majority of these.

TABLE 1   Examples of Muzzle Velocity

Weapon	Velocity (ft/sec)
.22 Long rifle	1,335
.22 Magnum	2,000
.220 Swift	2,800
.270 Winchester	3,580
.357 Magnum	1,550
.38 Colt	730
.44 Magnum	1,850
.45 Army Colt	850

TABLE 2   Common Sites of Injury: All Accidents

Site	%
Encephalon, skull, face	43
Chest	12
Abdomen, pelvis	9
Upper limbs	13
Lower limbs	23

Deceleration injuries are most often associated with high-speed motor vehicle accidents and falls from heights. As the body decelerates, the organs continue to move forward at terminal velocity, tearing vessels and tissues from points of attachment. Rotary forces also tend to cause tearing injuries from a tumbling type of action.

Shear forces have a tendency to produce degloving types of injuries, such as are apt to occur when the patient is run over by a large vehicle. As the vehicle passes over the body, the skin and subcutaneous tissues are pushed ahead, tearing nutrient blood supply from its muscular sources below. Subsequent extensive soft tissue loss is common following such injury.

Blunt trauma, under certain conditions, can result in a compartment syndrome, a syndrome of swollen necrotic muscle confined within a fascial compartment. The compartment syndrome can be caused by direct impact on the muscle or by continuous pressure, which produces tissue ischemia and necrosis. The continuous pressure can be generated by obtunded patients lying on their extremities in an awkward position; the pressure can also be generated with severe muscular exertion, metabolic disturbances, and toxicity syndromes.

The pathophysiology of compartment syndromes begins with local compression of muscle, decreased capillary flow, damage to capillaries, and eventually ischemic necrosis of the compressed muscle. This, in turn, leads to increased permeability of capillaries. Fluid leaks into the interstitium, compartment pressure builds up, and a compartment tamponade occurs.

The symptoms and signs of an early compartment syndrome include pain and tense swelling in the affected extremity. Skin edema is frequently minimal. If tissue damage is extensive enough, the patient develops a third-space loss of plasma resulting in an increasing hematocrit, progressive hypovolemia, and oliguria.

The sequelae of the compartment syndrome are muscle necrosis, nerve damage, and paralysis. Myoglobin and hemoglobin can be released into the plasma and can precipitate in the renal tubules and cause tubular necrosis.

Treatment includes early fasciotomy, excision of necrotic tissue, and volume resuscitation. An alkaline urine should be maintained by bicarbonate, and diuresis should be promoted with mannitol.

GENERAL APPROACH TO THE INJURED PATIENT

Prophylaxis Against Infection

Preoperative antibiotics are useful adjuncts in the management of the following injuries: (1) compound fractures, particularly grade 3, (2) dirty soft tissue wounds, (3) suspected small bowel or colon injuries, and (4) exposure of tendon and/or joint cartilage. The use of antibiotics in other trauma injuries has not been demonstrated to be efficacious. Suggested antibiotics are shown in Table 3. In the case in which antibiotics have been started for a suspected intestinal injury, but no injury is found at surgery, the antibiotics should be stopped in the immediate postoperative period; otherwise, the antibiotics should be given for a total of 48 to 72 hours.

Prophylaxis against tetanus should be considered for all open wounds. Guidelines have been developed by the American College of Surgeons (Table 4).

Assignment of Priorities

A team approach is often appropriate in the patient with multiple injuries and may include simultaneous decompression of a space-occupying intracranial lesion by neurosurgeons while general surgeons explore the abdomen. In the patient with massive abdominal injuries and associated widened mediastinum, exploration of the abdomen

TABLE 3   Antimicrobial Prophylaxis—72 Hours or Less

Suspected small-bowel or large-bowel injury
 Chloramphenicol, 60 mg/kg/day, IV in 4 divided doses*
  or
 Cefoxitin, 150 mg/kg/day, IV in 4 to 6 divided doses*
  or
 Clindamycin† 40 mg/kg/day, IV in 3 or 4 divided doses
  plus tobramycin or gentamicin, 5 mg/kg/day, IV or IM
  in 3 divided doses*
Traumatic wound (compound fractures, extensive soft-tissue
 injury)
 Methicillin, nafcillin, or oxacillin, 1 g IV three to four
  times a day
  or
 Cefazolin, cephalothin, or cephapirin, 1 g IM or IV three
  to four times a day

*Penicillin, 200,000 units/kg/day, in 6 divided doses may be added.
†Metronidazole may be substituted for clindamycin. Give 15 mg/kg over 1 hour (loading dose), then 7.5 mg/kg every 6 hours.

TABLE 4   Guidelines for Prophylaxis Against Tetanus*

I. Persons previously immunized
  A. When the attending physician has determined that the patient has been previously fully immunized and the last dose of toxoid was given within 10 years:
    1. For non-tetanus-prone wounds, no booster dose of toxoid is indicated.
    2. For tetanus-prone wounds and if more than 5 years have elapsed since the last dose, give 0.5 ml absorbed toxoid. If excessive prior toxoid injections have been given, this booster may be omitted.
  B. When the patient has had two or more prior injections of toxoid and received the last dose more than 10 years previously, give 0.5 ml absorbed toxoid for both tetanus-prone and non-tetanus-prone wounds. Passive immunization is not considered necessary.
II. Persons not adequately immunized
  A. When the patient has had no prior injection of toxoid or has received only one prior injection of toxoid, or when the immunization history is unknown:
    1. For non-tetanus-prone wounds, give 0.5 ml absorbed toxoids.
    2. For tetanus-prone wounds,
      a. Give 0.5 ml absorbed toxoid.
      b. Give 250 units (or more) of human TAT.
      c. Consider providing antibiotics, although the effectiveness of antibiotics for prophylaxis of tetanus remains unproved.

*Guidelines developed by the American College of Surgeons.

with repair of injuries is indicated first. Following laparotomy, an aortogram can be carried out and thoracic aortic rupture, if present, treated. If the patient has associated major vascular injuries to the extremities, control of these must be obtained prior to abdominal exploration. If the patient remains unstable, exploratory laparotomy should be carried out before definitive treatment of the peripheral vascular injuries.

Surgical Preparation and Exposure

The trauma patient must be prepared and draped widely so that the surgeon can gain access to any body cavity expeditiously and so that he can properly place drains and chest tubes, if needed. The entire anterior portion and both lateral portions of the torso should be prepared with iodine paint and draped off so that the surgeon can work in a sterile field from the neck and clavicles cephalad to the groins caudad, and from table top to table top laterally. Prepping should not involve more than a few minutes and is preferably carried out prior to induction of anesthesia so that, should deterioration occur, immediate laparotomy or thoracotomy can be carried out. If craniotomy is anticipated in the emergency room, the hair can be cut and the scalp shaved during the resuscitation to expedite the decompression.

For rapid access and wide exposure of the abdomen, the midline incision is the incision of choice. Only rarely will transverse or oblique incisions be appropriate for trauma. Surgeons should be prepared to extend the midline incision up the sternum as a sternal splitting incision or into the right or left chest if necessary. The chest should therefore be prepped along with the abdomen.

When the presence of abdominal injury is questionable or its site uncertain, it is usually best to start with an upper midline incision extending from just below the xiphoid to just above the umbilicus. The incision can be centered on the umbilicus if the injury is presumed to be in the lower abdomen. Most of the complicated problems, however, will lie in the upper abdomen—hence the xiphoid to umbilical exploratory incision.

When intra-abdominal injury is encountered, the incision should routinely be extended below the umbilicus to the pubis if the injuries appear major.

An abdomen filled with bright red blood indicates an arterial injury. The patient should be eviscerated, each corner of the abdomen rapidly inspected, and packs placed temporarily to absorb the free blood. All quadrants of the abdomen and the mesentery should be inspected on the first pass.

This can be done within a minute or two so that the most major source of hemorrhage can be located and dealt with first. The application of packs will control bleeding from many arterial injuries, and if the injury can be controlled by pack or direct pressure, this should be done while volume is restored. The injury should not be initially exposed directly because the vascular system may suddenly decompress; rapid bleeding in a previously hypovolemic patient frequently leads to cardiac arrest.

If the injury appears to be arterial and in the upper abdomen, the possibility of injury to the visceral portion of the aorta or one of its major upper abdominal branches should be considered and proximal control must be ensured. If a hematoma extends to the level of the diaphragm, the left chest should be opened and the aorta encircled. If the aortic hiatus is free of hematoma, the gastrohepatic ligament should be divided and the aorta encircled as it emerges through the crura of the diaphragm.

Minor injuries and minor sources of hemorrhage should not distract the surgeon from dealing with major ongoing hemorrhage, particularly venous hemorrhage. Venous bleeding may not be obvious, unless looked for, since it occurs under low pressure and may not be as dramatic or as evident as arterial hemorrhage. Almost all venous bleeding can be controlled by the judicious application of packs, permitting time for restoration of volume. If, during the initial exploration, retraction downward of the dome of the liver results in massive venous hemorrhage, injury to the hepatic veins or intrahepatic cava should be strongly suspected, and an intracaval shunt should be considered.

After the initial control of hemorrhage has been achieved with clamps or packs, an attempt should be made to control fecal soilage prior to definitive surgery. Obvious holes in small bowel or colon can be temporarily controlled by running suture or Babcock clamps.

In general, the supine position is preferred for all trauma surgery. One exception is the patient with demonstrated injury to the left subclavian artery between its take-off and the vertebral artery. In this injury, a right lateral decubitus position and left posterolateral thoracotomy are preferred.

After neurosurgical, thoracic, and abdominal injuries have been treated, maxillofacial and orthopaedic injuries are treated, in that order and often under the initial anesthetic. Exceptions to this general sequence may be necessary.

Penetrating Neck Trauma

The first problem in patients with extensive penetrating wounds to the neck is control of the airway. The swelling and hemorrhage associated with such injuries can make such control difficult and cause deviation of the airway to one side or the other owing to the expanding hematoma. In addition, airway control, difficult as it may be when the patient first presents, usually becomes more difficult as resuscitation and swelling progress. Thus, immediate control of the airway, either by endotracheal intubation or by emergency tracheostomy, is necessary.

The second problem in patients with severe neck injuries is control of bleeding. The bleeding can be formidable because of the rich vascularity of the region. Direct pressure, with avoidance of compression of the airway, is usually all that is required.

The third problem in neck injuries is that these patients may well have cervical spine injuries. Usually the neurologic damage has already been done, but every effort should be made to maintain axial orientation with traction.

In order to clarify the clinical approach to neck injuries we have divided them into zones I, II, and III. A zone I injury is injury to the thoracic outlet and extends from the clavicles into the chest. Zone II is the midcervical area and extends from the clavicles to the angle of the jaw. Zone III includes the entrance to the base of the skull and extends from the angle of the jaw cephalad. We generally recommend, in the stable patient, arteriograms on all zone I and zone III injuries. Arteriograms are also indicated in zone II injuries if the injury is posterior to the sternocleidomastoid muscle. In the hemodynamically unstable patient, arteriograms are impractical, and immediate surgery and control of the hemorrhage are indicated.

Zone I injuries have the potential for causing major vascular, tracheal, and esophageal injuries in the mediastinum. Ideally, arteriograms demonstrate the lesions and allow the surgeon to better achieve proximal control, which almost always necessitates sternotomy or thoracotomy in these injuries. Occasionally, removal of the medial half of the clavicle is all that is necessary to gain control and to surgically repair injuries to the subclavian artery and vein. If in doubt, proximal control through the chest should be obtained first. Subclavian vessels tend to be difficult to suture and may require bolstering with Teflon pledgets or graft replacement. Ligation of the subclavian artery can be carried out with minimal consequences to the patient.

Zone II injuries in the anterior neck do not usually require arteriogram. If the injury penetrates beneath the platysma muscle, we favor mandatory exploration. Arteriograms do not rule out significant venous injury, nor do they rule out injuries to the thyroid, trachea, or esophagus. For this reason we believe exploration to be the most conservative management. Injuries to the posterior neck in zone II may involve the vertebral artery within the intervertebral canal. Access to this area is extremely difficult, and alternative treatment modalities are available. For this reason, we favor arteriogram of all zone II injuries in the posterior neck. An alternative approach to surgery is embolization with polymer resins. They have not been a problem in embolization to the brain or the lung and yet control hemorrhage from arterial venous fistulas within the intervertebral canal.

Zone III injuries are hard to manage, since access to vascular injuries at the base of the skull can be extremely difficult. For this reason, we prefer arteriograms to demonstrate the lesion and to better plan the operative approach. Injuries involving the internal carotid artery at the base of the skull can be more easily approached by anteriorly dislocating the mandible after appropriate anesthetic and muscle relaxant have been administered. An alternative approach is to do an osteotomy of the mandible, sparing the lingual nerve. Lacerations involving branches of the external carotid can be approached directly, or if they are in the maxillary area, embolization can be done at the time of arteriogram.

THORACIC TRAUMA

Donald D. Trunkey, M.D.

Trauma to the thorax is present in 50 percent of all fatal accidents and is the primary cause of death in 25 percent. In general, blunt trauma is more common than penetrating trauma, except in urban areas. Significantly, only 15 percent of thoracic trauma patients require major surgery. The great majority (80 to 85 percent can be managed with relatively simple procedures, primarily tube thoracotomy.

The incidence of chest trauma is not well documented. We do know, however, that in one large metropolitan area in the United States (Cleveland) the trauma incidence rate is 197 per 1,000 population. This study is incomplete and does not tell us how many patients were admitted to the hospital. We do know from other studies that 9 to 14 percent of trauma patients seen in emergency rooms are admitted to the hospital. Data from Switzerland show that in a 1 million population base, thoracic trauma accounted for 12 emergency room examinations per day; four of these patients were admitted and there was at least 1 severe chest trauma every other day. We can thus assume that for every 1 million population there are at least 180 severe chest injuries annually.

TYPES OF INJURY

In a large urban area such as San Francisco, blunt trauma accounts for approximately 55 percent of all thoracic trauma, whereas, in suburban or rural areas, blunt trauma accounts for 80 to 85 percent of all thoracic trauma. The automobile accounts for the majority of blunt trauma injuries to the thorax, and it takes minimal kinetic energy to cause significant thoracic trauma. In studies by Stapp, a frontal impact to the steering wheel in a car travelling 16.8 miles per hour was sufficient to cause four rib fractures. A frontal impact at 19.5 miles an hour caused extensive fractures. The injury also depended on age, deceleration, skeletal deflection, and time.

Another source of chest trauma is blast injury, which occurs after an explosion or shock wave. The blast wave is propagated through the body as a pressure wave, and the degree of injury depends on the characteristics of the wave. The most vulnerable parts of the body are those containing air and gas, such as the ear drums, lungs, and intestines.

Penetrating trauma is dependent also on the kinetic energy imparted to the tissue; this is expressed as the formula:

$$KE = M \frac{(V_1 - V_2)^2}{2G} \quad \begin{aligned} M &= \text{Mass} \\ V_1 &= \text{Striking velocity} \\ V_2 &= \text{Exit velocity} \\ &\quad \text{(residual)} \\ G &= \text{Gravity} \end{aligned}$$

Since the lung is primarily a low-pressure system, low-velocity missiles and penetrating objects do not usually cause significant bleeding, particularly if the lung can be re-expanded to get pleural apposition. In fact, in most instances in which thoracotomy is required for bleeding after low-velocity injuries, a systemic vessel such as an intercostal artery or the internal mammary artery is found to be the cause. Occasionally, low-velocity weapons can cause significant bleeding when a hilar structure has been penetrated. High-velocity weapons and shotgun injuries, in contrast, cause devastating destruction to the lung parenchyma and chest wall, which almost invariably require major surgery. Low-velocity injuries to the mediastinum may require surgery, whereas high-velocity injuries to the mediastinal structures are not usually associated with survival long enough for the patient to be transported to a hospital.

INITIAL EVALUATION AND MANAGEMENT

As with any acutely injured patient, in the resuscitation of a patient with chest injury attention should first be directed to maintaining the airway and ventilation, controlling external bleeding, and resuscitating the cardiovascular system. Patients with direct trauma to the chest are particularly at risk for the development of ventilatory insufficiency. Specific signs of ventilatory insufficiency include air hunger, use of the accessory muscles of ventilation, and tachypnea greater than 30 per minute. Less specific signs include those of a generalized sympathetic discharge, such as anxiety, agitation, cold, clammy skin, and tachycardia.

The physician sometimes has time to confirm ventilatory insufficiency with arterial blood gases. A PCO_2 greater than 40 mm of mercury in an acutely injured patient who does not have a documented, chronic hypercarbia must be taken as absolute evidence of ventilatory insufficiency. Hypercarbia in patients with slow ventilatory rates is ominous because it implies depression of normal ventilatory drive. In patients with rapid ventilatory rates, hypercarbia implies that the patient is unable to eliminate carbon dioxide adequately even though he is working hard to do so.

In many cases of acutely injured patients, the physician does not have time to wait for the results of a blood gas determination. Lack of a confirmatory gas should not delay intubation and mechanical ventilation if the patient appears to have ventilatory insufficiency. Mechanical ventilation can be discontinued and the patient extubated later if he is proved to have adequate ventilatory function.

Eighty to 90 percent of all chest injuries, whether due to blunt or penetrating trauma, are adequately treated by insertion of one or more chest tubes and do not require open thoracotomy. Whether the injury produces hemothorax or pneumothorax, a chest tube is required to allow drainage of the intrapleural blood, monitoring of the rate of further bleeding, and evacuation of any air present. A large-bore siliconized tube (32 Fr to 40 Fr) is recommended for this, as blood may clot in smaller tubes, precluding their effective function. We prefer straight chest tubes because right-angle tubes are hard to place and position properly unless the chest is open.

If the patient's condition is stable after chest trauma, one should expeditiously obtain a chest film, upright if possible, to define the intrathoracic pathology. However, if the patient is in distress and clinical examination points to the possibility of hemo- or pneumothorax as the cause, a chest tube should be inserted in one or both pleural spaces, as clinically indicated, without waiting for the chest film.

In the trauma patient we insert the chest tube in the midaxillary line at the level of the nipple or higher. Insertion between the anterior and posterior axillary folds avoids the pectoralis and latissimus dorsi muscles and makes insertion technically much easier. Insertion at the nipple line or higher avoids the diaphragm and accidental puncture of intra-abdominal organs.

If the patient is conscious, the chest should be prepped and 1 percent Xylocaine injected into the skin at the insertion site. An attempt should also be made to anesthetize the parietal pleura. In the unconscious patient a local anesthetic is not necessary. An incision is made sharply about 3 cm long and is carried down through the deep fascia. I prefer to incise the intercostal muscles and parietal pleura directly to enter the chest cavity. This will not cause injury to the lung parenchyma, since it is usually collapsed or protected by clotted blood. An alternative method is to insert a large, blunt clamp after the initial skin incision. This is inserted through the musculature, through the pleural space, and opened to create a hole large enough for chest tube insertion. Prior to insertion of the chest tube, a gloved finger should be inserted into the pleural space and swept around to ensure that there are no adhesions, so that the chest tube can be inserted without entering lung parenchyma. After exploration, the chest tube is then grasped at the tip, with the clamp, and inserted through the hole and directed posteriorly and superiorly. The tube is inserted until the most proximal hole is well inside the chest and is tied in place. I prefer a horizontal mattress stitch of 2-0 or 0 Prolene with a single throw initially; then the suture is wrapped several times around the chest tube and the final ties are placed. When the tube is removed a few days later, this outer knot can be cut, the suture unwrapped, the chest tube removed, and a final throw placed in the suture. After the chest tube has been inserted it is connected, under sterile conditions, to a 3-bottle suction unit and 20 to 25 cm water suction is applied.

Chest tubes placed, as just directed, into the posterior pleural space effectively drain both fluid and air, and are universally effective in trauma, whereas anterior tubes are ineffective for fluid removal. The use of the second intercostal space anteriorly for chest tube placement should be condemned, as that is technically more difficult to place and position correctly and is less effective in the evacuation of fluid.

EMERGENCY THORACOTOMY

Emergency room thoracotomy offers the only chance for salvage in injured patients who have sustained, or are about to sustain, cardiac arrest. Closed chest cardiopulmonary resuscitation in trauma patients is doomed to failure because of inadequate venous return and limited thoracic blood volume. Open cardiac massage is also limited by inadequate venous return, but it does effectively empty the heart of the blood it does contain.

Occasionally, thoracotomy is also the best way to make a quick diagnosis of a life-threatening intrathoracic abnormality such as air embolism. A left thoracostomy permits the diagnosis, and treatment, of a left tension pneumothorax. A right tension pneumothorax is recognized because it pushes the heart and mediastinum into the left hemithorax. Pericardial tamponade can sometimes be recognized on opening the left chest and, in any case, can always be ruled out by opening the pericardial sac.

Emergency room thoracotomies succeed most often in patients with penetrating chest injuries. The patient may have a pericardial tamponade that is easy to relieve, intrathoracic bleeding that can be controlled with pressure, or a massive air leak that can be controlled.

Emergency thoracotomies occasionally succeed in patients with blunt thoracic trauma, particularly in cases of air embolism. The patient may have a controllable rupture of the thoracic aorta or the atrium, or may have a ruptured main stem bronchus which can be controlled by cross-clamping the pulmonary hilum. Emergency thoracotomies are not as successful in patients with penetrating extrathoracic trauma. Open cardiac massage may keep a young patient alive while he is being taken to the operating room for definitive control of an uncomplicated injury. Emergency thoracotomies almost never succeed in patients who have exsanguinated and experienced arrest from severe blunt extrathoracic trauma. The time involved in taking the patient to the operating room and then obtaining control of what is usually a complicated injury is almost always too long to allow salvage.

When trauma patients suffer arrest after penetrating injuries to the left chest, blunt thoracic injuries, and penetrating extrathoracic injuries, a left thoracotomy should be performed. The chest should be opened through the fourth or fifth intercostal space just beneath the nipple. The incision should be made from the sternum to the posterior axillary fold. If severed, the internal mammary vessel should be ligated. One or two of the costal cartilages at the sternum should be cut cephalad to the incision to facilitate exposure. The pericardium should be opened in a vertical direction, taking care to avoid the phrenic nerve. The physician should insert his right hand behind the heart and periodically compress it against the sternum. At the same time he should explore the hemithorax for correctable lesions. An adjunctive procedure is to control the descending thoracic aorta with the resuscitator's thumb or by cross-clamping, so that available cardiac output will be directed to the heart and brain.

In cases of penetrating injuries to the right chest, the physician should open that side. Although cardiac massage is difficult, the physician may find a correctable abnormality, such as a partially severed intercostal artery, a major air leak, or an air embolism. If air embolism is found, the hilum itself should be clamped with a vascular clamp to reduce the inflow of air. If necessary, the incision can be carried across the sternum into the left chest to initiate cardiac massage or treat left thoracic injuries.

DEFINITIVE MANAGEMENT OF IMMEDIATELY LIFE-THREATENING INJURIES

Injuries to the chest wall and parenchyma may be subdivided into two categories: immediately life-threatening and potentially life-threatening. There are seven immediately life-threatening injuries: airway obstruction, open pneumothorax, flail chest, tension pneumothorax, massive hemothorax, pericardial tamponade, and air embolism. The six potentially life-threatening injuries are: rupture of the tracheobronchial tree, pulmonary contusion, diaphragmatic rupture, esophageal perforation, myocardial contusion, and great vessel injuries.

Airway Obstruction

The airway can be obstructed by a foreign body, secretions, severe maxillofacial trauma, or a fractured larynx. Oropharyngeal obstructions can usually be removed by a sweep of the resuscitator's finger. Aspirated objects such as teeth or particles of food may require laryngoscopy or bronchoscopy for removal. With severe maxillofacial trauma, jaw lift or chin thrust should be tried initially if the bony structures are still intact. This maneuver lifts the tongue off the posterior pharynx and a temporary airway can usually be achieved. An alternate method is to grasp the tongue with a towel clip or a sponge to bring it forward if the bony structures are not intact. If these maneuvers fail, a cricothyrotomy should be performed (except in the patient with a complete laryngeal fracture). Classic tracheostomy through the second or third tracheal ring is rarely indicated and should only be performed by someone skilled in the method.

Open Pneumothorax

Either penetrating or blunt trauma can produce an open pneumothorax. The inability to generate negative intrathoracic pressure collapses the lung and leads immediately to ventilatory insufficiency. There may or may not be concomitant pulmonary parenchymal injury. Treatment entails immediate covering of the hole in the chest wall with petrolatum gauze or any other clean, air-tight dressing. A chest tube should be inserted through a separate counter-incision as soon as feasible. The most important aspect of immediate treatment is closure of the chest wall opening; re-expansion of the affected lung is of secondary importance. Once the chest wall defect has been closed, it is imperative to provide close monitoring to avoid the possibility of tension pneumothorax.

Flail Chest

Flail chest results from paradoxical movement of a portion of the chest wall when there are multiple rib fractures and usually when ribs are broken at multiple sites. The problem is analogous, in many ways, to open pneumothorax in that the lungs themselves are often not severely damaged, although there is usually a variable degree of pulmonary contusion in the lung beneath the fracture segment. Respiratory difficulty occurs because the chest wall is unstable, moving inward with inspiration and outward with expiration. The development of negative intrathoracic pressure is prevented; thus, the patient cannot move air in and out of the trachea normally. This is compounded by the severe pain and splinting associated with rib fractures. Knowledge of this fact also dictates the treatment: One need only stabilize the chest wall. In an emergency, simply preventing movement of the chest wall relieves the severe respiratory distress. This is most easily accomplished by turning the patient onto the affected side. If distress continues, immediate intubation and positive pressure ventilation are in order to achieve internal stabilization of the fractures and to ventilate the lungs adequately. In a few selected cases, massive flail chest has required an operative approach. In such instances, plates are wired across the fractured segments, usually on an alternative rib basis so as to stabilize the flail segment. This has allowed more rapid weaning from the ventilator.

Massive Hemothorax

Massive hemothorax usually results from injuries to the aortic arch, pulmonary hilum, or systemic vessels such as the internal mammary or intercostal arteries. Rupture of large vessels is usually incompatible with survival, but with rapid transport, many patients have been seen with continuing rates of blood of loss on the order of 500 to 1,000 ml per hour. Most patients with continuing pleural bleeding following thoracic injuries are not bleeding from the lung itself, as the pulmonary vasculature is a low-pressure system and the average pulmonary artery pressure is only about 17 mmHg, not much above venous pressure. As a result, the patient who continues to bleed is usually doing so from the systemic arteries in the chest: the intercostal or internal mammary arteries.

Early placement of chest tubes in any patient who has evidence of intrathoracic blood loss is essential. Monitoring of blood loss indicates how much blood volume replacement is needed and provides continuous assessment of the patient's hemodynamic status. Blood loss of more than 1,-000 to 1,500 ml total, or more than 300 ml per hour for 2 to 3 hours, usually indicates the need for thoracotomy. In addition, autotransfusion should be considered if the patient is bleeding massively.

Tension Pneumothorax

Lacerations in the pulmonary parenchyma sometimes act like flap valves and create a tension pneumothorax, as air enters the pleural space and cannot escape. Pleural pressure rises, the lung collapses, the mediastinum shifts toward the opposite hemithorax, and the vena cava is narrowed at the diaphragm and thoracic inlet, thus interfering with venous return. In addition, the remaining "good" lung is severely compressed. The combination of these two factors may lead rapidly to death. Treatment is immediate tube thoracostomy.

Pericardial Tamponade

Patients with pericardial tamponade typically present with shock and tightly distended neck veins. The only other conditions that present similarly in the injured patient are tension pneumothorax and myocardial failure, secondary to myocardial contusion or coronary air embolism. Of these, cardiac tamponade and tension pneumothorax are usually easy to treat, and the physician must be sure not to miss these diagnoses.

Fifty percent of penetrating cardiac injuries are instantly fatal. Another 25 percent of these patients die within the first 4 or 5 minutes of injury, and they rarely make it to a hospital alive. The remaining 25 percent of patients with penetrating cardiac injuries develop pericardial tamponade or exsanguinate into the hemithorax and are in profound shock, but do make it to a hospital alive and sometimes benefit from emergency thoracotomy.

Treatment of penetrating cardiac injuries has gradually changed from initial management by pericardiocentesis to prompt thoracotomy, pericardial decompression, and repair of the myocardial wound. Pericardiocentesis is reserved for selected patients in whom the diagnosis is uncertain or performed during preparation for thoracotomy.

The underlying cardiac injury with cardiac tamponade is usually easily repaired and does not require cardiac bypass. We prefer a nonabsorbable 2-0 cardiovascular suture. Adjunctive measures include tying the suture over Teflon pledgets. When suturing the wound, care must be taken not to compromise the coronary arteries with the repair sutures. This mishap can be averted, even when the wound is in close proximity to the vessels, by using a horizontal mattress suture to avoid tying the suture directly over the coronary artery. Postoperatively, the surgeon must also be aware of secondary complications, such as manifestations of injury to the papillary muscles, chordae tendinae, conduction system, and rarely the valve leaflets. Postcardiotomy syndrome is a not infrequent complication.

Air Embolism

Air embolism is caused by a fistula between a pulmonary bronchus and pulmonary artery or vein and can occur after either penetrating or blunt thoracic trauma. In our experience, 65 percent of air embolism is secondary to penetrating thoracic trauma and 35 percent due to blunt trauma. Diagnosis is difficult, at best, but should be strongly suspected in the following three conditions: (1) any patient who presents with penetrating chest trauma and focal neurologic findings without obvious head injury; (2) any patient who, after endotracheal intubation, with the first few breaths of positive pressure ventilation, develops cardiovascular collapse; and (3) any patient in whom air is found as froth in the initial set of arterial blood gas, this last condition being universally fatal in our experience. Confirmation of air embolism can sometimes be obtained by fundoscopic examination, in which air is seen in the retinal vessels.

Treatment of air embolism consists of emergency thoracotomy and cross-clamping the hilum of the damaged lung with a vascular clamp. Open cardiac massage may break up air bubbles in the coronary arteries; insertion of a needle in the apex of the left ventricle sometimes recovers air. Systemic administration of vasoconstrictors may increase the blood pressure enough to drive some of the air out of the arterioles and capillaries and into the veins. Definitive treatment for management of the damaged lung consists of oversewing of the laceration, segmentectomy, and even lobectomy.

DEFINITIVE MANAGEMENT OF POTENTIALLY LIFE-THREATENING INJURIES

Rupture of the Tracheobronchial Tree

Rupture of the tracheobronchial tree is characterized by ventilatory distress, subcutaneous emphysema, and hemoptysis. Some patients have obstruction of their airway, depending on the nature of the disruption. All patients have mediastinal air on chest roentgenogram, and many have a pneumothorax or tension pneumothorax.

Treatment consists of establishing an airway, if possible, by passing an endotracheal tube beyond the region of the tear so that the patient can be effectively ventilated and does not aspirate blood. A split endotracheal tube is preferable, but may be difficult to insert in the unstable trauma patient. A chest tube is inserted to evacuate the pneumothorax when indicated. The majority of patients require thoracotomy to control the tear. In 90 percent of cases the tear is within 2 cm of the carina or the bifurcation of main stem bronchi. Preoperative bronchoscopy is of benefit in establishing the location of the lesion.

Pulmonary Contusion

Pulmonary contusion is usually associated with rib fractures and represents a ''bruise'' of the lung. It is usually present on the initial chest roentgenogram in the ER, but typically progresses in size and density for 24 to 48 hours. CT scans are much more sensitive and specific for the lesion. Clinically, pulmonary contusion is often associated with an increase in shunt fraction and poor oxygenation.

Treatment regimens are controversial: diuretics, salt-poor albumin, and steroids all have their advocates. We would recommend that none of these agents be used, as all are ineffective in improving the pulmonary lesion, but may be harmful in other ways. Our management consists of pulmonary toilet and ventilatory support.

Rupture of the Diaphragm

Rupture of the diaphragm may be quite subtle and difficult to diagnose, and the clinician must maintain a high index of suspicion. Despite this awareness, more than one-third of ruptured diaphragms are missed initially, and secondary complications are common. Rupture that occurs after blunt trauma is always on the left side. It can occur in either hemidiaphragm when penetrating trauma is the cause.

Treatment is straightforward and consists of laparotomy with repair by interrupted, nonabsorbable suture. Horizontal mattress stitches may prevent tearing of the diaphragmatic fibers and ensure an airtight closure. A running locking stitch has also been advocated, particularly if the patient is unstable and has other injuries. Although diaphragmatic rupture can be repaired easily from above or below the diaphragm, we prefer the abdominal approach in the majority of cases. In extensive injuries in which there are large defects, such as shotgun wounds, it may be necessary to use prosthetic materials such as Marlex to cover the defect. This should be avoided if at all possible.

Esophageal Perforation

Esophageal perforation is almost always due to penetrating trauma. Depending on location, the symptoms vary. If the perforation is in the cervical area, the patient complains of difficulty in swallowing and pain on motion of the head. If it is in the thoracic area, the patient presents with fever, chest pain, and radiographic evidence of pneumomediastinum, a pleural effusion, or both. Definitive diagnosis is made by Hypaque swallow studies, endoscopy, or both.

Treatment of cervical perforation is primary repair and drainage. We prefer an absorbable suture for the mucosa and a nonabsorbable suture for the muscle layer. Interposition of strap muscles between the trachea and the esophagus may be a worthwhile adjunct if there is soilage in the wound. Thoracic perforation demands that the patient be explored, the laceration repaired, and the chest drained. Exploration is necessary to rule out associated injuries.

Myocardial Contusion

Myocardial contusion is analogous to pulmonary contusion and represents a bruise or intramural hematoma of the myocardial wall. It is probably underdiagnosed, and only recently has its incidence been appreciated with the advent of myocardial nuclear scanning. If the paramedics state that the patient was extricated from behind the steering column, there is at least a 20 percent chance that the patient has sustained myocardial contusion. It commonly presents with arrhythmias in the period immediately surrounding the injury. There is no set dysrhythmia pattern, but the one most threatening is ventricular tachycardia. These may be life-threatening, and procainamide (Pronestyl), given intravenously, is usually therapeutic. Frank cardiac failure is rare, but when present, it is treated by afterload reduction and inotropic support.

Great Vessel Injuries

Patients who suffer severe deceleration injuries or penetrating injuries in the vicinity of the great vessel are at risk for injuries to those vessels. The great majority of patients with rupture or penetration of the great vessels die at the scene of the accident, unless the hole in the artery is small or is tamponaded by the surrounding tissues.

If a patient with blunt trauma and possible great vessel injury arrives alive in the emergency room and is hemodynamically stable, work-up should proceed, consisting of a roentgenogram and, if indicated, a rapidly obtained arch aortogram. Most patients with rupture of the thoracic aorta secondary to blunt trauma have either a wide mediastinum or obliteration of the aortic knob on chest roentgenogram. Other radiographic signs include blood in the pleural cavities, apical capping, and rightward displacement of the trachea and main stem bronchi or esophagus (as seen by the position of the nasogastric tube). All of these signs arise because of thoracic bleeding, either intrapleural or extrapleural. An occasional patient has a well-contained periarterial hematoma, but none of these signs at presentation. The warning to the clinician in these cases is evidence of severe thoracic trauma with fractures of the posterior portions of the upper ribs, multiple rib fractures, or fractures of the scapula. Arch aortograms should be obtained in these patients as well.

Patients with blunt trauma, shock, and continuing bleeding from the left chest should be explored through a left posterolateral incision. Such patients usually have a transected aorta, this approach provides the best exposure for disruption of the aorta just distal to the take-off of the left subclavian. Besides being the most likely injury with blunt trauma, it is also the injury that the surgeon has the best chance of controlling. Controversy exists whether extracorporeal bypasses, or shunts, are useful in the surgical repair of the disrupted aorta. Although both techniques may allow more time for the procedure to be done, there is no evidence that it prevents paraplegia. Paraplegia is more dependent on the arterial anatomy to the spinal cord, and bypass does not avoid this complication. It has been our experience that patients with disrupted aortas also have other associated injuries, and it is prudent to avoid heparinization in these individuals.

Patients with blunt trauma, shock, and massive bleeding from the right chest should be explored through either a median sternotomy or a right anterolateral thoracotomy. The median sternotomy should not be used if it will delay exposure; the right thoracotomy usually is adequate. Patients with penetrating injuries of the great vessels which do not communicate with the pleural cavity frequently survive to reach the hospital, these penetrating injuries usually being at the base of the neck. In the hemodynamically stable patient, arteriography should be obtained to guide the surgeon in exposing the injured vessel. A left posterolateral thoracotomy should be used to expose injuries of the origin of the left subclavian artery; a median sternotomy with extensions into the neck should be used if necessary for the innominate artery or for the origins of the right subclavian and carotid arteries. If this determination cannot be made preoperatively, a median sternotomy is the incision of choice. If the left subclavian artery is involved between its origin and the vertebral artery, a "trap door" extension into the third intercostal space can be made to facilitate exposure.

Patients with penetrating injuries of the great vessels, which communicate with the pleural cavity, almost always exsanguinate into the pleural cavity, and only a small percentage reach the emergency room alive. If such a patient does reach the emergency room, the surgeon is alerted by a massive hemothorax and continued bleeding. If the wound is in the left supraclavicular area or in the left chest, an emergency left thoracotomy should be carried out, preferably a posterolateral thoracotomy with the patient in the lateral decubitus position. The posterolateral incision gives by far the best exposure of the origin of the left subclavian artery in the descending thoracic aorta. If the wound is in the right supraclavicular area or the parasternal regions, the median sternotomy gives the best exposure for the anterior surface of the heart, the ascending aorta, the innominate artery, and the origins of the right subclavian and common carotid arteries. A right anterolateral thoracotomy may be used, if necessary, and carried upward through the sternum or across the sternum if necessary. Repair of the injured vessel is usually by lateral repair, since larger wounds are rarely compatible with survival.

ABDOMINAL TRAUMA
Donald D. Trunkey, M.D.

Abdominal trauma continues to account for a large number of trauma-related injuries and deaths. In one large series, blunt abdominal injuries accounted for 6 percent of the total injuries, but contributed to 25 percent of the deaths. The incidence of abdominal trauma is higher with penetrating injuries—approaching 25 percent. The purpose of this chapter is to outline the treatment and priorities for treatment of abdominal injuries.

There are a number of controversies associated with abdominal trauma. Those surrounding penetrating abdominal trauma include: whether to explore or observe penetrating injuries; whether to explore or watch retroperitoneal hematomas; what is the best management for civilian colon injuries; whether to attempt splenic salvage; and when is it appropriate to use drains. Controversies surrounding blunt abdominal trauma include, in addition to the aforementioned, the management of retroperitoneal hematomas; whether to attempt splenic salvage; whether diagnostic techniques such as laparoscopy have a role; and what is the role of certain adjunctive procedures, such as hepatic artery ligation following major liver trauma. We will address these issues and other treatment problems in the following discussion.

DIAGNOSIS

Penetrating injuries present few diagnostic challenges. The real issue is whether or not to explore the abdomen. We have found the following guidelines very useful. If the penetrating wound obviously penetrates the peritoneal cavity, exploration is warranted. If the wound is located between the nipples and the pubis and the two anterior axillary lines, yet does not obviously penetrate the peritoneum, we would advise local wound exploration in the operating room under local anesthesia. If the wound penetrates the peritoneal cavity, full laparotomy is warranted. If the wound involves the flank of the abdomen between the anterior axillary line and the paraspinous muscles, exploration is mandatory to rule out a retroperitoneal colon injury and other injuries as well. If the wound is between the two paraspinous margins posteriorly, conservative management with observation in the hospital for 48 hours may be a worthwhile alternative to exploration.

Blunt abdominal trauma is more difficult to diagnose and presents in one of three ways: (1) the patient has obvious involuntary guarding and exploratory laparotomy is immediately warranted; (2) the patient presents with systemic signs of hypovolemic shock and no other source of hemorrhage can be found except the peritoneal space or retroperitoneal space; and (3) the patient has associated injuries such as pelvic fractures or lower rib fractures and an intraperitoneal injury or pelvic injuries are strongly suspected.

Diagnosis of intra-abdominal blunt tauma can also be aided by the history. If the clinician obtains a history from the paramedic or the patient that they were involved in a steering wheel type injury or that the patient was extricated from behind the steering wheel, this should strongly suggest duodenal or pancreatic trauma. Similarly, if there are rib fractures involving the left lower chest, there is a 20 percent incidence of associated spleen injury. If there is a history or finding of rib fractures on the right, there is a 10 percent incidence of associated liver injury. Physical examination can be notoriously misleading; approximately 40 percent of patients with significant hemoperitoneum may have no peritoneal signs. Distention of the abdomen has been interpreted by some as an excellent sign of intraperitoneal injury. Simple arithmetic, however, shows that the abdomen is a cylinder, and a 1-cm change in the radius of the typical 70-kg person's abdomen would account for approximately 2.9 liters of fluid. It is unlikely that any clinician can detect a 1-cm change in the radius of an abdomen.

A number of laboratory tests may aid the clinician in making a diagnosis of intra-abdominal injury. These would include serial hematocrit, serial white count, amylase determinations, and other special diagnostic studies. No patient who is hemodynamically unstable, however, should undergo any type of study, particularly if lifesaving laparotomy and control of hemorrhage are indicated.

The following represents an incomplete list of some special diagnostic studies that can be considered in the stable patient. If the patient has gross penile or urethral blood or an associated pelvic injury, a retrograde urethrogram should be considered. If the Foley catheter passes with ease and the patient has hematuria, a two-view cystogram should be obtained. This should include an AP and lateral or an AP voiding. Obtaining only one view will result in missing 40 percent of all bladder injuries. If the urethrogram and cystogram are normal and the patient has hematuria or if renal injury is strongly suspected after deceleration, the patient should undergo an intravenous pyelogram. If the history indicates epigastric blunt trauma, the minimum study necessary is a Hypaque study to rule out duodenal or pancreatic injury. Alternatively, a CT scan can be obtained of the upper abdomen. The need for arteriogram is somewhat limited and should be guided by the physical examination.

We have found the CT scan extremely useful in evaluating abdominal trauma. It is both qualitative and quantitative and allows assessment of the retroperitoneum, including the pancreas and duodenum. For all intents and purposes, it has replaced peritoneal lavage at our institution. CT is indicated for the patient who is unconscious, paralyzed, or uncooperative. It is also used for a particularly difficult diagnosis when history and physical examination cannot determine the need for laparotomy.

EARLY TREATMENT

Some of the early treatment to be considered in abdominal trauma includes the management of evisceration. In general, no attempt should be made to reinsert peritoneal contents, since such efforts may result in further damage to the intestines. Saline-soaked or petrolatum-impregnated gauze is put over the evisceration and covered with a clean or sterile towel. This should usually suffice until definitive treatment can be carried out.

Another area of concern is ballistics. It is unreasonable for most clinicians to assume that they can do forensic pathology. This requires an expert. Therefore, no attempt should be made to characterize the wounds as entrance wounds or exit wounds. It is far preferable to take a Polaroid or other photograph of the wounds, in case this is needed later for legal purposes. We have also found it useful to mark the wounds with a piece of tape and a paper clip, so that when x-ray studies are obtained these mark the entrance and exit wounds.

OPERATIVE APPROACH

Operative approach for abdominal trauma, whether penetrating or blunt, is very straightforward and simple. We advocate a midline approach, and there should be few reasons to deviate from this. This is a particularly good incision for the unstable patient, since it is rapid and safe. If there have been previous transverse incisions, there is no contraindication to going through the midline. An exception to the aforementioned rule is the neonate or infant with abdominal trauma. If the patient is stable, transverse incision may be preferable.

CONTROL OF HEMORRHAGE

Once the abdomen has been entered, there are a number of priorities. In the unstable patient with massive hemoperitoneum, control of hemorrhage is the number one priority. I place packs in all four quadrants, and this measure controls the hemorrhage in the majority of cases. I then remove the two lower quadrant packs, mopping up and cleaning up the blood, and then remove the left upper quadrant packs, examining the spleen carefully. If the spleen is the source of hemorrhage, it can be repacked temporarily in order to assess the right upper quadrant and to ascertain that there are no associated injuries that would militate against spleen salvage. I remove the right upper quadrant packs last, paying particular attention to whether there is bleeding when the dome of the liver is retracted inferiorly. If such is the case, one must assume a hepatic vein injury and decide early whether an intracaval shunt is warranted. If the bleeding from the liver is primarily arterial and fairly vigorous, temporary clamping of the porta hepatis may achieve the hemostatic control necessary to further assess the injury. If there are large retroperitoneal hematomas that are expanding or uncontained, a decision must be made whether control of the descending thoracic aorta is a worthwhile adjunct. In general, if the retroperitoneal hematoma is below the renal arteries, control is easily obtained at the crus of the diaphragm. If the retroperitoneal hematoma is higher in the midline, it is advantageous to perform an anterior thoracotomy and control the descending thoracic aorta in the chest.

The second priority is to control fecal contamination. Any obvious holes can either be sutured with chromic catgut or controlled temporarily with a Babcock or Allis clamp. The third priority, provided the patient has stabilized, is to do a thorough exploratory laparotomy assessing all injuries. I do this in a very methodical way, starting at the crus of the diaphragm and exploring the stomach and both sides of the spleen, splenic flexure, descending colon, sigmoid colon, pelvic organs, cecum, ascending colon, and liver. I then enter the lesser sac and explore the pancreas and consider a Kocher maneuver or taking down the ligament of Treitz to ascertain that there are no duodenal injuries. I then thoroughly examine the small bowel at least once. The diaphragm is thoroughly inspected for any possible penetration or rupture.

SPECIFIC INJURIES

Diaphragmatic Injuries

Following blunt abdominal trauma the diaphragm is involved in 4 percent of all injuries. It is frequently missed as a diagnosis and yet all must be repaired or there are long-term consequences that may be fatal to the patient. Penetrating injuries between the nipple and below the costal margins should be assumed to have penetrated the diaphragm. At the time of an exploratory laparotomy, the entire diaphragmatic surface should be explored thoroughly to rule out injury. Simple holes can be repaired with interrupted horizontal mattress stitches of nonabsorbable suture. Larger lacerations and rents obviously require more sutures, and I prefer interrupted sutures unless the patient

is unstable, in which case a continuous locking stitch is warranted. If a significant defect exists in the diaphragm secondary to blast injury, such as with a shotgun, Marlex may be used as an acceptable tissue substitute. It is unnecessary to drain diaphragmatic injuries, but tube thoracostomy is often indicated to drain the pleural cavity on the involved side.

Splenic Injuries

The spleen is an important organ and has important functions including that of filter for particulate matter, a source of opsonins, a source of IgM, and regulator of T- and B-lymphocytes, and it is a source of intrauterine hematopoiesis. The spleen is the most common solid organ to be injured by blunt trauma. The controversy involving spleen injuries is whether to salvage the spleen. I believe the evidence is very convincing that spleen salvage is worthwhile in the prepubertal child and is probably worthwhile in the adolescent and adult. Overall risk of postsplenectomy sepsis is 0.5 percent, yet the mortality, once postsplenectomy sepsis occurs, is 50 percent.

The key to operative repair or splenectomy is to mobilize the spleen into the midline. The spleen started out as a midline structure, and it is relatively easy to mobilize unless there has been previous surgery or infection with subsequent adhesions. Barring these problems, it is easy to mobilize the spleen either bluntly or with some minimal sharp dissection. I place my hand over the diaphragmatic surface and then develop a plane between the pancreas and Gerota's fascia. With surprisingly little effort, the spleen can then be brought into the center of the wound, where it can be inspected and repaired or partially or totally removed.

If the wounds are simple and involve primarily the capsule and superficial parenchyma, control of bleeding can usually be achieved by the application of microcrystalline collagen or the electrocautery unit. Alternative therapy available in some European countries includes infrared diathermy or a ''hot air gun.'' The latter may be particularly useful in controlling parenchymal bleeding, but has not yet been tried in this country.

Deeper lacerations to the parenchyma usually require control with horizontal mattress stitches buttressed with Teflon pledgets. I prefer 0 chromic catgut on a large needle. This glides easily through the parenchyma, and the majority of moderate lacerations can be controlled by means of this technique. If there is avulsion of hilar vessels or if the laceration is extensive, a partial or hemisplenectomy must be considered. The arterial blood supply of the spleen lends itself very well to the resection, since the arteries are end arteries and parallel each other. I usually grasp the spleen with one hand and with the scapel remove the involved segment. This usually leaves one or two, sometimes more, bleeding arterioles within the parenchyma, and these can be controlled with 4-0 silk suture ligatures. I then place multiple horizontal mattress stitches of 0 chromic through the capsule and parenchyma and tie over Teflon pledgets. This will control the parenchymal bleeding in about 90 percent of all cases. In the remaining 10 percent, the electrocautery unit, microcrystalline collagen, or a viable pedicle of omentum may be placed over the stump.

Splenic artery ligation has been described as a useful adjunct. In my experience it has had variable results, the primary complication being infarction of the spleen. If the splenic artery is to be ligated, it must be ligated centrally so as to preserve collateral blood supply from both the short gastrics and the pancreatic branches. There is some evidence that clearance of streptococcus pneumonia is impaired after the splenic artery has been ligated. In all preservation procedures, at least 40 percent of the spleen mass must be preserved in order to preserve function. Autotransplantation is of no proven benefit. Splenectomy should be carried out immediately if it is obvious that the spleen is not salvageable because of massive injury, or if there are associated injuries that would militate against the time necessary to salvage the spleen. If the patient is in profound shock, splenectomy may also be warranted. There is no indication for drainage of spleen injuries.

A highly controversial area involving the management of spleen injuries is whether to treat them conservatively without operation. In my opinion, this is unacceptable. In most large series, splenectomy and spleen salvage have an operative mortality rate of less than 1 percent. The surgeons proposing conservative management have an operative mortality rate of 5 percent. Some of these children have required as much as twice their blood volume in replacement, which hardly can be termed conservative treatment. Furthermore, these children are treated with intensive care management for 3 days, complete bed rest for an additional 2 weeks, and no activity for 6 to 8 weeks. Following splenorrhaphy or splenectomy, a child is usually discharged on the fourth or fifth postoperative day, returns to school immediately, and can resume all physical activity at 4 weeks. Spleen salvage has been less likely in patients requiring surgery after a period of conservative management.

If splenectomy is indicated or required, postoperative prophylaxis is an issue. There are no randomized series showing the benefit of prophylactic antibiotics or pneumococcal vaccine. At present, the best prophylaxis would be a bracelet or necklace of the Medi-Alert type, identifying the patient at risk for postsplenectomy sepsis.

Hepatic Injuries

The liver is a very important organ with the following functions. It detoxifies substances, synthesizes many of the important proteins, serves as an immunologic organ, and is extremely important in fat, carbohydrate, and protein metabolism. The liver is the second most common organ to be injured following blunt trauma and is more commonly injured than the spleen following penetrating trauma. Approximately 70 percent of all liver injuries can be managed quite simply, either by direct suture ligation of the bleeding points or by hemostasis with the electrocautery unit or microcrystalline collagen. Some of these wounds probably would not even require exploration if diagnosis could be ascertained prior to exploration. This may be possible in the near future with CT or NMR scans. Simple lacerations, as already described, do not require drains.

Some injuries continue to bleed despite attempts at local control. In these instances the wound must be opened or tractotomy performed. The depths of the wound must be explored in detail and each vessel and biliary radical individually ligated. If bleeding continues to be a problem, the porta hepatis should be dissected free and selective clamping of the portal veins and the hepatic arteries carried out. If selective clamping controls the bleeding, one of these vessels can be safely ligated. This should be needed in less than 1 percent of all liver injuries. The common hepatic artery can also be safely ligated, but the proper hepatic must never be ligated.

An alternative treatment for deeper lacerations with continued bleeding is resectional debridement of that segment of the liver. This usually implies removing, sharply and with finger fracture technique, devitalized liver or a portion of a segment to allow access to the deeper bleeding. Each biliary vessel and radical should be individually ligated. It is prudent to drain after such injuries. I prefer a closed system with a sump catheter, using an in-line air filter on the sump inlet drain.

In approximately 5 to 8 percent of all major liver injuries, resection is required. This consists of either a lobectomy or a segmentectomy, depending on the nature of the injury. Most of these injuries are large stellate lacerations, extending deep into the parenchyma and involving more than one segment. Another indication for resection is injury to the hepatic veins or to the intrahepatic inferior vena cava. Knowledge of anatomy is imperative, particularly the relationships of the hepatic veins. I prefer sharp division of the capsule and finger fracture technique for the parenchyma. As vessels and biliary radicles are encountered, they are encircled with 2-0 silk, double-tied, and divided. Major hepatic veins can either be suture-ligated or closed with a running cardiovascular stitch of 2-0 or 3-0 nonabsorbable suture. In approximately one-half of all major liver resections, the gallbladder must also be taken because of its dependence on blood supply from the cystic artery, which comes off the hepatic artery in a significant number of cases. A closed drainage system is indicated for all major resections.

In less than 1 percent of all liver injuries, intracaval shunt should be considered. We reserve this primarily for hepatic vein injuries and intrahepatic caval injuries. The sternum is split and a purse-string of cardiovascular silk is placed into the right atrium. A 38 or 40 Fr chest tube is inserted through the atrial appendage and is guided into the inferior vena cava distally, making sure that the holes in the chest tube lie distal to the renal veins. The suprarenal cava and intrapericardial portion of the inferior vena cava are encircled with vascular tubing and Rommel type tourniquets. After the chest tube is in position it is withdrawn approximately 2 inches, side holes are cut, and the tube is reinserted. After application of the two tourniquets and a vascular clamp to the portal triad, a relatively avascular operative approach to the liver can then be performed. Special tubes with balloons are available which can be passed through the right atrial appendage, through the inferior vena cava, or through a groin incision and a femoral vein. After the lobectomy is performed and

the hepatic veins and inferior vena cava are repaired, the shunt is withdrawn in the reverse order that it was inserted. Drains are always indicated after a major resection or use of the intracaval shunt.

Rarely, liver injuries may be so devastating and so extensive that resection is impossible. Examples would include bilobar involvement or a hospital setting in which blood resources and other adjunctive measures are not available. In such instances, packs may either be definitive therapy or provide time wherein the patient can be transferred to a facility where resection can be carried out.

Following major liver surgery, the patient is kept in the intensive care unit and cardiovascular support is provided. We prefer to give patients D10W to provide additional nutritional support and start them on enteral or total parenteral nutrition early. Coagulation abnormalities are frequent and may require the use of relatively fresh whole blood and fresh frozen plasma. If the patient develops hematobilia in the post-injury state, arteriography is indicated with selective embolization to the offending arterial bleeder.

Pancreatic Injuries

Pancreatic injuries are relatively infrequent following abdominal trauma, but if missed, they have a high mortality and morbidity. If the pancreatic injury involves a duct and treatment is not instituted within 24 hours, there is essentially a 100 percent mortality.

Diagnosis of penetrating injury is usually not a major problem. If the patient is being explored for a penetrating abdominal injury, the question only arises as to whether the missile or knife involved the pancreatic gland. This demands a thorough exploration of the pancreas, including a Kocher maneuver, taking down the ligament of Treitz, entering the lesser sac, and exploring around the splenic hilum. If there is a capsular hematoma, this must be entered and a diligent search for ductal injury carried out. If no ductal injury occurs, treatment is usually confined to drainage, either by Penrose or by sump, of the immediate area.

In more extensive penetrating injuries, involving ducts, several options exist. If the ductal injury is in the body or tail, a distal resection is prudent. If the injury is in a prepubertal child, it is worthwhile to consider preserving the spleen. A second option is to simply ligate, with horizontal mattress stitches of nonabsorbable nylon or polypropolene, both ends of the gland including the duct. One accepts atrophy of the distal exocrine tissue, but preserves endocrine function. Pancreatic fistulas are rare and usually close within 4 to 6 weeks following such treatment. If the injury is more extensive and involves the head, resection or "diverticulization" may be necessary. Resection is usually reserved for patients who have combined pancreatic or duodenal injuries and extensive devitalization of tissue. Diverticulization is the treatment of choice for most other pancreatic injuries. This consists of gastrojejunostomy, closure of the duodenum, tube duodenostomy, and drainage of the wounds. Choledochostomy is not recommended.

Blunt trauma to the abdomen causing pancreatic injury is sometimes extremely difficult to evaluate. There is often a paucity of anterior peritoneal signs, and missed diagnosis is common. A threefold elevation of amylase is indicative of pancreatic injury, but not diagnostic. Recently, our experience with CT scan shows a relatively high sensitivity in diagnosing pancreatic injuries. The minimum test necessary is Hypaque swallow to rule out significant duodenal or pancreatic injury.

The principles of pancreatic management following blunt abdominal trauma are similar to those for penetrating trauma. If there is only contusion of the gland, drainage is appropriate. If a duct has been injured, resection of the distal segment or ligation of the proximal and distal segments is indicated with appropriate drainage. Diverticulization is the treatment of choice for most injuries involving the head of the pancreas, and resection is reserved for devitalizing extensive injuries.

Small Bowel Injuries

The treatment principles for small bowel injuries are straightforward. Repair when possible, resect if necessary. The overriding general principle is to preserve as much small bowel as possible.

Colonic Injuries

Colonic injuries are potentially the most devastating intraperitoneal injury, since they have a high morbidity and mortality unless properly treated. The mortality from colonic injuries has progressively declined from 90 percent during the Civil War to 13 percent during the Vietnam Conflict. In civilian practice we are seeing a trend toward more gunshot wounds and, surprisingly, about 15 percent of all colonic injuries are due to blunt trauma.

Considerable controversy currently exists over the best management of civilian colonic injuries. Many series have described primary closure of the wounds with varying results. Many criteria have been developed in order to help the surgeon decide which wounds need to be treated with diversion of the fecal stream and which can be treated with primary closure. I believe in a very conservative approach and would do a primary closure or anastomosis *only* if there is no contamination, no shock, and no major associated injuries. This will only account for approximately 15 percent of all colonic injuries. The majority, or 85 percent, must be treated with diversion of the fecal stream, repair, or resection.

All rectal injuries should be treated by diversion of the fecal stream, repair of the injury if possible, and insertion of presacral drains. The latter is done at the end of the abdominal procedure. The patient is put in a lithotomy position, a curvilinear incision is made beneath the anus, dissection is carried up bluntly to the levators, and presacral Penrose drains are placed. A controversial issue is whether the distal segment should be irrigated with antibiotic solutions or saline. If the rectal injury has been repaired, it makes sense to irrigate feces from the distal segment. If the rectal injury has not been repaired, it makes no sense to irrigate and further contaminate the presacral space.

Uterine Trauma

The uterus subjected to trauma may be either nongravid or gravid. In the nongravid uterus, repair should be carried out with absorbable suture, if possible. For the patient in the child-bearing age it is reasonable to spend a little extra time trying to salvage reproducibility.

There is a primary axiom associated with trauma to the gravid uterus. *The mother always takes primary priority, the fetus is secondary.* Obviously, if both can be salvaged, this should be done. Often, however, it is necessary to sacrifice the fetus and the uterus to control hemorrhage, which can be extensive, particularly during the third trimester. If hemorrhage is massive, there should be no hesitation in performing a hysterectomy to save the mother's life.

Genitourinary Trauma

Trauma to the urethra, bladder, and kidneys are relatively common, whereas trauma to the ureter is uncommon. Urethral trauma is commonly associated with pelvic fractures and straddle injuries. Emergency repair of the urethra should be avoided, since there is a higher incidence of impotence after such repair. Temporary control can be achieved by suprapubic cystostomy and drains if necessary. If it is a partial injury and a urethral catheter can be passed safely, this is an acceptable alternative approach.

Injuries to the bladder necessitate repair of the injury, suprapubic cystostomy, and drains to the space of Retzius. In rare instances, with extensive injuries such as shotgun blasts, proximal diversion by bilateral nephrostomy may be necessary.

Injuries to the ureter are usually easily repaired by end-to-end anastomosis with fine suture, much like a vascular anastomosis. I prefer not to drain and I do not use internal stents. In lower ureteral injuries, it may occasionally be necessary to do a ureteroneocystostomy. However, the indications for this are uncommon. If there has been segmental loss of the ureter, nephrostomy is a temporary measure until a later date when ureterostomy can be performed or ileal conduit substituted.

Pelvic Injuries

Pelvic injuries can be the most difficult abdominal injuries to treat. Hemorrhage can be devastating and uncontrollable. Pelvic fractures are among the few injuries that may require *immediate* resuscitation with whole blood in the emergency room. Blood losses of over 10 units are common and may exceed 50 units in severe type I fractures. Associated injuries to the genitourinary tract are the rule rather than the exception. It is imperative to rule out other intraperitoneal injuries, such as ruptured spleen or liver, before assuming that the blood loss is entirely from the pelvic fracture.

The majority of pelvic bleeding is venous in origin. This represents the shearing off of large veins as they enter the sacral foramina. Treatment is confined to blood replacement and resuscitation. It is prudent to leave the pelvic hematoma alone; it will contain the bleeding in most instances. If there is ongoing or continued bleeding, an arteriogram is indicated. If the arteriogram is positive, showing bleeding arteries, the surgeon has two

options. One is to have the radiologist embolize the offending vessel with Gelfoam or a similar substance. The second alternative is to directly ligate the bleeding vessel. Ligation of both hypogastrics is inadvisable, since this will eliminate the possibility of future embolization. Furthermore, ligation of the hypogastric artery for pelvic bleeding has universally been unsuccessful in controlling pelvic hemorrhage. If the arteriogram is negative, the surgeon must assume that the bleeding is due to venous causes, in which case three options exist: (1) my preference—application of external fixation devices such as the Hoffman or the AO apparatus; this could be done in conjunction with orthopedic surgery; (2) application of a hip-spica cast, to immobilize the fracture and minimize ongoing bleeding (also immobilizing the patient, unfortunately, and aggravating some of the pulmonary complications that occur in the post-injury state); and (3) application of the pneumatic antishock garment for periods of 3 to 4 hours at pressures of 40 torr. In some instances, the last-mentioned has proven effective in controlling venous hemorrhage.

Compound fractures of the pelvis are particularly vexing, and all must be treated by diversion of the fecal stream, even if the rectum is not injured. This measure is necessary to minimize contamination of the open wound and prevent pelvic sepsis. Patients with compound pelvic fractures treated with fecal diversion have a 25 percent mortality rate, whereas, if fecal diversion is not accomplished, the mortality rate is increased to 50 percent. It is also imperative to debride devitalized tissue and provide adequate drainage. The latter is best accomplished with multiple sump drains.

Abdominal Vascular Injuries

Major abdominal vascular injuries occur in about 5 percent of all abdominal trauma, most commonly after penetrating injury. The primary vessels involved are the aorta, vena cava, hepatic vein, portal vein, renal vessels, and pelvic vessels. Most of these wounds do not involve segmental loss or they would be rapidly fatal. Often there is some containment of the hematoma, but usually there is rapid exsanguination. Most injuries can be treated by lateral repair, ligation, or, occasionally, a patch angioplasty. I prefer autogenous patch angioplasty, if at all possible.

The key to repair of vascular injuries is access to the injury. For central retroperitoneal hematomas that are expanding, pulsatile, or uncontained, I prefer to take down the right colon, including the duodenum, and to mobilize everything toward the midline. This will usually expose the infrarenal cava, aorta, and bifurcation of both. If, on the other hand, an aortic injury is suspected, an alternative approach is to take down the left colon, including the spleen and pancreas, with the option of bringing up the left kidney, if necessary. This may even expose some of the suprarenal aorta. If the injury is at the diaphragmatic crus, it may be necessary to extend the incision into the chest to control the descending thoracic aorta.

Suspected injury to the renal vessels should always be approached through the midline to gain central control first. This is usually done very easily with vascular tubing encircling the vessels at their origins.

The portal vein can create difficulties of access. If the injury is at the junction of the splenic vein and superior mesenteric vein, it may be necessary to divide the body of the pancreas to gain control of the injury and to repair it. If the injury is extensive, ligation of the portal vein can be carried out with acceptable morbidity to the patient. It is obviously optimal to repair it. Hepatic vein injuries have been previously discussed under liver trauma, and pelvic vessel injuries have been discussed under pelvic trauma.

In summary, abdominal injuries continue to be a challenge to the general surgeon. Treatment is usually straightforward and based on the principle of salvaging as much as possible of the organ involved with minimal morbidity to the patient. If necessary, resection may be the only alternative in order to salvage the patient's life.

TRAUMA TO THE EXTREMITIES
Robert E. Markison, M.D.

This chapter will focus on trauma to the soft tissues of the upper and lower extremities. Special emphasis will be placed on injuries to the hand. Optimal results are obtained when a single team manages problems related to soft tissue cover, peripheral nerve injuries, vascular compromise, and musculotendinous disruption.

General considerations include history, physical examination, imaging, and preoperative care. Separate sections follow on the treatment of breaks in soft tissue cover, vascular injury, peripheral nerve problems, and musculotendinous trauma. Consideration will then be given to selected problems involving combinations of these issues, including a discussion of follow-up and rehabilitation.

GENERAL CONSIDERATIONS

Routine history-taking provides an essential base for evaluation of the injured extremity. When one or both hands have been injured in a conscious patient, the completeness of history is of prime importance. Information must include the following: (1) age, (2) height and weight (these indicate how the part is stressed), (3) handed dominance, (4) occupation, (5) avocations, (6) employment history, (7) previous extremity injuries, (8) allergies, (9) medical problems, (10) current medications, and (11) precise time of last food or drink. This will serve as background for the following questions regarding the injury itself: (1) what happened? (2) when did it happen? (3) how did it happen? (4) how much blood did the patient lose? (5) how has the patient treated the part since the injury? (6) date of last tetanus immunization? and (7) other questions, as appropriate, for specific injuries, such as the identity of a biting animal, nature of substance injected, and status of missing parts.

The completeness of physical examination will be determined by the patient's overall status. Injured extremities find a relatively low priority in the unstable patient with multiple wounds. The resuscitation of such an individual typically involves observation of physiologic imperatives during the primary survey, which, on occasion, will lead to immediate transport to the operating room, with minimal imaging. More often, however, even in the severely traumatized person, there is time for a secondary survey, which consists of complete head-to-toe physical examination. The flow of this portion of the evaluation should not be interrupted by prolonged specialty-type examinations if the patient is unstable. When time is short, the examining extremity team must reduce its immediate concern to questions of viability and gross deformities of the extremities. Further direct investigations are carried out after central problems are corrected. For purposes of this discussion, we will assume that the patient is stable and able to communicate with the examiner.

Full exposure of all four extremities is necessary, prior to inspection. This requires removal of clothing and of rings and other potentially constricting forms of jewelry. Fingers are occasionally lost from neglect of simple ring removal prior to massive fluid resuscitation. Observation of the extremities then begins with (1) appreciation of grossly visible wounds, (2) attitude in which the affected part is held, (3) shape and relative size of the affected part, (4) color. (5) spontaneous movements, and (6) patient's subjective response to the injured part. Rapid bleeding from wounds should have been recognized during the primary survey and controlled by pressure. The need for tourniquet control of bleeding extremity wounds is rare, and exceptional cases are traumatic proximal amputations. During this overview, obvious extremity wounds are seen as landmarks to direct attention distally. Attitude of the proximally injured extremity may reflect fracture or dislocation, depending on the presence of angular and/or rotational distortions. Further assessment of attitude, i.e., posture, of the hand and foot may provide valuable information regarding disruption of musculotendinous units. For example, the supinated hand in repose has a gentle increase in curve to the fingers, proceeding from the index to little finger, and minimal interphalangeal flexion of the midpositioned thumb. The hand should look as if it were holding an egg. If, for example, this expected attitude is disturbed by the combined presence of a distal palmar surface forearm laceration and an extended finger, the diagnosis of divided flexor tendons is confirmed. This immediately obviates exploration of the wound in the emergency room, since complete operative exploration is required.

Perception of shape and relative size of an injured extremity is of particular value in proximal injuries wherein blood loss may be massive. Femur fractures, for example, can result in 3 to 6 units of bleeding into the thigh. Color assessment of distal parts defines the time frame for ordering of imaging studies (if necessary) and performance of definitive repairs. A cyanotic finger, for example, with division of both flexor tendons requires immediate repair to include digital arteriorrhaphies, digital neurorrhaphies, and flexor tenorrhaphies. This is in stark contrast to the patient who has divided flexors but a pink fingertip, and who might be treated with simple skin closure and elective repair of flexors within 7 days with a good result. The presence or absence of spontaneous movement in a proximal or distal part can be very revealing relative to the presence of proximal nerve lesions or musculotendinous disruptions. Finally, observation is not complete without perceiving the patient's subjective response. One must never subject the patient to additional discomfort when adequate information has already been gained from visual scanning to make an informed decision about the complexity of the problem and the timing of repairs.

Depending on the information gathered from visual inspection, the second step may consist of auscultation with a stethoscope, supplemented by the use of a Doppler. If, for example, a pale fingertip is seen, it is reasonable to apply a Doppler to the finger pad for assessment of the digital arterial distribution. Similarly, posterior knee dislocation with distal pallor and diminished Doppler pulses marks the need for acceleration of the care process. Auscultation is also essential for stab and gunshot wounds to the extremity, to determine the presence of arteriovenous fistulas.

Functional testing, the next step in the examination, should proceed from proximal to distal

upper and lower extremities; the patient is asked to move parts through a range of motion at each joint. When pain limits active motion of parts distal to forearm, hand, leg, or foot lacerations, one depends on the flexor and extensor tenodesis effects. Tenodesis refers to the position assumed by distal parts when tendons are stretched by passive movement of a joint. Upper extremity extensor tenodesis effects are demonstrable by stabilizing the elbow and flexing the wrist. With 70 to 90° of passive wrist flexion, the thumb pulls into full extension with the index, and the remaining fingers lack 10 to 20° of extension at the metacarpophalangeal joints, but are fully extended at the proximal interphalangeal and distal phalangeal joints. Therefore, a laceration at the wrist or hand dorsum that caused an increased drop in any of the fingers would signal the presence of an extensor tendon division. Upper extremity flexor tenodesis effect is seen when the elbow is stabilized and the wrist is cocked back into 60 or 70° of extension. Tenodesis then brings the fingers in convergence toward the scaphoid, the interphalangeal joint of the thumb is flexed 45°, and pads of the long ring and middle fingers touch the palm, but the index fails the thenar eminence by 2 to 3 cm. Failure of the interphalangeal joint of the thumb to flex in this instance, e.g., in the presence of a palmar wrist laceration, would signal division of the flexor pollicis longus tendon. Employing the tenodesis effects, which are equally applicable in the foot, spares the patient the discomfort of active attempts at moving musculotendinous units through zones of injury.

If findings on observation of tenodesis effects are equivocal, functional testing proceeds with evaluation of individual motor units, from proximal to distal extremity. Throughout the functional testing sequence, the examiner must be aware that distal motor deficits may be the result of motor nerve division, substance division of musculotendinous units, or both. Therefore, a review of major upper and lower extremity motor nerves is appropriate here.

There are 4 upper extremity motor nerves, the first of which is the musculocutaneous, C5 to C6, and this supplies the coracobrachialis, long and short heads of the biceps, and the brachialis. A palsy of this nerve will lead to loss of forearm flexion and reduction of the power of supination of the forearm. The deep radial (posterior interosseous) nerve, C6 through C7, innervates the thumb, wrist, and finger extensors, and a classic posture of radial palsy is easily recognized. The ulnar nerve, C8 through T1, innervates several extrinsic hand motors, consisting of flexor digitorum profundus to the ring and little fingers and flexor carpi ulnares, as well as 15 of the 20 intrinsic muscles of the hand. Ulnar palsy therefore results in a clumsy hand with weak grip, inability to cross the fingers, and flexion of the thumb interphalangeal joint (Froment's sign) to assist a weak pinch. The median nerve, C6 through C7, innervates all the superficial finger flexors, the index and long finger profundus flexors, flexor carporadialis, and the muscles of the thenar wad. Median palsy, depending on its level, at the very least causes thenar motor deficit by inability to pronate and oppose the thumb or, at higher levels, failure of thumb and finger flexion.

Three principal motor nerves serve the muscles of the thigh. The femoral nerve innervates the anterior muscles, and palsy is reflected by weakness in thigh flexion and leg extension. Medial thigh muscles are innervated by the obturator nerve, and a palsy results in adduction deficit. The tibial nerve innervates the posterior thigh muscles and reflects its palsy by loss of thigh extension and leg flexion. The tibial nerve continues as the posterior tibial and innervates the plantar flexors and toe flexors. Foot dorsoflexors and toe extensors are the motor territory of the deep peroneal nerve. Intrinsic foot muscles are innervated primarily by the medial and lateral plantar branches of the posterior tibial nerve.

Palpation, the next step in examining the extremities, involves consideration of (1) temperature, (2) pulses, (3) presence or absence of sweat, (4) turgor, (5) sensation, and (6) pain on passive motion. Temperature and sweat both reflect perfusion as well as sympathetic nervous system activity. Sweat is also an important indicator of peripheral nerve division. Within seconds of nerve transection, sweating is eliminated through the nerve's sensory territory. Since patients are often diaphoretic from anxiety, the contrast of a dry, denervated field can be dramatic. Sidelighting of the part will show the absence of beads of sweat, and a simple test, called "pen drag," can be very useful. This consists of drawing the body of a non-textured, plastic ballpoint pen across the sensate area and the area in question, comparing the amount of friction in each. Sensate areas will grip the pen, whereas dry, denervated areas will allow it to slip across, as if the pen were drawn across silk. Two-point discrimination is also valuable and

can be done with a paper clip. Either of these tests is far preferable to sticking pins into the extremities of patients and causing needless anxiety. Sensory denervation in the hands and feet of small children can be assessed by soaking the part in warm water: insensate areas will not wrinkle.

Pulse examination proceeds from proximal to distal and is on a scale of 0 to 4+, with 4+ as normal. Diminution or absence of pulses requires historical questioning relative to vascular disease, including claudication, and further evaluation of deficits by use of the Doppler. The Allen test in the hand and its equivalent in the foot are very useful in determining the balance of flow between radial and ulnar arteries, and anterior and posterior tibial arteries, respectively. The test can be performed in a conscious or unconscious adult by exsanguination of the part, occlusion of both arteries, and comparison of filling times when they are opened in turn. Normal hand filling is symmetrical from ulnar and radial vessels and takes 2.4 seconds on the average. Similarly, anterior and posterior tibial arteries contribute roughly symmetrical filling of less than 3 seconds to the foot. Tissue turgor should also be assessed, since it may warn of a developing compartment syndrome (to be discussed). Pain on passive motion may add additional support to this impression.

Direct probing of wounds is seldom required if adequate physical examination, including careful observation and thoughtful palpation, has been completed. It should be remembered that the goal of physical examination of the injured extremity is to confirm, as early as possible, with minimal trauma, the presence or absence of structure division below skin level that requires operative repair. If questions remain, tourniquet examination is appropriate. Optimal examination is carried out by a physician who will be part of the operating team. After the sensory examination has been performed and recorded on paper, anesthetic is placed in the wound if it is proximal on the extremity, and in the neighborhood of appropriate digital nerves if it is distal. Great care must be taken to avoid placement of digital blocks beyond the distal palm of the hand or distal plantar surface of the foot in instances in which capillary filling of the pad of the finger or toe is compromised. Anesthetic volume placed in the base of such a digit may shut off existing flow for a sufficient period to cause necrosis. Cast padding is then applied to the proximal extremity and a blood pressure cuff is wrapped over this. The part is elevated for one minute, and the cuff is then inflated to 250 mmHg. Even the most compliant patient cannot be expected to tolerate this for more than 10 or 15 minutes of examination. Therefore, skin preparation drapes, instruments, lighting, and expertise must all be adequate. Minimal wound extension is made along proper lines to gain adequate visualization of structures. A minimum of $2\times$ loupe magnification is required. Depending on findings, definitive care may involve simple placement of skin sutures or simple approximation of skin edges to allow for later repair of divided structures. Dressings and splints are applied after closure, and the blood pressure cuff is released.

Imaging of the wounded extremity begins with plain radiographs. The value of these films extends well beyond the simple exclusion of fractures. One should remember, when obtaining radiographs of hands and feet in children, to request bilateral studies in order to avoid confusion between injury and normal patterns of development. Prior to sending the patient for x-ray films, one must also consider the application of radiopaque markers to the wound surface. This should be done as a matter of routine in gunshot wounds and other deep penetrating injuries of any etiology. Several points should be considered in obtaining films. Multiple views may be required, since shards of glass in particular may be difficult to locate in the hand or foot. In every significant injury related to glass wounding, x-ray study should be obtained, since glass is well demonstrated radiographically in 90 percent of cases. Earlier thinking that only leaded automobile glass was visible has been proved untrue in recent years. Animal and human bite wounds to the extremities should also be imaged radiographically; sometimes surprising findings are revealed, such as the presence of teeth in the joints or soft tissues. Plain films are also helpful in the evaluation of high pressure injection injuries from paint or grease. Most commonly, these problems occur in the hand and have as their entry point the palmar surface of the finger. They tend to travel the flexor sheaths of the fingers and may break through into one or more of the deep spaces of the hand. Grease can be seen as radiolucent and paint as radiopaque. In either case, immediate exploration is required, and incision planning is aided by the extent of spread seen on x-ray studies.

Angiography often plays a vital part in the assessment of blunt and penetrating extremity trauma. The presence of distal pulses is reassuring, but does not in any way rule out the possibility of proximal vascular disruption. It has been estimated that 20 percent of arterial divisions are associated with normal distal pulses. A high index of suspicion will promote the finding of vascular problems before complications occur. Indications for angiography include: (1) posterior knee dislocation, which is associated with 60 percent incidence of popliteal artery disruption. (2) gunshot and penetrating wounds in proximity to major vessels, (3) extremities injured in multiple levels with distal ischemia, in which multiple vascular exposures would be impractical and injurious, (4) certain fractures, particularly supracondylar fractures, of the humerus, major femur fractures, and some tibial and fibular fractures, (5) complex injuries of the hand in which microvascular repairs may be necessary, (6) acute ischemia from arterial drug injection injuries, which may benefit from interventional radiologic techniques, such as the use of thrombolytic or spasmolytic agents. Osmotic diuresis amounting to 7 ml urine output per milliliter of angiographic dye is an important consideration, since the average study may promote the urine output of up to 500 ml. This volume should be replaced, and the possibility of urinary retention should be addressed by close surveillance or insertion of a urinary catheter.

Preoperative care of patients with injured extremities involves four major areas of concern: (1) total physiologic support, (2) immediate wound management, (3) antimicrobial prophylaxis, including tetanus, and (4) patient information. Total physiologic support relates to care priorities as established in the primary and secondary surveys of the multiply injured patient. As mentioned previously, the extremities may run a low priority, but must not be neglected. Perfusion status generally indicates the timing of repairs. For example, an automobile passenger may be in shock from central injuries and may also have a pale hand from division of most of the palmar surface wrist structures. Total care in this unstable patient is best effected by simultaneous attention to the central problems while a single wrist artery is rebuilt. Once perfusion to the hand has been restored, the skin is closed and definitive repairs may be deferred for a day or two, pending total patient stability. Immediate wound management depends on the nature of the injury and the anticipated delay before definitive operative care can be rendered. Untidy wounds are best treated by generous normal saline irrigation and sterile dressings with splints, as appropriate. Antimicrobial prophylaxis includes the use of tetanus toxoid and tetanus immune globulin (TAT), when appropriate. The previously immunized patient in whom more than 5 years has lapsed since the last dose should receive 0.5 ml of adsorbed tetanus toxoid. Individuals who have not been adequately immunized and those whose immunization history is unknown should receive 0.5 ml of adsorbed toxoid for the non-tetanus-prone wound; for tetanus-prone wounds, they should receive 250 units or more of human TAT at different injection sites. Antibiotic prophylaxis is most useful for wounds that (1) are associated with fractures, (2) include tendon divisions, and (3) disrupt joint capsules. First-generation cephalosporins are generally used for this purpose. Cultures should be taken of all open fractures and heavily contaminated wounds prior to the initiation of antibiotic therapy.

Adequate patient information is perhaps the most important element of preoperative care. Severe injuries require a clear understanding between the surgeon and the patient that a substantial period of rehabilitation may be required. If communication breaks down in the beginning, the best surgical efforts may be thwarted. A discussion of the extent of injury is often enhanced by showing the patient his x-ray films, drawing simple diagrams, and obtaining an inclusive consent. The patient with multiple injuries of the extremities should be told of the possible need for vein grafts to repair arteries, tendon grafts to replace segmental losses, and nerve grafts, when necessary. An estimate of the period of extremity immobilization should also be discussed. Once the consent is obtained, the patient should be medicated appropriately for pain after consultation with the anesthesiologist. Close family members should be included in these discussions whenever possible, since a great deal of assistance may be required in the activities of daily living after major limb compromise.

DISRUPTION OF SOFT TISSUE COVER

The responsibilities of extremity soft tissue cover include sensibility via specialized micro-end-organs of the system, tissue homeostasis by way of venous and lymphatic outflow channels, insulation and heat exchange, and simple protection. The value of vital, durable cover is greatest in areas of major vascular structures and in the hand, where a high density of covering, gliding, and skeletal structures is present. Therefore, the seriousness of soft tissue disruption is governed by location and coincidence with the division of associated structures. Restoration of surface continuity must not proceed at the expense of overall function. This simple fact is sometimes ignored when extravagant procedures are undertaken to restore cosmetic integrity at the expense of function. The spectrum of soft tissue disruption runs from simple abrasion to complete degloving.

Abrasions and tattooing injuries are best treated by adequate debridement, which may require proximal field blocks to scrub away loose embedded particulate matter, followed by the application of nonadhering gauze dressings. Immobilization of the part is generally unnecessary in this circumstance. Full healing without skin grafting is expected. Tidy incised wounds involving skin and fat without major sensory nerve division do not require prophylactic antibiotics, and may be approximated by a minimal number of interrupted simple or vertical mattress sutures. Subcutaneous and subcuticular sutures are avoided on the extremities, since they result in a higher incidence of wound sepsis, and the reaction caused by them may impair the gliding of underlying musculotendinous units. The treatment of flap type injuries depends on whether the base of the flap is proximal or distal. Proximally based flaps should be thought of as random pattern in distribution, and if the length is greater than 1½ to 2 times the width, there is only a marginal chance of flap survival. Perfusion of distally based flaps is generally estimated by visual inspection of color, but may be additionally resolved in marginal flaps by Wood's lamp examination following peripheral venous injection of sodium fluorescein.

A newly created device, the digital dermofluorometer, has proved useful, as it gives an actual numerical readout of tissue fluorescence following peripheral injection of 1 to 2 mg/kg of sodium fluorescein. Nonviable flaps should be debrided back to bleeding or adequately fluorescing tissue. Closure with a minimal number of simple interrupted sutures may then be attempted, but only if the perimeter of the proximal wound edge can be mobilized safely. Two alternatives are to defat the distal portion of the flap and create a full-thickness skin graft, or to full-thickness debride the nonviable tissue and close the gap immediately, or in a delayed fashion with split-thickness skin. Secure coverage is vital over major vascular structures and distal gliding structures, and in these circumstances, marginal flaps should not be retained. In these cases, the use of remote or local pedicle or free flap is preferred.

Degloving injury refers to the loss of skin and fat down to the fascia, and the seriousness of this problem is dependent on the location. The degloved tissue, when present, is often of poor quality, since fasciocutaneous circulation has been disrupted. Full-thickness losses overlying muscle bellies proximal to the wrist and ankle are very well tolerated and are best treated by initial debridement followed by moist dressings over a period of several days, until early granulations appear. Split-thickness skin grafts may then be applied. One must guard against premature resurfacing of these regions, since attempts may fail, and even a brief period of immobilization can impair ultimate functional recovery. It is better to encourage a full active range of motion of an extremity that has suffered a proximal degloving injury than to tie up the part with extravagant early restoration of surface continuity.

Degloving injuries distal to the wrist present special problems. Fingertip tissue losses can be treated in one of three ways: (1) Defects measuring 1 cm square may be left open and will heal within 8 weeks with minimal residual difficulty. (2) Split-thickness skin grafting from the proximal upper or lower extremity provides immediate simple coverage for tip injuries, including those in which bone is involved. Grafts contract at a rate of 40 to 50 percent within 8 weeks, leaving minimal disability. (3) Flap procedures, including thigh axial V-Y advancement (Kutler) or palmar surface V-Y advancement (Kleinert), or cross-finger pedicle tissues may be helpful, but have significant drawbacks of technical difficulty in V-Y advancement flaps, and donor as well as recipient stiffness in cross-finger flaps. The majority of patients therefore benefit from simple split-thickness coverage of these wounds. Major finger degloving injuries in which minimal skin bridges remain at the base of the finger are best treated by amputation most of the time. A small fraction of these are amenable to microvascular anastomosis, provided neurovascular bundles have not been significantly crushed. The "red line sign" refers to red streaks over the distribution of the digital arteries, reflecting major crush and breakdown of distal vascular integrity, with subsequent extravasation of blood into tissues. The presence of this sign is an absolute contraindication to attempts at microvascular repair. In the absence of crush, microvascular repair may be attempted, if suitable veins and arteries can be found in the distal tissues. Volar forearm vein grafts and antebrachial cutaneous sensory nerve grafts are useful in such procedures. Primary anastomosis without grafting is seldom secure. Degloved thumbs pose a more serious problem, since the thumb constitutes 40 percent of the value of the hand, according to disability ratings. Debridement, followed by microvascular repair if appropriate or abdominal pedicle flap, should be considered as part of a major effort to salvage thumbs. Palmar hand degloving wounds may cause substantial disruption of neurovascular structures. Occasionally, microvascular jump grafts are run from the intact portions of vascular arch to distal vessels of the fingers. Time should not be wasted during such salvage procedures by adding nerve grafting, since this can be accomplished later in the patient's course. Often, wounds may be left open without any biologic coverage, moist dressings are applied, and some minimal active motion is encouraged within a day or two following injury. Split-thickness skin grafts, abdominal pedicles, or free flaps are applied 2 to 7 days after the initial injury. Supervised early motion of openly wounded hands often provides the best chance of functional recovery.

Dorsal degloving injuries of the hand, in which the paratenon is intact, are simply treated by debridement and subsequent split-thickness skin grafting. When tendons are exposed or disrupted, extensor function will depend on the presence of subcutaneous fat to permit glide. Therefore, abdominal pedicle or groin flaps are preferred. Early granulations must be present on the tendons before such reconstructions are attempted. Dorsal foot degloving injuries require debridement and subsequent split- or full-thickness skin graft coverage. Subsequent reconstruction of the toe extensors is seldom of functional importance.

VASCULAR INJURIES

A list of arterial injuries ranging from the most critical to the least critical of injuries, as determined by the incidence of distal gangrene, is as follows: (1) femoral artery, (2) popliteal artery, (3) combination of anterior and posterior tibular arteries, (4) brachial artery proximal to profunda brachial, (5) superficial femoral artery, (6) iliac artery, (7) axillary artery, and (8) brachial artery distal to the profunda brachial. Ligation of the common femoral results in a 70 to 80 percent incidence of distal gangrene, and ligation of the brachial artery distal to the profunda results in a 10 to 15 percent incidence of distal gangrene. Ligation of either the radial or ulnar artery results in 1 to 2 percent incidence of distal gangrene, and ligation of both results in gangrene in 10 to 30 percent of cases. Venous injuries are coincident in 60 percent or more of cases of arterial disruption and should be repaired when possible. Popliteal venous injuries pose the greatest threat to the distal extremity if left unrepaired. Preoperative care of the patient with arterial injury includes rapid control of external bleeding, resuscitation from shock, adequate imaging of the artery and associated arteriovenous fistula, minimizing the time lag from injury to repair, and a consent that includes the possibility of vascular grafting.

Technical considerations common to all vascular repairs include the following: (1) incision planning, (2) proximal and distal control, (3) irrigation of the wound, (4) debridement, (5) repair, and (6) soft tissue coverage. Skin preparation and draping must include the entire extremity and, in many cases, expose the surface of another limb for harvest of autogenous graft material. Whenever possible, a well-padded, pretested tourniquet should be applied to the proximal aspect of the extremity and left uninflated. This will permit immediate control if unexpected major hemorrhage occurs; it also allows a dry field for repair of nerves and musculotendinous structures, as indicated. Incisions generally run over and parallel to the course of the underlying vessels to be repaired, and then cross joint creases at a 45° angle or less, to the transverse axis in order to avoid scar contracture. The direction of an incision may also be influenced by the possible need to temporarily divide major muscular structures, as in the case of axillary artery repair, which is facilitated by division of one or both pectoralis muscle tendons near their origins.

Proximal and distal control are seldom gained by application of clamps through the original wound. First, temporary control of major hemorrhage is gained in the operating room by direct finger pressure while the extremity is being prepped and draped, by inflation of a 33 ml balloon-tipped Foley catheter within the wound, or by temporary tightening of a proximally placed tourniquet while the incision is being made. Proximal control is gained first as the operating surgeon works from known to unknown regions and iso-

lates vessels in uninjured tissues. Silastic tubing should be used to encircle vessels whenever possible, since it is less traumatic than the application of clamps. When clamps are needed, they should be applied with minimal force to avoid crushing of the vessels. Back bleeding should be noted prior to securing distal control, and if there is none present, the extremity should be milked in the direction of the wound by pressure over the distribution of the injured vessel. Often, this measure releases clots and back bleeding increases. It should be noted, however, that back bleeding confirms only patency of the nearest collateral branches into a vessel, and the distal vascular tree may contain clot. Therefore, use of a Fogarty catheter of the correct size, with several gentle passes, is strongly recommended. Heparinized saline may then be injected into the distal end of the vessel before the Silastic loop or clamp is applied. Collateral vessels should be spared whenever possible, and these are occluded by temporary application of silver clips.

The goal of irrigation is to remove clot and debride. Once the surrounding structures have been cleared, the exposed lumina of the vessels are cleansed to allow direct inspection of vessel walls and determine whether additional intimal damage is present. Debridement is then carried out to freshen surrounding tissues as well as the vascular wounds themselves. Tidy incised arterial and venous wounds need not be debrided. However, untidy wounds and, in particular, blast injuries often require careful excision of vascular segments. Contused arterial segments are sometimes challenging, and these require debridement back to the point at which subintimal hemorrhage is no longer noted.

The repair itself consists of either end-to-end anastomosis, lateral repair, vein patch, or interposition of a vascular graft. Useful sutures include Teflon, Dacron, nylon, polypropylene, and silk. The suture technique itself may be a running or interrupted technique. Lateral repair of large vessels is usually accomplished by running sutures; however, the smaller the caliber of the vessel, the more imprecise this technique can be. We favor the general use of an interrupted technique in end-to-end anastomosis, consisting of anterior and posterior stay sutures, which are placed 180° apart and held in various positions in order to rotate the vessel for subsequent placement of the remaining interrupted sutures. The final two or three sutures in the smaller-caliber vessel may be laid in and tied subsequently, to permit continuous visualization of the lumen and avoid capturing the back wall with the passage of the needle. This also facilitates assessment of back bleeding, which should always be checked prior to tying the final suture. Pulses should return immediately in the distal extremity after clamps or vessel loops are removed. Absence of distal pulses following repair must be investigated by operative arteriogram. When repairs have been performed distal to the wrist and ankle, perfusion is assessed by color, capillary fill, Doppler, and digital dermofluorometry.

Vascular grafts are sometimes needed when end-to-end anastomosis is not possible without undue tension. The saphenous vein is the best source for such a graft and should be taken from the contralateral extremity in the case of leg and thigh repairs. This is important in order that additional incisions in a wounded part can be avoided, and potentially important venous outflow of the affected limb is not compromised. The upper extremity cephalic vein is also useful as a graft source, but its relatively smaller caliber limits its usefulness in the proximal thigh or arm. If suitable graft sites are not available, polytetrafluoroethylene (Gortex) is very useful, provided adequate muscular soft tissue cover is available. Synthetic grafts are anastomosed with polypropylene suture. Small grafts are sometimes required for use in palmar and digital wounds of the hand. These may be harvested from volar forearm or the foot dorsum. Optical loupe magnification, $2.0\times$ to $6.0\times$, is used for repairs in the arm between the elbow and wrist, and in the leg between the knee and ankle. A microscope is used for more distal repairs. Suture caliber at the wrist level is 6-0 or 8-0 nylon; in the palm, 8-0 to 9-0 nylon; and in the digits, 10-0 nylon. The vessels are held by microvascular clamps, and repairs are performed with the use of specially ground jeweler's forceps, which have silicon-coated handles to permit rotation of the instruments between the surgeon's fingers. Patency of anastomosis is tested by applying both pairs of forceps to the distal artery just beyond the anastomosis, milking out the blood from the vessel with one forceps, then releasing the proximal one while the distal forceps occludes the lumen. The vessel should instantly fill and be seen to pulsate.

Soft tissue coverage is vital to the survival of vessels that have been exposed and injured by trauma. An understanding of vascular anatomy as it relates to muscle flaps, myocutaneous flaps, and fasciocutaneous flaps has increased tremendously in recent years. This has promoted the acceptability of synthetic graft materials for extremity use. Rectus abdominis muscle flaps, for example, are useful in proximal thigh disruptions of the femoral vessels. Similarly, pectoralis major muscle flaps can be used to cover axillary and brachial artery injuries when blast injuries have compromised cover by local muscles. Muscular coverage of vascular repairs allows the surgeon to pack open the soft tissues for later delayed primary closure by flap approximation or split-thickness skin graft coverage.

Postoperative care following vascular repairs will depend on the composite nature of the extremity injury. A period of immobilization for arteriorrhaphy and venorrhaphy alone should be minimal, and certainly no more than a few days. Substantial muscular repairs in conjunction with vascular reconstruction require one week of immobilization proximal to the elbow and knee; two weeks of immobilization between wrist and elbow and ankle and elbow; and three weeks when tendon and nerve injuries distal to the wrist are repaired in addition to vascular repairs. Low-molecular-weight dextran is sometimes useful when significant devitalization of structures surrounding the repaired vessel has occurred and is believed to pose some threat to the distal microcirculation. However, in most cases, adequate hydration is sufficient to maintain patency of vascular repairs.

Upper and lower extremity fasciotomies may be important adjuncts to vascular reconstruction. They are performed for the relief of compartment syndromes and are effective only if performed early. Compartment syndrome occurs as a result of fluid extravasation from capillaries consequent to refilling after a period of ischemia, and this causes an obstruction of venous return within tight fascial compartments. A vicious cycle is then begun, which can only be relieved early, before myonecrosis occurs, by opening of the appropriate compartments. Generally acknowledged circumstances in which fasciotomy should be seriously considered are: (1) prolonged hypotension, (2) delay of more than 6 hours between injury and repair, (3) crush injuries with massive soft tissue trauma, (4) massive edema, and (5) combined arterial and venous injuries. Clinical indicators of compartment syndrome in the upper extremity are numbness and tingling (particularly in the nerve distribution), pain on passive motion of the fingers and thumb, and an increased flexion attitude of wrist and fingers due to flexor spasm. In the lower extremity, the first nerve to suffer ischemia is the deep peroneal, which supplies the dorsal web space between the great toe and second toe. Pain on passive motion of the ankle and, particularly, the great toe, may also be present. Compartment pressures are best measured by connecting a wick catheter to a standard pressure transducer and inserting it into the appropriate muscle compartments. Fasciotomy should be seriously considered when pressures are between 30 and 40 mmHg, and should definitely be performed when pressures exceed 40 mmHg in the forearm and the leg. Upper extremity fasciotomy requires four incisions: (1) A lazy S-shaped incision which extends from the proximal palmar ulnar forearm, gently curves across to the radial palmar forearm, returns to the ulnar side, and then extends into the midpalm just ulnar to the thenar crease. This allows freeing of superficial and deep flexor wads and decompresses the median nerve by carpal tunnel release. (2) A dorsal, linear longitudinal forearm incision is made between the mobile extensor wad and the extensor digitorum communis muscle bellies. These are two separate discrete compartments which must be opened individually. (3) and (4) Two linear, longitudinal hand dorsum incisions are carried over the second and fourth metacarpals, and the extensor tendons are retracted, allowing access to the dorsal and volar interosseous compartments which are separate. These compartments are opened by longitudinal slits. Dorsal incisions can generally be closed primarily, and delayed primary closure, with or without skin graft, is required for the volar surface incision.

Lower extremity fasciotomies must decompress the anterior and lateral compartments as well as the superficial and deep posterior compartments. A single incision opens the anterior and lateral compartments, and a posteromedial incision permits release of the posterior compartments. Primary closures are occasionally possible here, but more often delayed closures are required. A high level of clinical suspicion and the means for monitoring pressures are the keys to avoiding tissue necrosis from compartment syndromes.

PERIPHERAL NERVE PROBLEMS

Injuries to peripheral nerves may result in neuropraxia with eventual complete return of function, severe crush without hope of functional return, partial disruptions, or complete nerve divisions. Careful sensorimotor testing is the first step in planning treatment. Accurate diagnosis depends on a knowledge of normal and anomalous patterns of upper and lower extremity innervation. Timing of repair will then be determined by (1) the nature of the wound and wounding agent, (2) relative sensorimotor importance of the nerve(s) division(s) to patient and extremity function, and (3) availability of experienced surgeons and proper equipment. Tidy incised wounds in which nerves have been divided should be explored, and repairs should be performed as soon as conveniently possible. When these are associated with tendon divisions at the level of the wrist, repairs should be undertaken within a day or two, because of the great tendency of the flexor and extensor tendons to retract well up into the forearm. Another strong argument for repair within this time period is the ease with which freshly divided nerve ends can be accurately coapted. Within several days of injury, wallerian degeneration reduces the diameter of the distal nerve stump. Meanwhile, the proximal nerve end begins its axonal budding within a few days, and consequently increases in caliber. Budding also distorts the normally crisp definition of fascicular bundles in the proximal nerve stump. While loupe magnification of 3.5 to 6× is generally sufficient for nerve repair, delayed repairs may require use of a microscope in order to accurately join the differing diameters of the two ends. Repairs should not be performed when total hand function might be compromised, as in the case of digital nerve divisions proximal to nonpinch and nonprotective finger territories in the hand of an arthritic.

Repairs are also contraindicated in the presence of untidy wounds, such as blast and crush injuries. When nerve ends are visible in such wounds, they should be tagged with nylon sutures and secured into surrounding tissue in as close an apposition as possible. Repairs may be accomplished weeks or months after the primary wounds are healed. The actual zone of injury in a nerve that has been blast divided may not become apparent for several days, and premature repair would be doomed to failure by inclusion of a devitalized segment. Sensory nerve repair can yield good results with delay of up to 2 years between injury and neurorrhaphy. Motor nerves, however, depend on viable motor end-plates for functional return, and after 12 to 18 months, irreversible loss of neuromuscular junctions can occur, making repair a futile exercise.

The relative sensory and motor importance of divided nerves in the periphery must be considered prior to undertaking repair. The most important sensory nerve of the hand is the median nerve, which has been referred to as the "eye of the hand." This is so because it innervates the pinch surfaces of the thumb, index, and long fingers, and therefore governs tactile sensation for the manipulation of objects. The "eye" of the foot is the posterior tibial nerve, which innervates the entire plantar surface, including the heel, by way of its calcaneal, lateral plantar, and medial plantar branches. Priority would therefore be given to posterior tibial nerve repair in an incised ankle wound associated with plantar hypesthesia. Priorities of digital nerve repair in the hand relate to protective borders and pinch surfaces. Border nerves are thumb radial digital, index radial digital, ring ulnar digital, and little finger ulnar digital. Pinch nerves of importance are thumb ulnar digital, index radial digital, and long finger radial digital. Digital nerves of lower priority are therefore the index ulnar digital, long ulnar digital, ring radial digital, and little finger radial digital. Since repair of peripheral nerves requires 3 weeks of immobilization for healing, the financial burden of this time away from work is often too great to recommend repair of the lesser nerves to patients whose vocations and avocations do not demand sensation in those areas.

Priority assignment to the repairs of upper extremity motor nerves is difficult and depends on the level and identity of the nerve(s) injured. Nerve divisions above the level of the elbow often require subsequent tendon transfers. Motor nerves should be repaired in this region, but there is less than 50 percent chance of useful motor function in the future. Prognosis, from best to worst following motor nerve repair, is radial, median, and ulnar. Children may regenerate motor nerves at a remarkable rate and therefore should be simply observed following repair for a period of at least 6 months. Adults, however, often benefit from early tendon transfers within 3 months of nerve repair (to be discussed).

Lower extremity motor nerve divisions cause a disturbance of stability against gravity, as opposed to the dexterity and range of motion compromised by upper extremity motor divisions. Femoral nerve division causes the least disturbance, provided strong hip extensors are present. Walking up stairs is difficult for these patients, due to loss of quadriceps function. Common perineal palsy causes the well-known foot drop, and primary nerve repair is indicated whenever possible. Even so, tendon transfers and orthoses may subsequently be required. Similarly, divided tibial nerves should be repaired whenever possible, and again, may require subsequent reconstructive procedures.

Operative techniques in peripheral nerve repair have been a subject of recent controversy. Bold claims regarding the superiority of one type of nerve repair over another should be considered with caution, since our knowledge of the basic physiology of nerve healing lags well behind the capabilities of microtechnique. The best approach is a flexible one by an operator who is trained in microsurgery. Tourniquet control is essential for repairs at or distal to the elbow and knee. Well-padded, pretested arm tourniquets are inflated to 250 mmHg for a maximum of 2 hours, with an interval of 15 minutes between inflations if more time is needed. Thigh tourniquets are inflated to 300 mmHg. A minimum of $2 \times$ optical loupe magnification is used for the anatomic exposure of peripheral nerves. Exposures are generous, but mobilization of the nerve is minimal, particularly in the case of tidy transections. In the case of untidy transections, such as blast and crush-avulsion injuries, it is best not to attempt primary repair, and delayed treatment is facilitated by tagging the nerve ends with nylon sutures and sewing them into neighboring muscle or fascia, with the ends in close approximation. These tag sutures are cut 1 cm long for easy retrieval. Fresh, tidy divisions of peripheral nerves without segmental loss seldom require mobilization greater than 2 cm of each stump. Motor nerves are tested intraoperatively by a disposable nerve stimulator set at one-half to 2 milliamps of current. Repair of large peripheral nerves begins with inspection of the posterior wall of the stumps and alignment of the longitudinal vasa nervorum. Three 6-0 nylon epineural sutures are then laid in 60° apart, and are serially tied after alignment is rechecked. The ends are cut long so that these may act as stay sutures. This provides an excellent display of the fascicular bundles when the nerve is viewed from the anterior side. If the fascicular bundles are well contained within the epineural envelope, loupe magnification is used for the remaining repair (3.5 to $6 \times$), and if the bundles are splayed, the microscope is brought into the field. In the former case, epineural repair continues with interrupted 9-0 nylon sutures, the first of which rejoins the anterior vasa nervorum. When the microscope is used for splayed fascicular bundles, 10-0 nylon intraneural sutures are used to coapt the fascicular bundles, but no additional dissection is performed to allow individual fascicular repairs. We feel that each additional bit of dissection causes devascularization of the nerve and provides anatomic juncture at the expense of microcirculation. When fascicular bundles are repaired under the microscope, no more than two 10-0 nylon sutures are used per bundle. Partial nerve divisions occasionally cause difficulty because the traction of the semi-divided nerve stumps may cause buckling of the intact portion of nerves when they are brought together. Minimal buckling is acceptable; however, significant nerve distortion, as in the case of injuries that are a week or two old, is best avoided by interposition of a graft. Favored sites of nerve grafts are the medial and lateral antebrachial cutaneous sensory nerves of the proximal forearm or the sural nerve of the leg. Fascicular groups are matched for size, and segments are interposed with 10-0 nylon under the microscope.

The most important adjunctive procedures following nerve repair are those that anticipate obstacles to regeneration. Ulnar nerve division, just proximal to or within the cubital tunnel, is benefited by cubital tunnel release. The next point of entrapment for the ulnar nerve is the loge of Guyon at the wrist, and ulnar divisions just proximal to or within the loge, are accompanied by release of this compartment. The median nerve is often divided at the wrist, and divisions at the proximal lip of the carpal tunnel are accompanied by carpal tunnel release. Similarly, the radial nerve passes beneath the supinator muscle at the arcade of Frohse, and nerve divisions just proximal to or beneath the arcade require arcade release. Such considerations reduce the uncertainty of follow-up by eliminating questions of entrapment as a cause of failed sensorimotor return after repair.

Follow-up of peripheral nerve injuries is concerned with re-education of sensibility and evaluation of results. Following 3 weeks of immobilization for nerve healing, the first priority is to regain full range of motion of all joints. During this period, the anesthetic sensory fields must be protected from accidental thermal, crush, and incising injuries. Smokers are particularly prone to secondary problems in this regard. Patients are told that regeneration will be slow and steady, and often will involve a wide range of dysesthetic sensations, including "pins and needles," cold intolerance, and occasional pain. Cutaneous sensibility is refined by instructing the patient to practice reaching into a paper bag full of objects of varying shapes and textures and to identify them without looking at them. Sensory recovery should be graded and reported in a standard manner, and the system in widespread use is S_0 through S_4: S_0 = absence of sensibility in the autonomous area; S_1 = recovery of deep cutaneous pain sensibility within the autonomous area of the nerve; S_2 = return of some degree of superficial cutaneous pain and tactile sensibility within the autonomous area; S_{2+} = stage two, but with permanent paresthesia; S_3 = return of superficial cutaneous pain and tactile sensibility throughout the autonomous area with disappearance of any previous over-response; S_{3+} = stage 3, with some recovery of two-point discrimination in the autonomous area; and S_4 = complete recovery. Good sensory return is considered to be an S_3 or greater, and this can reasonably be expected in 70 percent of patients under the age of 40. Good fingertip two-point discrimination following neurorrhaphy is 10 mm or less.

Motor recovery is graded on the basis of M_0 through M_5: M_0 = no contraction (complete paralysis); M_1 = flicker of contraction; M_2 = contraction only with gravity eliminated; M_3 = contraction against gravity; M_4 = contraction against gravity and some resistance; and M_5 = contraction against powerful resistance, and normal power. Good results in this regard refer to M_4 to M_5, and may be reasonably expected in 40 to 50 percent of patients under the age of 40. The importance of long-term follow-up by the same examiner cannot be overemphasized, and evaluation should not be considered final before 2 to 5 years have passed. During this period, nerve conduction studies are occasionally indicated for apparent failure of regeneration.

Finally, mention should be made of early tendon transfers as internal splints following peripheral motor nerve divisions. The goal of such early tendon transfers is to improve overall hand function by avoiding external splinting devices. The most successful internal splint is the anastomosis of the median innervated pronator teres to the extensor carpi radialis brevis and longus for radial nerve palsy. This acts as a dynamic internal cock-up splint, allowing a more efficient use of the flexors for grasp. We often perform this transfer at the time of radial or posterior interosseous nerve neurorrhaphy. Low median nerve palsies cause a deficit in thumb pronation and opposition. This can be remedied within 3 to 4 months of injury, if no function is returning to the abductor pollicis brevis, by some form of opponens plasty as an internal splint to overcome the supinating forces of the extrinsic thumb extensor and the abductor pollicis longus. Ulnar claw hand can be reconstructed, with subsequent improvement in power grip, 3 to 4 months following nerve division, by extending the extensor carporadialis longus via grafts that pass proximal and volar to the intermeticarpal ligaments and enter the proximal phalanges of the ring and little fingers as a dynamic intrinsic transfer.

MUSCULOTENDINOUS TRAUMA

Repair of divided muscles and tendons makes special demands of the surgeon's judgment and technical skills. The challenge of restoring glide within a bed of injured tissue increases as the location of wounds proceeds from axilla to fingertip and from groin to toe. This discussion will consider (1) the nature and level of injury as related to timing of repairs, (2) techniques of repair, and (3) postoperative care, rehabilitation, and evaluation of results. Tidy incised wounds of less than 6 hours duration, which merely open the superficial fascia over muscle bellies proximal to the midforearm and ankle, may be managed in the emergency room. Such wounds are copiously irrigated with a balanced salt solution, and the fascial layer is longitudinally opened in a proximal and distal direction and the skin is closed. Fascia is not closed in these wounds for fear of development of compartment syndrome. Skin edges are coapted with interrupted nylon or Prolene vertical or horizontal mattress sutures. Subcutaneous sutures are avoided. Deeply incised tidy wounds at the same levels are managed in the operating room. A proximal tourniquet is applied whenever possible; it is of enormous benefit in achieving identification and subsequent anatomic reapproximation of the deep fascial envelopes of divided muscles. Repairs of pure muscle units are performed with 3-0 or 4-0 polydioxanone sutures (PDS), which are placed as horizontal mattress sutures, and all the sutures are laid in before any are tied. The laying-in technique avoids tearing of muscle bundles. Serial tying of these sutures is facilitated by the assistant snugging down the knot as the operating surgeon ties his suture. Repair continues from the depths of the wound to the surface, and the superficial fascia is

left open. Again, skin edges are coapted with nylon or prolene, and subcutaneous sutures are avoided, since these encourage reaction and ultimately impair the gliding of underlying muscles. Muscle-tendon junctions in the forearm and leg have a diminished local vascular supply available for healing following repair. For this reason, nonabsorbable monofilament sutures, such as nylon or Prolene, are used for repair to provide a longer period of tensile strength during the repair phase. Horizontal mattress sutures are used, and knots are buried within the substance of the juncture. Timing of muscle belly and muscle-tendon junction repairs is very important, owing to the extreme retraction of these units which occurs after 24 to 48 hours. Beyond this interval, anatomic repair is extremely difficult. On occasions when such delay is required, it is best to irrigate the wound and coapt the skin edges with interrupted sutures to avoid desiccation of the muscle bellies.

Untidy wounds of muscle bellies and muscle-tendon junctions should not be repaired primarily. Such wounds are irrigated, debrided generously, and packed open with sterile dressings. The patient is given prophylactic cephalosporin, and 2 to 5 days after admission, the patient is returned to the operating room for delayed primary closure only if the severed units are critical to function. Skin grafts are applied for coverage.

Timing the repair of tidy upper extremity flexor tendon divisions depends on the level of injury. Between the distal third of the forearm and midpalm, the tendons are not tethered proximally, and retract a significant distance immediately following division. With each passing day, tension-free repair becomes increasingly difficult. Therefore, in this region, tenorrhaphy should be performed within 3 days, and certainly within one week. This requires immediate irrigation and skin closure of the fresh wound if delay is anticipated. Slash wounds of the wrist with multiple tendon divisions are included in this category. The technique is as follows: (1) A well-padded, pretested tourniquet is applied to the upper extremity, and the arm is abducted onto two arm boards. (2) The extremity is painted with povidone-iodine solution and draped in the usual sterile manner. (3) Circumferential pressure is applied as the tourniquet is elevated to 250 mmHg. The wound is irrigated free of clots with normal saline. (4) An incision is extended distally as a formal carpal tunnel release. (5) An ulnar or radial border longitudinal proximal extension is made, to raise a flap for the retrieval of proximal stumps. (6) Proximal stumps of deep and then superficial flexors are retrieved by following clots proximally and milking the forearm to help deliver these structures into the wound. As each stump is delivered, it is grasped with toothed Bishop-Harmon forceps and held very gently as an anterior to posterior stay suture is passed through the stump, 1 cm from the cut end. Small hemostats are applied to the individual stay sutures to follow the proximal stumps. Next, the distal stumps are identified with ease since the carpal tunnel has been opened, and the ends are similarly tagged. Each pair of hemostats is then held together by a towel clip, and the system of identification is therefore complete. All flexors are repaired in the wrists of children when the divisions are tidy. Priorities of repair in adult wrists are (1) all of the profundus tendons, (2) flexor pollicis longus, and (3) flexor digitorum superficialis to the index. Our policy has been to repair all tendons, even in adults when the divisions are tidy, with the understanding that the ultimate independence of the profundus and superficialis functions will be variable. Repairs proceed from one side of the wrist to the other, as 4-0 nylon sutures are used for tenorrhaphy by the modified Kessler technique, in which the knot is intratendinous. The flexor pollicis longus and the superficial flexors are next repaired. Wrist flexors are generally the last structures repaired, and 3-0 nylon sutures are used for these. The skin is closed with interrupted horizontal mattress sutures of 5-0 nylon, and the short arm splint or circumferential plaster dressing with foam padding is applied, holding the wrist at 35° flexion. The elbow is immobilized at 90° in a long arm cast if wrist flexors have been divided.

Untidy injuries of the wrist are best treated by initial debridement and passage of simple 4-0 nylon sutures through proximal and distal stumps of the profundus tendons, the flexor pollicis longus, the index superficialis, and the radial wrist flexor. These sutures should be cut long for easy identification and should leave the tendon ends within less than 1 cm of each other. Continuously moist dressings are applied, and definitive repairs are made within 3 to 7 days. Reconstruction by simplification is the rule in such injuries.

Tidy wounds dividing the flexor tendons between the level of the carpal tunnel and the entry to the fibro-osseous sheath (first annular pulley) are straightforward and, provided the skin has been closed, can be repaired within 1 to 3 weeks with good results. The proximal profundus tendon is easily found because the radial side origin of the lumbrical muscle prevents proximal retraction. Similarly, the divided superficialis is easily found because it has a filmy yolk around the profundus tendon. Modified Kessler suture technique is used for tenorrhaphy of these structures. Lumbrical muscles are repaired with horizontal mattress sutures when they have been divided.

Zone II ''no man's land'' refers to the region between the distal third of the palm and the midportion of the midphalanx, in which the superficialis and profundus tendons travel close together in the fibro-osseous sheath. Good results can be achieved following meticulous repair of both tendons if divisions are tidy in patients under age 40. Similar results will be gained when such repairs are done within one week of injury. Technique of zone II flexor tendon repairs involves extension of the wound by a palmar zig-zag (Bruner) incision, if the laceration is oblique, or an ulnar border axial incision, if the palmar laceration is transverse. Radial border axial incision is used for the little finger. Proximal retraction of stumps requires a longitudinal distal third of the palm incision, just proximal to the first annular pulley. Proximal stumps are then retrieved by passage of No. 5 pediatric feeding catheters from the original wound, out through the proximal palmar counter-incision. These are sutured separately to the superficialis and profundus tendons, and the tendons are then drawn sequentially out through the original wound. When annular pulleys must be opened, they are flapped to the radial or ulnar side of the sheath and subsequently repaired with interrupted 6-0 nylon suture following tenorrhaphy. Tendon repairs are performed with 4-0 nylon modified Kessler suture to the profundus, and 5-0 nylon modified Kessler or horizontal mattress sutures individually to the radial and ulnar slips of the superficialis tendons. A running 6-0 nylon suture is then carried around 270° of the anterolateral aspects of the profundus repair, in order to smooth it for improved glide. Flexor sheath is repaired, and tendon glide is checked by passive finger motion. Skin edges are coapted with interrupted 5-0 nylon sutures, and short arm splint or circumferential plaster is applied with the wrist in 35° of flexion with the thumb excluded.

Only the profundus is vulnerable distal to the midportion of the middle phalanx (zone I). Standard tenorrhaphy with intratendinous 4-0 nylon and anterior basting suture of 6-0 nylon are performed if the distal stump is adequate. Otherwise, a 4-0 suture is passed through the proximal stump and run out through the distal pad just beyond the fingernail and tied over a foam-padded button. Untidy divisions of flexors within the digital sheath and beyond will not be discussed in this chapter.

Upper extremity extensor tendon divisions follow similar principles of timing, out to the distal third of the hand dorsum. Repair as early as possible is favored in this region because of the tendency of proximal stumps to retract upward into the forearm. The extensor/retinaculum consists of 6 dorsal compartments, and when tendons are divided within these, retrieval is facilitated by the pediatric feeding catheter technique. If repairs do not glide well through their compartments, they should be re-done outside the tunnel in the subcutaneous position. Bow-stringing will be visible, but function is very good in this circumstance. Juncturae tendinum (conexus intertendineus) prevent proximal retraction of extensor tendons divided beyond the distal third of the hand dorsum. These tether one tendon to another. Depending on the flatness of the tendons in this region, horizontal mattress sutures are used (for flat tendons) and modified Kessler sutures are used for thicker tendons. Distal to the MP joints, the tendon flattens as an extensor hood, and paired horizontal mattress sutures of clear 5-0 nylon are used for repair. Black sutures may show through the skin in fair individuals and are therefore avoided. The terminal extensor tendon over the DIP joint, if cleanly incised, is repaired with clear 6-0 nylon paired horizontal mattress sutures or simply splinted across the joint for 6 weeks. Untidy divisions proximal to the PIP joints may be repaired in a delayed fashion, up to one week, as long as skin covering is adequate. Untidy PIP joint divisions are splinted for 6 weeks to avoid boutonierre deformity, and untidy DIP joint level tendon divisions are splinted for 6 to 8 weeks to avoid mallet deformity. Immobilization of extensor tendons involves wrist extension at 70° and metacarpophalangeal joint flexion at 45°, so that the rays of the fingers and dorsal forearm are parallel. PIP and DIP joints are held in 20° of flexion for tendon divisions proximal to the MP joints, and are kept as straight as possible if divisions are distal to the MP joints. Repair of flexor and extensor tendons of foot will not be discussed here, but general techniques are similar.

Postoperative care of muscle and tendon divisions requires close attention to elevation of the injured part. If edema is allowed to occur by dependency, results are invariably poor. Immobilization of muscle divisions proximal to the elbow requires one week in a sling. Between the elbow and the distal third of the forearm, 2 weeks in a long- or short-arm splint are sufficient. Thumb and finger flexors are immobilized in a short-arm splint or circumferential plaster dressing for 3 weeks. Four weeks are required if wrist flexors are involved, and the immobilization here is long-arm, as already noted, to avoid disruption of the lateral-based structures by pronation and supination. Short-arm immobilization is adequate for both wrist extensors and extensors of the thumb and fingers, and should be continued for a 4-week period. The extra week is added to allow some additional tensile strength, since the overwhelming power of the flexor tendons can easily disrupt an extensor tenorrhaphy after 3 weeks.

Rehabilitation is usually carried out by the patient, without formal physical therapy, under the surgeon's continual guidance and close supervision. First, the elbow and wrist are mobilized, then hand rehabilitation is effected by having the patient squeeze a sponge in warm water three or four times a day, for 5 minutes. Office visits at a frequency of three times per week are not unusual for the first 2 weeks after cast removal. Functional return after flexor tenorrhaphies is assessed by angle measurements of all involved joints in flexion and in extension, with calculation of range of motion and the differences between hands. Grip and pinch strength are measured at regular intervals, when appropriate. Angle measurements are supplemented by the patient's ability to straighten his fingers to the plane of a table when the hand is resting supine, and the distance by which the flexed finger(s) fail(s) to touch the proximal, mid, and distal palm. This is measured in centimeters. Steady recovery may continue for as long as 2 years; therefore, great optimism must be projected to the patient.

SELECTED PROBLEMS

Replantation

Replantation of amputed parts requires careful patient selection. Enthusiasm for widespread application of these expensive surgical techniques to all patients should be tempered by a careful history regarding the mechanism of injury, close scrutiny of the amputed part, and an overview of the patient's total hand requirements. A recent survey of nearly 200 surgeons worldwide, who had lost one or more digits that were not replanted, revealed that more than 95 percent of these individuals continued to work and claimed no significant disability.

Poor candidates for replantation include: (1) drug or alcohol-dependent individuals, (2) transients, who are not likely to maintain the close follow-up required, (3) unemployed individuals who are not actively seeking work, (4) patients who have lost single digits, except for the thumb, (5) victims of severe crush injuries, and (6) patients whose medical condition will not tolerate 4 to 12 hours of anesthesia. The influence of age on outcome following replantation has undergone reassessment in recent years, and the best approach is a careful review of the patient's needs for total hand function.

All primary care physicians should be aware of the "red line" sign. This refers to red streaks over one or both neurovascular bundles within an amputated part, and represents diffuse blood extravasation from severe crush injury to the distal arterial tree. Reanastomosis of such vascular segments is doomed to failure, and this finding therefore represents an absolute contraindication to replantation. False expectations and costly patient transfers can best be avoided by recognition of the red line sign.

Replantation should be considered for amputations involving: (1) multiple digits, (2) the thumb, (3) partial hand (through the palm), (4) wrist or forearm, (5) sharp amputations at or above the elbow, and (6) almost any body part in a child.

Once the decision to replant a part has been made, transportation of the patient and part to the appropriate facility should be as rapid as possible. Management of the amputated tissue prior to replantation consists of wrapping the part in gauze moistened with saline or Ringer's lactate solution, placing it in a plastic bag, and placing the bag on crushed ice. Parts handled in this way will survive 12 hours, and occasionally 24 hours, but the best results are obtained after the shortest time intervals. Patient care involves: (1) complete physical examination to ensure that 4 to 16 hours of surgery will be well tolerated, (2) placement of intravenous line, with administration of antibiotics, (3) tetanus prophylaxis, and (4) maintenance of NPO status.

Expectations following replantation include: (1) active range of joint motion, approximately 50 percent of normal, (2) nerve recovery comparable to that which is achieved following repair of isolated peripheral nerve divisions, (3) cold intolerance, which generally resolves by 2 years, and (4) an acceptable cosmetic result.

Gunshot Wounds

Most gunshot wounds seen in civilian practice involve low-velocity missiles, generally ranging from .22 to .38 caliber. All tissue types may be injured, but priority is given to assessment of the vascular tree. Arteriography is performed for wounds that have traversed regions of major blood vessels. It is remarkable how seldom these low-velocity injuries involve tendons and nerves. In most cases, debridement of 1 or 2 mm of devitalized skin and subcutaneous tissue, in addition to fixation of fractures, constitutes sufficient treatment. Vessel, nerve, and/or tendon injury requires exploration. Primary repairs of all three structures are often possible in low-velocity wounds. However, if there is any question as to degree of contamination and viability of structures, it is best to tag nerve and tendon stumps and return several days later for definitive repairs. Delayed primary closure or split-thickness skin grafting is best for the re-establishment of cover following appropriate repairs, provided there is adequate muscle protection over the part.

High-velocity missile wounds of speeds greater than 2,000 feet per second uniformly require exploration and debridement. The principles of treatment are similar to those for low-velocity wounds, except that wider debridement is often necessary, and it is uncommon to perform primary nerve and tendon repairs at the first operation. A second-look procedure at 24 to 72 hours is mandatory and, depending on the wound environment, may permit repair of essential tendons and nerves. Abdominal pedicle flaps are useful in providing durable coverage of the hand following major tissue losses, but these should not be performed until 3 to 5 days have elapsed, permitting time for improvement of tissue equilibrium.

High-velocity gunshot wounds to the hand require prolonged hospitalization, which includes early range of motion of the fingers whenever possible, supervised by the surgeon and physical therapist. Pain is most often the limiting factor in this type of treatment; peripheral nerve blocks are often very helpful in reassuring the patient.

Crush Injuries

Crush injuries may be open or closed. Open wounds have the obvious potential for greater bacterial contamination, but both share the risks of local myonecrosis and compartment syndrome. Additionally, myoglobinuria may occur and should be treated by alkalinization of urine and promotion of osmotic diuresis in order to spare the kidneys. Sodium bicarbonate, one ampule, and sodium mannitol, 12 g, are added to each liter of 5 percent dextrose and water, and the solution is administered at a rate of 200 ml/hour until brisk diuresis is obtained; the rate is then reduced to 100 ml/hr. Urine is checked frequently for the presence of myoglobin.

Injection Injuries

These injuries call for special mention since they cause great threat to the hand and are often treated inadequately and after too much delay. High-pressure grease and paint-guns are the most common causes, and the site of injury is often the pad of the thumb or index finger, or the palm. The injected substance passes rapidly through the subcutaneous tissue and enters the flexor tendon sheath. From here, it passes into one or more of the deep spaces of the hand. The thumb and index finger conduct substances into the thenar space, and the long ring and little fingers conduct injected material into the mid-palmar space. These two spaces may communicate with each other, and they also refer material proximally into Parona's space. All three spaces are deep to the profundus tendons. Proper treatment involves emergency debridement within 2 hours, consisting of (1) opening of the fingers along nonpinch, nonprotective border surfaces, (2) dorsal thumb web incision to debride the thenar space, and (3) midpalmar incision to open the midpalmar space. The midpalmar incision is often extended proximally to allow carpal tunnel release. Failure to perform adequate wide debridement emergently will result in necrosis of parts. Plain radiographs are often useful in evaluating this injury; they reveal the spread of paint, which is radiopaque, or change in tissue planes by the spread of radiolucent grease. Second-look operations within 24 to 28 hours are sometimes required.

POSTOPERATIVE CARE AND REHABILITATION

The mainstays of postoperative care for the patient with extremity injury are: (1) steady psychologic support, (2) comfortable dressings which support the injured part in an appropriate position, (3) elevation when appropriate, particularly in the case of the hand, which should be kept above the level of the heart by the use of pillows or by a tubular stockinette that is tied around the trunk, run up over the arm and hand, and secured to an IV pole (this latter means of immobilization is safe only when the elbow is well supported), and (4) appropriately timed wound inspections which are coordinated with analgesia.

Physical therapy is often helpful, but also very expensive, and should never supplant the surgeon's responsibility for direct communication of graded exercises and the maintenance of goal orientation, including the patient's return to work. Re-education of the nondominant hand is often beneficial for patients who will be passing through a long care sequence with significant ultimate disability from the injured part. The best results following complex injuries are gained in motivated patients who understand at each stage of recovery precisely what is expected of them. This often involves daily visits to the office during the early post-hospital phase. The patient should also be encouraged to call at any time if there are any questions regarding progress. In contrast to the automaticity with which injured internal organs are re-integrated into the patient's total function, the injured hand requires great expenditure of physical and emotional energy by all involved, to find its way into productive activity.

The annual cost of disability from hand and upper extremity injuries is approximately 30 billion dollars in the United States. This figure exceeds the cost of head injury by a factor of 3. Cost containment is best effected by: (1) early assessment of the individual patient's functional extremity needs, (2) appropriate timing of interventions, (3) single team management of soft tissue cover, neurovascular structures, and musculotendinous units, (4) close personal follow-up with appropriate guidance and goal setting, and (5) physical therapy, when needed, with emphasis on proper balance of exercise, elevation, and rest. Numerous expensive adjunctive therapies are currently available and, in our experience, find a limited place in the care of most patients with extremity injury.

FRACTURES

Peter G. Trafton, M.D.

The purpose of this chapter is to alert the general surgeon to recent advances in the management of musculoskeletal trauma. Emphasis is on the therapeutic decisions that must be made during the early period after injury. It is my belief that knowledgeable, aggressive, early management of the trauma patient's musculoskeletal injuries will contribute significantly to his overall care, and to his ultimate rehabilitation. This is not a "how-to-do-it," but a plea for immediate collaboration with an experienced orthopaedic traumatologist. The care of musculoskeletal injuries can be dealt with only briefly and arbitrarily in a chapter like this. Several alternative treatments exist for most fractures. Controversy is unavoidable.

Skeletal injuries cannot be managed safely in isolation. The treating physician must always think beyond the broken bone, and include in his assessment the associated soft tissue trauma, the status of the rest of the injured limb, and the whole affected patient—his other injuries, his age and anticipated activity level, his pre-existing musculoskeletal resources, and his ability to contribute to a rehabilitation program. The choice of management for fractures and joint injuries may depend on whether an injury is isolated, or is one of several problems affecting a multiply traumatized patient. Treatment is also affected by the resources available to the surgeon. In the absence of a well-stocked operating room, effective radiographic monitoring, and an experienced team, modern techniques of internal fixation are likely to come to grief. The advice offered in a book must always be interpreted carefully in the light of the responsible surgeon's experience. Finally, no book is a substitute for consultation, which can be invaluable for appropriate management of trauma to the musculoskeletal system.

EARLY CARE OF MUSCULOSKELETAL INJURIES

Injuries of the musculoskeletal system may appear dramatic, but rarely pose immediate threats to life or even limb. As described in the chapter on Emergency Room Care, initial attention is directed toward the patient's resuscitation. During these efforts, one must heed the possibility of an unstable fracture or dislocation of the spine, especially in the neck. History and physical examination, if possible, are rarely adequate to exclude such injuries. Radiographs are essential, beginning with a cross-table lateral film that shows the entire cervical spine, down to T1. Such a radiograph is mandatory for all patients with head or face injuries, unconsciousness, neck pain, or abnormal neurologic findings. Most unstable cervical spine injuries are evident on this x-ray study, but its normality does not guarantee a stable spine.

If manipulation of the head or neck is necessary before radiographs, it should be done in a way that minimizes the risk of damage to the spinal cord. Flexion, hyperextension, and rotation of the neck away from the midline must be avoided. Gentle (5 to 7 lb) traction on the head with hands or a cervical halter will stabilize the neck. If the head is adequately supported, the patient may be rolled "like a log," to permit examination of the back. A patient who is alert enough to be moving his head and neck voluntarily has little risk of injuring himself. Poorly tolerated restraints add little protection. The patient with a painful neck and an acute unstable injury usually appreciates immobilization with sandbags taped together over the forehead, or traction by means of head halter or tongs.

In an acutely injured patient, the thoracic and lumbar spine and the pelvis cannot adequately be evaluated by physical examination alone. If the injury is due to a significant fall, a vehicular accident, or to other high-energy trauma, and if the patient is unable to deny pain in back and pelvis, and cannot demonstrate normal active motion of back and legs, AP and lateral radiographs of the entire spine and an AP film of the pelvis must be obtained. However, these studies should not interrupt more urgent early evaluation and treatment. Until they have been obtained and reviewed, spine precautions are maintained.

Extremity injuries may be obvious or occult. Initial care of obvious injuries includes control of bleeding with pressure dressings, splinting unstable injuries in an acceptable position, and urgent identification and treatment of arterial occlusion.

Once resuscitation is under way and the patient is responding, a thorough and systematic search must be made for more occult injuries. Inspect all skin surfaces, from digits to trunk, for deformity, swelling, ecchymosis, and laceration. Skin abrasions are significant. If in the region of a musculoskeletal injury, they require that any needed operation be done promptly or else delayed until the abrasion heals. Palpate each bone and joint for swelling, deformity, and tenderness (if the patient is responsive). Stress each bone to confirm stability. Move each joint to demonstrate normal range of motion, and absence of abnormal motion. When emergency surgery is a part of the resuscitation or early care of a trauma patient, extremity examination should always be completed before terminating the anesthetic. Confirm presence of peripheral pulses. Obtain radiographs of all abnormal areas.

When the patient is conscious and able to cooperate, active voluntary motion of each joint must be assessed to check motor nerve and myotendinous integrity. Check sensation in the isolated sensory area of each major peripheral nerve. For critically ill patients who are unable initially to cooperate, completion of this evaluation may take several days. Such follow-through is mandatory to avoid the embarrassment of missing injuries. Resuscitation of the multiply injured patient necessarily places diagnosis and treatment of musculoskeletal conditions at a relatively low priority. Many injuries are not initially appreciated. Repeated examinations during the early recovery period are frequently rewarded by the discovery of additional diagnoses in time for effective treatment.

OPEN FRACTURES

Classification

Open fractures require special attention to minimize the risks of clostridial and pyogenic infection. Treatment is guided by classification of the severity of injury, primarily according to the extent of soft tissue trauma, and level of contamination.

GRADE I   Small wounds caused by low-velocity trauma, with minimal contamination and soft tissue damage, e.g., skin laceration by a bone end, or a low velocity gunshot wound.

GRADE II   Wounds extensive in length and width, but with little or no avascular or devitalized soft tissue, and relatively little foreign material.

GRADE III   Moderate or massive wounds with considerable devitalized soft tissue, foreign material, or both.

Identification of an open fracture is the first step of early management. Although usually obvious, open fractures occasionally are not appreciated because of incomplete examination. Posterior surfaces must be checked. Seemingly superficial wounds may communicate with underlying bone or joint injuries. Whenever the pelvis is fractured, perineal, vaginal, and rectal lacerations should be ruled out. Neurovascular status, myotendinous function, and the possibility of multiple injuries must be checked. When totally satisfactory examination and treatment of a wound near a fracture cannot be carried out in the emergency ward, assume that the fracture is open, and proceed to the operating room where adequate anesthesia, assistance, hemostasis, and lighting usually confirm suspicions and facilitate treatment.

Once an injured limb has been examined, control of bleeding is achieved with sterile compression dressings, and a splint is applied before transportation to the radiology department or the operating suite. If a patient arrives with a well-described open fracture already covered, the dressing should be removed only in the operating room.

Roentgenographs of injured or suspect areas are essential for evaluating the trauma patient. Unfortunately, the quality of emergency studies is quite variable, and it is risky for the patient to languish, poorly monitored, in the radiology department. The responsible surgeon must be prepared at any moment to conclude that the films already obtained are the best possible, and that the patient should proceed to surgery. Chest and cervical spine films are of highest priority. Those of extremities are necessary for a complete evaluation. Without adequate radiographs, the fracture surgeon operates at his peril. For example, views centered on joint rather than the diaphysis may be needed to define fully an intra-articular injury. Of course, such films may be obtained during surgery once the patient has been stabilized.

Management of Open Fractures

I feel strongly that each open fracture should be cared for in a well-prepared operating room, with adequate anesthesia, as soon as is safely possible.

Immediate Wound Care

The basic aspects of surgical wound care have changed little since their description by Desault in the late eighteenth century. Medical adjuncts have been added. Tetanus prophylaxis is administered immediately. I urge the use of an appropriate intravenous antibiotic promptly upon the diagnosis of an open fracture. The value of this *adjunct* to surgical treatment has been shown by several comparative studies. We currently use 1 g IV cefazolin every 6 hours, beginning in the emergency ward, and continuing through the first 48 hours after injury, whether or not the wound is left open. Alternative antibiotics are required for allergic patients.

The properly evaluated patient is brought to the operating room as soon as team and equipment are assembled. Adequate anesthesia is induced, and following or concurrent with higher priority surgical treatment, definitive care of the open fracture is begun.

This starts with a careful reassessment of the injured limb—an examination under anesthesia. Is salvage warranted or must primary amputation be considered? If amputation appears to be a possibility, we attempt to discuss this with the patient preoperatively in the emergency ward.

A pneumatic tourniquet is applied, but inflated only if necessary to control bleeding or to assess tissue viability with postischemic hyperemia. In principle, the cleansing of an injured limb should not be allowed to contaminate further the wound of an open fracture. However, in practice it is hard to scrub the limb adequately while a sterile occlusive dressing is kept over the usual wound. Most detergents and soaps are injurious to tissue. Therefore, avoid the wound itself with scrub solution. The scrub is done with the limb lying on a sterile waterproof disposable drape, which is replaced twice during the 10-minute wash. Detergent suds are rinsed and the skin is dried with sterile towels. Then the entire limb, including the wound, is painted with iodophor antiseptic solution, and new waterproof sterile drapes are applied.

Irrigation and Debridement

Next irrigation and debridement are performed. It is often necessary to enlarge the wound to permit adequate inspection and cleansing. This should be carefully planned so as not to devitalize skin flaps or interrupt superficial veins, which might be essential for blood return. If possible, incisions should avoid contused skin and preserve a healthy flap of tissue to cover the fracture site and any implanted internal fixation device. With adequate exposure, all foreign material and dead or questionable tissue are removed, while sparing nerves, major vessels, and as much bone as possible. Small free fragments of cortical bone are discarded. Grossly contaminated bone surfaces are removed with rongeur or curette. All joints that have been penetrated are opened and inspected for debris including osteochondral fragments. We leave questionably viable skin, which can readily be assessed during the days following injury. Subcutaneous fat, fascia, and injured muscle are aggressively removed if dead or dirty, although it is important not to undermine excessively a viable skin flap. Contractility, consistency, and especially the presence of bleeding from small intrinsic vessels are more helpful than color as indicators of muscle viability.

A pulsatile irrigation system enhances cleansing of injured tissue. This generally permits use of less than the 10 or more liters of irrigant previously recommended. I use at least 5 liters of normal saline or Ringer's solution for the average Grade II open fracture. I use 0.2 percent kanamycin solution as a final antibiotic rinse (2 g kanamycin in 1 liter, with 2 ampules of sodium bicarbonate to ensure an alkaline solution).

During debridement, decisions must be made about two other aspects of care for the injured limb: fracture stabilization and wound closure. Complications arising from either of these controversial areas can considerably increase the patient's period of disability, and can jeopardize his eventual result. Avoidance of grief is perhaps best achieved by the surgeon's use of techniques with which he is thoroughly familiar, and for which he is completely equipped. Although no rules apply unequivocally, the safest general course is to avoid both primary wound closure and primary internal fixation of open fractures. Adequate stabilization is important, however, and fixation may both reduce the risk of infection and facilitate overall management. Meticulous wound toilet and delayed primary closure are essential if internal fixation is used.

Reduction and Fixation

Whereas articular surface fractures should be reduced anatomically, extra-articular fractures generally require only adequate restoration of angular and rotational alignment, with preservation of length. How to stabilize an open fracture remains controversial. Traction, plaster cast, external skeletal fixation, and the several forms of internal fixation are all useful, individually and in combination. The problems that must be solved anew for each fracture patient are: (1) How much stability is necessary, or even possible? and (2) What is the most beneficial and least hazardous way of obtaining that stability? No direct comparative studies document the unequivocal superiority of one form of stabilization over another.

For certain injuries and certain patients, *internal fixation* may yield improved results. Therefore, it seems indicated selectively. Patients with intra-articular fractures, multiple injuries, segmental fractures, or acute spinal cord injuries, and some with significant bone loss, are candidates. Those with severe soft tissue wounds over fractures that can be stabilized better with internal than external fixation are also more easily managed this way, although infection is likely. This use of internal fixation should be recognized as an attempt at salvage of a limb that might otherwise be amputated. Primary internal fixation of fractures adjacent to arterial anastomoses is not necessary to protect the vascular repair.

External skeletal fixation must be coordinated carefully with wound management and bone grafting. It offers a powerful and adaptable technique for stabilizing open fractures without additional exposure or devascularization of bone, and without the encumbrance of plaster casts or traction. If delayed wound closure or the use of a muscle pedicle or myocutaneous flap is anticipated, an external skeletal frame is preferable to pins and plaster, but familiarity with the technique and the specific device is necessary to avoid complications. When-

ever possible, I prefer to use half pins inserted through the subcutaneous surface of a bone. External skeletal fixation is especially applicable to unstable open fractures of the pelvis, which have a mortality rate of up to 50 percent. External fixation devices can also maintain fixed traction across an injured joint, thus permitting mobilization of a patient who might not tolerate recumbency.

Skeletal traction often provides a safe provisional or definitive means of stabilizing open fractures for the patient with an isolated injury. Variations on traditional traction techniques can be valuable for the management of open fractures. *Plaster casts* are satisfactory for many open fractures. Military surgeons have popularized open wound treatment under plaster for open fractures. Functional use of the limb is stressed. Wounds can be closed later through a window, or with a cast change, or they can be left open until they heal. However, it is difficult and unpleasant to manage large soft tissue wounds this way in a civilian orthopaedic practice. Early coverage with split-thickness skin is appreciated by patients with large granulating wounds.

Wound Coverage

Whether, when, and how to close an open fracture wound are as controversial as the question of stabilization. Once again, comparative clinical trials do not exist to guide us. Skin closure is dangerous when a wound is contaminated. When host defenses are further compromised by the implantation of foreign material, primary suture seems even more risky, and failure is nearly assured if skin tension is produced by the closure.

It is easy to say that the early goal of open fracture care is to convert the initially contaminated open wound into a clean closed one. Several techniques are advocated for this, ranging from leaving the wound open until it heals secondarily to primary closure with any of a variety of plastic surgical procedures, if simple suture is not possible. While military surgeons maintain their hard-learned tradition of open wound management, a number of civilian traumatologists have presented examples of early closure techniques, which are said to promote wound healing and even fracture union. Several types of pedicle flaps may be used: skin and subcutaneous tissue, muscle alone, or muscle with overlying subcutaneous tissue and skin. Most recently, one or the other of the last two flaps has been done "free," with microvascular anastamoses to local vessels. Split thickness skin graft can be used to cover healthy wound tissue at any time, though it is unsatisfactory over exposed blood vessels, tendons, and bare cortical bone. The multiple perforations produced by a meshing device minimize fluid accumulation under split-thickness grafts.

It is entirely possible to manage severe open fractures without the use of elaborate plastic surgical procedures. Open fractures heal successfully in spite of bone and hardware remaining exposed for periods of several months or more. Furthermore, the severely traumatized limb is usually in no condition for early extensive plastic surgical procedures. Waiting may permit better definition of the "zone of injury," which must be bypassed completely by microvascular anastomoses.

COMPARTMENT SYNDROMES

A variety of injuries can cause progressive elevation of tissue pressure within the confines of "compartments" formed by the normal fascial envelopes around groups of skeletal muscles. Once compartment pressure is elevated sufficiently to block microvascular perfusion, muscle and nerve ischemia leads to necrosis of the involved tissue. Eventually the pressure recedes to normal levels, leaving behind dead muscle and nerve, the cause of Volkmann's contracture.

The key to effective treatment is early diagnosis. This requires suspicion of compartment syndrome whenever an extremity sustains a crushing or severely contusing injury, with or without a fracture. Conscious patients with compartment syndrome develop pain and firm swelling of the entire involved compartment, and soon lose function of the muscles and nerves that lie within it. Pulses and skin perfusion are often normal.

Every two hours, at least, patients with significant extremity injuries must be monitored for inordinate pain and for loss of sensation or motor function distal to the area of injury. Release of any constricting bandage or cast is the essential first step in treatment of a suspected compartment syndrome, to permit examination, and to allow maximal elasticity of the involved compartment. This may reduce pressure sufficiently to restore tissue perfusion and prevent necrosis. If the patient is unconscious or has an associated nerve injury that prevents clinical assessment, compartment pressures are measured with a commercially available wick catheter (or "slit-wick," made from polyeth-

ylene tubing with the terminal end slit about 1 mm longitudinally in several places). This is connected to a sterile strain gauge, as used for monitoring intra-arterial pressure, and is introduced through a large-bore needle into the suspected compartment. A satisfactory measurement system will respond promptly to manual pressure on the compartment, and will fall to a reproducible level soon after such external compression is released. It is important to measure the pressure in *each* compartment of the involved area. For the leg, this means anterior, peroneal, deep posterior, and superficial posterior spaces. In the forearm, both flexor and extensor groups should be assessed at multiple sites.

If neuromuscular findings are perfectly normal, a patient with elevated pressure may be monitored clinically or by repeated pressure measurements. If sensation or contractility is impaired, or if both are unassessable and the compartmental pressure is over 30 to 40 mmHg, fasciotomy is required. All involved compartments must be released. To release the fascial compartments of the leg, I use two incisions. One is anterolateral with identification and preservation of the superficial peroneal nerve, for release of anterior and peroneal compartments. The second is just posterior to the medial tibial shaft, for the deep and superficial compartments. Skin incisions 8 to 10 cm long should permit adequate decompression with minimal tissue damage, with longer fasciotomies using partially opened scissors as a fasciotome. Usually the skin is left open for delayed closure by suture or split-thickness graft. If an associated fracture is present, fixing it at the time of fasciotomy simplifies wound management. Either external or internal skeletal fixation may be used, depending on fracture configuration and the degree of additional soft tissue dissection required.

Compartment syndromes that are recognized after necrosis is far advanced are probably best left closed rather than treated with fasciotomy, because of their very significant risk of infection and the lack of potential benefit from decompressing dead tissue.

FRACTURES AND DISLOCATIONS OF THE SPINE

Initial and subsequent evaluations must deal with two fairly separate issues. The first area of concern is the status of the neural elements: spinal cord and nerve roots (see chapter on Neurologic

Injury.) The second is structural damage to the spine. An injury may involve bone, ligaments, or both. Spine injuries may be stable or unstable. Unstable injuries risk early neurologic damage and/or subsequent mechanical failure with excessive mobility or progressive deformity, either of which might cause late neurologic damage or pain.

Principles of Treatment

The principles that guide treatment of spine injuries are:

1. Consider all injured spines unstable until assessment is complete.
2. Identify unstable injuries, and treat them so as to minimize the risk of neurologic damage and persisting instability.
3. Identify and carefully follow neurologic deficits. Provide treatment that maximizes the potential for neurologic recovery and best facilitates rehabilitation of the patient.
4. Generally speaking, correction of spinal deformity is essential to prevent further mechanical damage to an injured spinal cord. Debridement of the spinal canal anterior to the neural elements may also be required to eliminate continuing compression and promote maximal recovery of an incomplete injury to cord or roots. Laminectomy is of no benefit.
5. If a cord injury is neurologically "complete," attention should be directed toward achievement of a stable well-aligned spine, rather than toward decompression of the neural elements, since no currently available treatment improves neurologic recovery in these patients.
6. Patients with significant spine and cord injuries should be transferred to a spinal cord injury center as soon as this can be done safely, preferably within the first 2 days.

Dislocation or significant angulation can usually be improved by longitudinal traction, which also splints the injured area, minimizing motion that might further damage the cord. If traction is not successful within several hours, open reduction should be considered promptly. After correction of angulation and displacement evident on AP or lateral x-ray films, persisting canal compromise anterior to the cord may be caused by retropulsion of vertebral body bone fragments. These are clearly demonstrated by CAT scans. It is tempting to conclude that they are the cause of any neurologic deficit, and thereby to justify their removal.

Our review of such cases, with and without neural injury, reveals a poor correlation between the degree of canal occlusion and the extent of cord or root injury. This is consistent with the belief that neural injury is due primarily to crushing and contusing sustained at the moment of impact when deformation is greatest. The initial radiographs do not show this maximal deformity, but reveal instead the final resting position of bone fragments and spine once all forces have dissipated.

Cervical Spine

Stabilization

Patients with potentially unstable cervical spine injuries should be transported with the head secured to a spine board. In the emergency room, bilateral sandbags, joined by a strip of 3-inch wide cloth adhesive tape over the forehead, provide the most secure stabilization of the neck. Skeletal traction should be instituted immediately if a cervical cord injury is present, or if an unstable fracture is evident radiographically (angulation greater than 11 degrees or displacement over 3.5 mm at a single level on the lateral radiograph). Five pounds of traction is sufficient to immobilize most injuries in the upper cervical spine, progressing to 10 to 15 pounds for lower cervical injuries. Significantly greater traction, increased in stages with careful radiologic and neurologic monitoring, may be required to reduce a fracture or dislocation. Alignment must be monitored with radiographs, with special attention to the possibility of overdistraction of upper cervical injuries, and to loss of alignment with postural changes.

Gardner-Wells tongs can readily be applied in the Emergency Room by a single surgeon without significant assistance. No shaving is needed. Hair and scalp are soaked with iodophor solution, and the tongs are applied according to the attached instructions with the pins centered over the auditory meati, below the maximal circumference of the head. Lidocaine (1 percent) anesthesia is first injected into the scalp and down to the skull in the appropriate sites. Once the tongs are secure, traction is applied with a rope through a pulley attached to the head of the bed or stretcher. If this is unavailable, the rope is merely passed over the rail at the top of the stretcher.

Although its application is more complicated, the cranial halo is a most valuable device for skull traction, as it can be used not only for traction, but also to provide immobilization by attachment to a plastic vest, or plaster body jacket. This technique provides the most secure external support available for cervical spine injuries and may permit early sitting and ambulation. However, it does not maintain fixed traction. Alignment that requires traction or recumbency can be lost in a halo-vest.

Injuries of the upper cervical spine may be extremely unstable and threaten the medullary respiratory and circulatory centers. Forceful traction may cause additional neural injuries. Patients resuscitated at the scene of injury may have *occipitoatlantal dislocations,* with subtle radiographic signs. Halo-vest immobilization should be applied as soon as possible, and careful radiologic monitoring is needed to identify displacement that may occur even with this support. Arthrodesis will be required, but probably offers little additional early stabilization.

Burst Fractures of the Atlas

Burst fractures of the atlas (Jefferson fractures) may disrupt the transverse atlantal ligament and remain unstable even after the ring fractures unite. Generally, I prefer halo-vest immobilization for 12 weeks, followed by assessment of stability with flexion-extension radiographs, in hopes that if C1–C2 instability persists, union of the posterior arch of C1 will permit fusion at this single level, rather than to the occiput as well.

Odontoid Fractures

Fractures of the odontoid process are controversial. If they involve the narrow waist (sometimes called "base") of the dens, and are displaced, the incidence of nonunion is significant, so that early C1–C2 fusion is often advised. If an anatomic reduction is achieved and maintained with 12 weeks halo-vest or halo-body cast immobilization, a trial of nonoperative treatment seems reasonable, deferring arthrodesis until failure to unite is demonstrated. Fractures of the true base of the dens, which involve significant amounts of the cancellous bone of the C2 vertebral body, usually unite during halo-vest or cast immobilization for 12 weeks. *Fractures of the pedicles of C2* (Hangman's fractures) unite reliably with similar treatment.

Lower Cervical Spine Fractures

Fractures and dislocations of the lower cervical spine can usually be satisfactorily reduced in traction and maintained in alignment until bone and ligament healing are secure enough to provide stability, which must be proved by flexion/extension radiographs following removal of immobilization and restoration of normal neck mobility. Halo-vest treatment with fairly early patient mobilization may be possible. Open reduction may be required, particularly with incomplete posterior ligament disruptions and a unilateral jumped facet joint. A posterior approach provides direct access to the fracture, and permits local posterior fusion once reduction is achieved. Even grossly unstable fractures usually become stable after healing. If the injury is predominantly ligamentous, late instability is more likely, and early arthrodesis deserves consideration to prevent this possibility and the attendant need for arthrodesis and continued restriction of activity while it heals.

Thoracolumbar Spine

Associated thoracoabdominal and extremity injuries may be present and may require immediate treatment. Since physical examination may not reveal the presence or degree of injury to the spine, good-quality radiographs, carefully interpreted, are mandatory. Injuries range from stable wedge compression fractures, through bursting vertebral body fractures with more or less ligamentous disruption, to fracture dislocations that are grossly unstable. Such dislocations may appear deceptively well aligned on a single radiographic projection.

Significant instability is present in thoracolumbar spine injuries if the anterior portion of the vertebral column is so disrupted that it is unlikely to be able to support the compressive load of body weight, or if the posterior complex of bone and ligaments is unlikely to sustain the tensile loads that will be placed on it by normal forward flexion. Instability clearly comes in varying degrees, rather than "all or none."

Surgical treatment for thoracolumbar spine injuries is controversial. Unreduced fracture dislocations and marked angular deformity are certainly reasonable indications. If a neurologic deficit is present, surgery is easier to justify, especially to maximize cauda equina recovery if the neural canal is compromised, as well as to facilitate rehabilitation, to prevent late deformity that may interfere with wheel-chair sitting, and possibly to decrease the risk of late pain. Most thoracolumbar fractures will become stable in 3 months. If no neurologic deficit exists, surgery may only provide mobilization a few weeks earlier.

The gross instability of a *fracture-dislocation* mandates anatomic reduction of the vertebral column and maintenance of alignment during healing. Initially, I attempt this with halo-tibial traction, applied as soon as possible. For adults, 15 to 20 lbs is applied to the halo and a similar weight to each tibia, with careful attention to ensure that traction attachments do not press against insensible skin. Halo-tibial traction is usually best managed on a turning frame, upon which the patient can be anesthetized and operated without additional traumatic transfers. This traction technique provisionally stabilizes the thoracolumbar spine during emergency treatment of associated injuries, which are disturbingly frequent in our patients.

The need for halo-tibial traction can usually be judged from AP and lateral radiographs. A detailed demonstration of the injured area, and of residual deformity, is best provided by a CAT scan, which I prefer to obtain with the patient in traction if marked instability is present. Although the routine transaxial views clearly show retropulsed body fragments, the scout-view or appropriately chosen computer-reconstructed views may be needed to demonstrate angulation and displacement or posterior element injuries. Routine myelography does not appear to be helpful.

When displaced thoracolumbar injuries are initially treated with halo-tibial traction, alignment is usually fairly well achieved. The improved alignment and effective splinting facilitate surgery, which is often indicated for patients with highly unstable spines. Posterior open reduction, stabilization with Harrington instruments, and arthrodesis should generally be performed as soon as the patient's overall condition permits and appropriate personnel and equipment are available.

Postoperatively, halo-tibial traction is discontinued. When wounds are healing, ileus is resolved, and sufficient stability is present, the patient may get up in a plaster or molded plastic body jacket.

Unstable thoracolumbar injuries without marked displacement usually become stable after bone and ligaments have healed—a process that might require 3 or more months. External support alone often fails to provide satisfactory immobilization for these injuries, so that bed rest should also be advised. Individualized treatment is necessary, but I generally plan 6 weeks recumbency, followed by gradually increased ambulation and

sitting in a body jacket or cast. Radiographic monitoring and eventual confirmation of stability are necessary during recovery.

PELVIC RING INJURIES

The pelvic ring consists of the sacrum, both innominate bones, and their sacroiliac and pubic symphysis articulations. Disruptions may be caused by (1) sideways compression, (2) by anterior forces that tend to open the pelvis like a book, and (3) by vertically directed shearing forces, typically a fall from a significant height. Although the anterior ring disruption through pubic rami or symphysis pubis tends to be obvious on an AP pelvic radiograph, more careful inspection is necessary to identify the site of posterior injury. Yet such posterior disruption must be present for the ring to be displaced anteriorly. The posterior injury is generally the more significant, and its precise identification is necessary to permit appropriate treatment; 45-degree downshot ("pelvic inlet") and 45-degree upshot ("tangential") radiographs demonstrate displacement clearly. A CAT scan shows the posterior lesion especially well, but does not reveal longitudinal displacement. Posterior pelvic ring injuries may involve, singly or in combination, the sacral wing, the ilium, or the sacroiliac joint. The SI joint can be totally disrupted or merely hinged open on its stout posterior-superior ligaments.

Instability of a pelvic ring injury can be inferred from radiographs that show gross displacement. Even minimally displaced injuries can be significantly unstable, however. Physical examination is required to evaluate ring stability. Significant instability is present if either or both iliac wings can be moved by manual force applied mediolaterally to the anterior iliac crests.

Pelvic ring injuries pose several problems. Retroperitoneal bleeding from the fracture surfaces and adjacent blood vessels may be life-threatening. Associated abdominal and thoracic injuries are common and often serious. Urologic trauma, especially ruptures of bladder or posterior urethra, may be present. Neurologic injury, usually involving the sacral nerve roots, may occur as well. In addition to the sequelae of these injuries, pelvic deformity and pain may persist to cause permanent disability. Open pelvic fractures have exceptionally high morbidity and mortality.

Initial management of a pelvic ring injury requires hemodynamic monitoring and stabilization, with identification and appropriate treatment of associated injuries. Catheterization, preceded by urethrography, if indicated, and a cystogram are routine. If one hemipelvis is displaced proximally, 15 to 30 lbs skeletal traction should be applied via a Steinmann pin in the tibial tubercle. Done early, this decreases motion at the site of injury and usually restores pelvic symmetry.

External Skeletal Fixation

Unstable pelvic ring fractures should usually be treated by early stabilization. The traditional pelvic sling fails to provide this and may increase deformity if medial displacement is possible. A spica cast offers considerable external support, but it is cumbersome and interferes with mobilization of the patient. Internal fixation is advocated by some authors, but it is not always possible and is accused of frequent failures. External skeletal fixation permits early, rapid, and minimally invasive stabilization of most pelvic ring injuries. By controlling motion at the site of injury and by restoring the normal close confines of the true pelvis, bleeding may be staunched. Pain relief is often dramatic. Unless posterior disruption is complete with obvious vertical shear displacement, traction is omitted, and early mobilization of the patient may be possible. However, with an anteriorly attached pelvic external fixator, vertical shear injuries can displace. To avoid this, additional protection is generally required, with bed rest and traction on the involved side for several weeks.

I believe that external pelvic fixation significantly facilitates the management of patients with unstable pelvic ring injuries, and I recommend that it be used whenever examination demonstrates pelvic instability or radiographs show significant displacement. The fixator should be applied as early as possible, immediately after any indicated laparotomy, or as soon as initial evaluation is complete and before development of an extensive retroperitoneal hematoma, which it may help to contain.

One must occasionally choose between application of an external fixator and arteriography with embolization to control arterial bleeding, if it is seen. Unless rapid volume replacement shows little or no response, I would recommend external fixation first, because bleeding from fracture and veins often responds to external fixation and volume replacement. If this fails to control hemorrhage adequately, arteriography is the next appropriate step and it is not compromised by the presence of the fixator.

The fixator must be applied in the operating room with sterile preparation and draping. Depending on the ease of demonstrating the iliac crests, the exact insertion site chosen, and the surgeon's experience, pins may be placed percutaneously or with small insertions to permit placement of thumb and index finger on opposite sides of the ilium for precise control of the pins. I prefer at least three (5-mm diameter) pins, inserted deeply into each ilium. They should not tent the surrounding skin, which may be left open, if needed to avoid this problem. A number of configurations have been proposed for the external frame used to connect the iliac crest pin clusters. It should be as rigid as possible and must not impinge on the abdomen or the skin near the pin insertion sites. Triangular cross-bracing helps to prevent displacement, as does adjustment of the frame to maintain a compressive force across the posterior ring injury, which must be reduced as well as possible at the time of fixator application.

In contrast to reports of late pain and disability following significant pelvic ring injuries managed with traditional techniques, external pelvic fixation appears to offer an improved long-term result. In our experience, anatomic reduction of pelvic ring injuries has not always been maintained by external fixation, but no significant complications have so far resulted from our use of the technique.

SHOULDER INJURIES

Shoulder trauma may cause neurovascular injuries. A careful physical examination is as necessary as high-quality radiographs for complete assessment of the patient with an injured shoulder.

Clavicular Injuries

Sternoclavicular Dislocations

Sternoclavicular (SC) dislocations are either posterior or anterior. Although they are not obvious on routine radiographs, physical examination demonstrates asymmetry, swelling, and tenderness. Signs of respiratory or vascular compromise may be present in some patients with posterior SC dislocations. A closed, manipulative reduction is almost always possible, although anesthesia and muscle relaxation may be required. The technique is as follows. Lateral traction is applied to the clavicle. With a narrow sandbag between the scapulae of the supine patient, backward pressure on the anterior aspects of the shoulders produces scapular retraction and distraction of the overriding sternoclavicular joint. Percutaneous manipulation of the clavicle with a stout sterile towel clip may be required. Posterior sternoclavicular dislocations that do not respond to closed manipulation should be reduced open, with appropriate thoracic surgical assistance, because associated mediastinal complications are common and may persist if the clavicle remains dislocated. Once reduced, posterior SC dislocations are usually stable. A figure-of-8 dressing is worn for 4 to 6 weeks to prevent shoulder protraction.

Reduction of anterior sternoclavicular dislocations is usually easy with forcible retraction of the shoulder, but may be difficult to maintain. The complications of internal fixation exceed the problems of a chronic dislocation, however. Therefore, I attempt an initial reduction, but counsel the patient to accept redisplacement of an anterior SC dislocation, deferring resection of the medial end of the clavicle for those few cases that remain symptomatic after several months of rehabilitation.

Clavicle Fractures

Clavicle fractures practically always heal unless open reduction is performed. Deformity is common, but while occasionally unsightly, almost never compromises function. A figure-of-8 bandage and sling usually provide enough support to minimize early discomfort and can be discarded as soon as the patient wishes. Efforts should be directed toward early and complete shoulder rehabilitation.

Acromioclavicular Separations

Some authors advocate repair of complete AC separations. I am unimpressed with the functional deficit that results from this injury. Primary surgical repair, with or without reconstruction of the coracoclavicular ligaments, is not free of complications, including failure to achieve the desired result. Therefore, I prefer to accept the anatomic deformity, unless it is severe, and concentrate instead on shoulder rehabilitation, which usually takes only a few weeks. Those few patients who remain symptomatic may be candidates for sub-

periosteal resection of the distal clavicle, with careful reefing of the local soft tissues to minimize residual prominence.

Shoulder Dislocations

Anterior dislocations are usually obvious by their asymmetry, deformity, and typical AP radiographic appearance. Posterior dislocations, while much less common, are frequently overlooked, perhaps because the deformity is less obvious, but primarily because of overreliance on the AP radiograph, which looks deceptively normal. A crucial physical finding in posterior shoulder dislocation is absence of external rotation of the humerus. If external rotation is limited, posterior dislocation must be excluded with an adequate lateral radiograph.

Once diagnosed, a shoulder dislocation should be reduced as soon as possible. Many techniques are described. Closed manipulation almost always suffices, but the total muscle relaxation provided with general anesthesia may be required. I usually reduce anterior dislocations of the shoulder by manual traction on the humerus, using countertraction on the chest with a sheet, if needed. Preliminary analgesia and muscle relaxation are valuable aids.

Following reduction, shoulder alignment and integrity are confirmed by adequate AP and lateral radiographs, a sling and swath or commercial shoulder immobilizer is applied, and the patient is observed until he is clearly recovered from any medications. The length of immobilization for a first dislocation depends primarily on the age of the patient. Because of their high risk of recurrence, 6 weeks is appropriate for young adults. Older individuals are more at risk of limited motion and should be mobilized sooner (within 3 weeks if over 40), beginning with pendulum exercises, but avoiding external rotation stresses for several weeks after injury. Recurrent dislocations need be immobilized only long enough for comfort. If redislocations are frequent enough to trouble the patient, elective shoulder repair should be advised.

Posterior shoulder dislocations can usually be reduced with traction along the humerus, similar to that for anterior dislocations, after muscle relaxation is adequate. Immobilization after reduction is best done with a wide adhesive tape that surrounds the supracondylar region and is attached to the back so that the elbow cannot move anterior to the coronal plane of the body.

Fractures of the Proximal Humerus

These injuries may be isolated or associated with dislocation. A number of factors influence treatment, including amount of comminution and of displacement, whether or not soft tissue attachments to the humeral head are sufficient to maintain its blood supply, and whether or not bone quality is sufficiently adequate to permit surgical fixation. Dislocations require urgent treatment. If the problem is a fracture, temporary mobilization of the multiply injured patient can be obtained by supporting his shoulder with a sling and swath, deferring definitive care until the patient's general condition permits, although delay beyond 7 to 10 days increases the difficulty of surgery and may compromise the result. *Proximal humerus fractures with little or no displacement* usually heal reliably with sling and swath immobilization and proceed quite rapidly to the rehabilitation phase of treatment. Fortunately, most proximal humerus fractures fall into this category. Many displaced fractures of the neck of the humerus can be aligned satisfactorily with skeletal traction, applied to a screw or threaded pin inserted in the olecranon. Care must be taken to avoid the ulnar nerve and the elbow joint and to ensure secure bone fixation. The traction is arranged so that the forearm hangs over the head of the supine patient, supported by an additional fixed sling. The pull is adjusted so that the shoulder girdle is just barely lifted off the mattress. This technique usually provides satisfactory alignment of proximal humeral fractures, but it requires several weeks of recumbency and may compromise the overall care of the multiply injured patient. A similar position can be maintained, though not quite as stably, with a shoulder spica cast, which is rarely acceptable for a non-ambulatory patient or one with additional injuries. The remaining options for such patients are open reduction and internal fixation (ORIF), primary proximal humeral replacement with reconstruction of the rotator cuff and its attachments to the humeral shaft (Neer hemi-arthroplasty), closed reduction with percutaneous pinning, and deferral of treatment of the shoulder injury until the patient's condition permits definitive treatment.

Comminuted fractures and fracture dislocations of the proximal humerus that remove all soft tissue attachments from the humeral head (four-part, displaced fractures) have a significant risk of avascular necrosis of the humeral head, with resulting pain and limited motion. Reconstruction-arthroplasty is advisable primarily for most patients with these injuries. Displaced fractures of greater or lesser tuberosities require repair to prevent impingement and to restore rotator cuff integrity.

The ultimate result of a serious shoulder injury is often determined by how soon and how effectively the patient is able to begin range-of-motion exercises. Any treatment that requires prolonged immobilization of the arm is likely to result in permanent loss of mobility. When comminution is marked or bone is osteoporotic, internal fixation offers unreliable stability. Avascular necrosis and nonunion may follow extensive stripping of soft-tissue attachments in an effort to improve fixation.

HUMERAL SHAFT FRACTURES

Fractures of the shaft of the humerus can be accompanied by radial nerve palsy. This usually occurs at the time of injury, but may develop subsequently if the injured limb is inadequately splinted and occasionally after manipulative reduction. In our experience, these radial nerve palsies resolve during closed treatment of the humeral shaft fracture.

Almost all humeral shaft fractures are amenable to closed treatment. If the injury is isolated and the patient ambulatory, a light-weight hanging-arm cast or a U-shaped coaptation splint, changed frequently to maintain fit and alignment, provides adequate fracture control during the 3 or 4 weeks required for consolidation. Difficulties arise when the patient is multiply injured or must remain recumbent. Gravity no longer helps to keep the fracture reduced. Malunion and perhaps nonunion become more likely. Overhead olecranon traction, as described for proximal humerus fractures, offers a possible solution, but interferes with mobilization and nursing of a multiply injured patient. Intramedullary nailing, with open or closed reduction of the fracture, is a possible answer for some patients. Open reduction with plate fixation is another alternative. It offers an opportunity to explore the radial nerve (if this is believed indicated), to obtain secure rotational control, and to bone graft an extensively comminuted fracture. Because plating of the humeral shaft requires significant stripping of the fracture site, it may hinder bone union. Yet another alternative for the management of humeral shaft fractures in polytraumatized patients or those with significant soft tissue injuries is external skeletal fixation. Half-pins are inserted laterally, taking care to avoid the axillary nerve and posterior humeral circumflex artery proximally and the radial nerve distally. Open pin placement may be required for safety. Such external fixation is minimally invasive, does not significantly encumber the patient, and usually provides satisfactory fracture control. It is generally my first choice for humeral shaft fractures in multiply injured patients who cannot be treated satisfactorily by nonoperative means.

ELBOW INJURIES

Elbow fractures and dislocations may have associated neurovascular injuries and may cause forearm ischemia due to arterial occlusion, compartment syndrome, or both. Resulting Volkmann's contracture is seriously disabling and should be prevented by careful attention to early diagnosis and appropriate treatment of neuromuscular ischemia. Forearm pain, impaired sensation, and loss of motor function are the important signs of problems. They should not be ascribed to nerve injuries until it is clear that perfusion is adequate (p. 5). Elbow injuries should be splinted in moderate flexion, since forced extension or flexion may compromise the nerves and vessels crossing the joint. No attempt at reduction is appropriate until satisfactory radiographs have been obtained. If skin damage is present, the possibility of early operative treatment must be considered, because intra-articular elbow fractures frequently do require surgery, and delay may compromise the result.

Elbow dislocations should be reduced promptly, with adequate analgesia and muscle relaxation. An assistant holds the humerus stable while the surgeon exerts manual traction on the forearm, with the elbow moderately flexed, and corrects medial or lateral displacement as required. Following reduction, stability is assessed by checking range of motion and exerting varus and valgus stress on the extended elbow. If the medial collateral ligament is intact and the joint remains located throughout its range, a long-arm splint is needed only briefly. If mobilization can begin within a few days, when the patient is comfortable, recovery is swifter and possibly more complete.

If the elbow is unstable, movement must be deferred until soft tissue healing is well under way— usually 3 weeks after injury. Furthermore, there is some risk of early redislocation unless the joint is immobilized in more than 90-degree flexion. A long arm cast or splint actually offers marginal protection for an unstable elbow injury. Increasing flexion and preventing shoulder motion by securing the arm to the chest augments its effectiveness. Before applying any radiopaque splint or cast, postreduction films should be obtained to confirm satisfactory reduction and to check for any associated fractures.

Displaced fractures of the elbow joint are often best treated by surgery. Those of the distal humerus can offer formidable challenges. Postoperative complications, including inability to achieve sufficient fixation for early motion, may lead to a result no better than that achieved by overhead olecranon traction and motion as tolerated in such a device. In the absence of extensive experience with internal fixation of distal humerus fractures, when comminution is extreme, or when extensive soft tissue injury is also present, traction deserves serious consideration. If multiple injuries preclude its use, external fixation across the elbow joint may maintain alignment while permitting the patient (but not the elbow) to be mobilized.

Olecranon fractures tend to separate because of the pull of the triceps on the proximal fragment. If displacement occurs, repair is advisable with either ORIF or excision of proximal fragments and triceps reattachment. Olecranon fractures associated with subluxation or dislocation of the elbow joint are much more extensive injuries. The distal humerus has been driven posteriorly through the olecranon: ligaments are disrupted, and there is often marked comminution of the distal olecranon, which may involve the coronoid process. Incongruity of the radiocapitellar joint is evident on the lateral radiograph. A radial head fracture may be present. Treatment of these injuries must be directed at restoration of elbow alignment and maintenance of stability during the first few weeks of healing. Internal fixation is often tenuous. Radiographs should be monitored to ensure that redisplacement, if it occurs, is identified promptly.

Radial head fractures are painful injuries that usually respond well to early active mobilization. Aspiration of a tense painful elbow hemarthrosis and injection of a local anesthetic provide immediate relief. A splint and sling applied for the first few days should be removed as soon as possible to encourage early movement. Only comminuted displaced radial head fractures are candidates for early excision.

FOREARM FRACTURES

Open reduction and internal fixation with plates and screws constitute the standard treatment for displaced *fractures of the radius and ulna* in adults. Satisfactory initial immobilization is usually obtainable with a well-padded splint or cast, and unless the fracture is open or ischemia develops, fixation can be done semi-electively during the week or so after injury, but becomes progressively more difficult with much further delay.

It is important to assess the elbow and wrist of a patient with a forearm fracture. If a *displaced fracture of either radius or ulna* is present without fracture or plastic deformation of the adjacent forearm bone, there must be damage to the proximal or distal radioulnar joint. With ulnar fractures, dislocation is at the elbow, with displacement of the radial head from the capitellum as well—the so-called Monteggia fracture. Isolated radial shaft fractures may have associated injuries of the distal radioulnar joint—Galeazzi's fracture. Successful treatment of both these injuries reduces the joint disruption, as well as the fracture, and maintains alignment during healing and mobilization. In adults, ORIF of the diaphyseal fracture and, occasionally, open joint repair are necessary.

Isolated radial shaft fractures, even without distal radioulnar joint disruption, are poorly controlled with casts, and therefore should generally be repaired. External fixation is an option for severely contaminated wounds. Intramedullary nailing is possible, but not always technically satisfactory. Functional bracing has also been proposed as an alternative when the distal radioulnar joint is intact.

Isolated ulnar shaft fractures may require surgery, but I believe that most can be managed more efficiently in other ways. A long arm cast significantly impedes use of the arm and seems to delay union of these fractures. With minimal immobilization, most will unite rapidly. For isolated minimally displaced fractures of the distal two-thirds or so of the ulna, I apply a long arm splint for the first few days until swelling has receded, and then support the forearm with a snugly molded sleeve of plaster from below the elbow to the wrist. This is applied with the forearm fully supinated. Activity, including wrist and elbow motion, is encour-

aged, and healing generally occurs within 6 weeks. For more proximal fractures or those with more intrinsic instability, intramedullary nailing often provides a satisfactory means of control. The need for postoperative support is usually minimal.

WRIST INJURIES

Fractures of the distal radius are the most common injuries in this region, but other less obvious ones may prove equally disabling. Careful examination and thorough interpretation of adequate AP and lateral radiographs are essential to distinguish fracture-dislocations from purely metaphyseal injuries, and to avoid missing distal radioulnar dislocations as well as fractures and dislocations of the carpals. Since the initial physical findings of a wrist injury may appear minimal in patients with other serious trauma, and because their arms rapidly become encumbered with IVs, wrist radiographs must be obtained upon the slightest suspicion of injury.

Fractures of the distal radius range greatly in severity. If comminution is marked or either radiocarpal or distal radioulnar articular surfaces are involved, poorer results are likely. Although closed reduction and appropriately molded plaster cast suffice for the less severe cases, pins and plaster, external fixation, or, rarely, internal fixation might be required to maintain nearly normal anatomy. Casts applied to severely injured wrists frequently need to be loosened to accommodate swelling. During this period, maintenance of reduction is secondary to preservation of blood flow. If an initial closed reduction proves unstable, it can be followed later by a more extensive procedure. If there is palmar or dorsal displacement of the carpus and an attached fragment of distal radius, ORIF may be necessary.

Carpal dislocations usually involve the lunate and its attachments to radius, capitate, or both. An associated scaphoid fracture may be present or the scapho-lunate ligaments may be ruptured. Dislocation is best diagnosed on the lateral wrist radiograph. A prompt closed reduction is usually successful with fingertrap distraction and manipulation. This should be done as soon as possible to minimize swelling and neurovascular compromise. These are unstable injuries, however, so that open reduction and internal fixation often are needed to maintain alignment as well as for reduction if closed manipulation fails.

Carpal fractures without dislocation or persistent displacement should be managed closed initially. A short arm splint alone is sufficient for the first few days. The thumb is included for scaphoid fractures. If reduction is satisfactory, the splint is replaced with a cast once swelling has abated.

FRACTURES AND JOINT INJURIES OF THE HAND

Hand injuries are readily ignored in polytrauma patients. Yet their inadequate early treatment can result in significant permanent disability. Therefore the hands must be carefully evaluated for fractures and joint injuries as well as damage to skin, neurovascular structures, and tendons. Stiffness, the most common complication after hand fractures, is best avoided by the early achievement of skeletal stability and prompt range-of-motion exercises. Closed treatment is often possible with isolated injuries. More severe, multiple, or intra-articular fractures may require internal fixation. If immobilization is employed, it should be in a safe position, with the metacarpophalangeal joints flexed nearly 90 degrees, the interphalangeal joints nearly extended, and the thumb in opposition, anterior to the hand. The fate of the whole hand should not be compromised by ill-advised immobilization to treat a single joint or digit.

Interphalangeal dislocations can usually be reduced closed, but may be unstable and require splinting for a brief period. Dislocations of the finger metacarpophalangeal joints usually require open reduction. Those of the thumb might. The metacarpophalangeal joint of the thumb is prone to sprains, especially of its ulnar collateral ligament. If the joint is unstable, ligament repair may be required. The carpometacarpal joints of the thumb and of the little and ring fingers are quite unstable after dislocation or fracture-dislocation. Closed reduction is usually possible, but percutaneous pinning may be needed to maintain it.

HIP INJURIES

Acetabular Fractures

Acetabular fractures are a major area of interest in orthopaedic traumatology. Traditional reluctance to undertake open reduction and internal fixation is being challenged, but treatment remains controversial. Like pelvic ring fractures, which

may also be present, acetabular fractures are usually caused by high-energy trauma and can be accompanied by life-threatening hemorrhage and other serious thoracoabdominal or extremity injuries. The whole patient must not be obscured by concern for the acetabular fracture. The presence of an acetabular injury is generally evident on the routine screening AP radiograph of the pelvis, if not on physical exam. Its precise definition requires 45-degree right and left oblique views of the entire involved innominate bone and is greatly facilitated by CAT scans with appropriate parasagittal and paracoronal reconstructions.

If the femoral head is dislocated—posteriorly, centrally, or, rarely, anteriorly—a closed reduction is performed as soon as possible. I prefer to do this under general anesthesia, with adequate muscle relaxation. Skeletal traction is instituted via a pin in the tibial tubercle. Radiographic assessment is then completed. If there is incongruity of the weight-bearing portion of the hip joint, if traction cannot maintain a satisfactory reduction, or if fragments of bone are interposed between the articular surfaces, open reduction and internal fixation must be considered. These procedures require extensive exposure, with risk of infection, hemorrhage, and neurovascular injury. An alternative to ORIF is continued traction for the 3 months generally required for union, followed by total hip arthroplasty if and when the patient's symptoms warrant. If displacement is severe, there can be significant problems anchoring the acetabular component of a total hip prosthesis, a factor that should be considered in the choice of early treatment.

Nonoperative treatment is appropriate for undisplaced acetabular fractures. I prefer traction for those that have an intact weight-bearing articulation or are in older patients with adequate bone stock for total hip arthroplasty. For others, I advise ORIF by a well-prepared team of experienced surgeons. This should be delayed until the patient's overall condition permits, but it becomes significantly more difficult with increasing delay, especially after 2 weeks.

Hip Dislocations

Hip dislocations without acetabular fractures should also be reduced as soon and as gently as possible to minimize the risks of avascular necrosis and further damage to the articular surface. If at all possible, I prefer general anesthesia with muscle relaxation, which permits reliable assessment of stability as well. The dislocated hip can be reduced immediately after endotracheal intubation and minimally delays any other necessary procedures. On those rare occasions when closed reduction is unsuccessful, prompt open reduction is required. Postreduction x-ray studies must confirm anatomic reduction of the femoral head. If there is any sign of incongruity, I obtain a CAT scan to search for intra-articular fragments that will require arthrotomy for removal.

If the hip is stable after reduction, rest in 5-lb Buck's traction with the hip extended is advised until the patient is able to control the limb comfortably. At this point, crutch walking is begun, with progressive weight bearing. If the hip is not stable, several weeks of traction will be required before mobilization.

Proximal Femur Fractures

Hip fractures are often the results of a minor fall. They tend to be more severe in the victims of high-energy accidents and, until internally fixed, significantly compromise the patient's mobility. Even in closed injuries local blood loss may cause shock.

Femoral Neck Fractures

Femoral neck fractures may occur in isolation or together with a fracture of the femoral shaft. Often initially undisplaced, they must be looked for carefully on the pelvic x-ray examination of every multiply injured patient. Especially in young persons, femoral neck fractures have a high incidence of nonunion and of avascular necrosis of the femoral head. Treatment is surgical, with the hip protected in splint or traction until it can be carried out. I attempt closed reduction and fixation with multiple pins or cancellous screws inserted under fluoroscopic control. If an adequate closed reduction cannot be obtained, arthrotomy and open reduction, possibly with posterior bone graft, should be performed in those under 50 years of age whereas older patients are more appropriately candidates for hemiarthroplasty.

Intertrochanteric Fractures

Intertrochanteric fractures are also best managed by internal fixation, as soon as possible in multiply injured patients. Union and femoral head survival rarely are problems, but difficulty in nursing the patient in traction for 3 to 4 months and malunion of fractures mobilized earlier can be avoided if internal fixation is used. Modern compression hip screw devices have proved reliable in our hands. After fixation, the wound should be debrided of traumatized muscle, irrigated copiously, and closed over suction drains to minimize the risk of infection.

Subtrochanteric Fractures

Subtrochanteric fractures must be considered separately because of their association with high-energy trauma and because of their well-recognized incidence of nonunion and fixation failure. These fractures involve the proximal femur from the trochanteric region down to an arbitrary 10 cm below the lesser trochanter. Below this level, intramedullary nailing techniques for femoral shaft fractures are usually reliable. Treatment of a subtrochanteric fracture must be individualized, and the patient must be followed until bone union is secure, for failure, when it occurs, is often not seen until 4 to 6 months after injury. In healthy individuals with isolated injuries, traction may be considered for subtrochanteric fractures if a satisfactory alignment is achievable. It is usually followed with a 1½ spica cast or a single abducted spica cast-brace for the several months required to complete healing. Internal fixation generally facilitates early management and is preferable for the multiply injured patient. Several techniques are available. Condylocephalic nailing appears attractive, but in our experience often requires opening the fracture site to obtain reduction and to permit passage of the nail into a satisfactory position. When the trochanteric region is intact, the Zickel nail provides good fixation and is stout enough to outlast a delayed union. However, comminution of the greater trochanter zone is frequently present. For this reason, I think the compression hip screw is the most adaptable device for these injuries. It must be used carefully, with achievement of a stable reduction or with supplementary bone graft.

FEMORAL SHAFT FRACTURES

These injuries are usually due to significant force. The possibility of associated trauma must always be remembered. A radiograph of the pelvis is mandatory to avoid missing a fracture or dislocation involving the hip. Tenderness, swelling, or radiographic abnormalities may indicate injury to the knee. Blood loss into the fracture site may cause shock. The considerable pain of a femoral shaft fracture can be controlled partially by traction-splinting. If operative treatment will not be carried out within a few hours, skeletal traction should be instituted via a Steinmann pin in the tibial tubercle, or the distal femur if the knee is injured. Twenty to 30 lbs are required, depending on the muscularity of the patient.

Several options are available for the definitive management of femoral shaft fractures. The traditional use of skeletal traction until consolidation occurs, followed by a spica cast until union is secure, is rarely acceptable in adults. Early use of a cast brace, perhaps with intermittent traction via an incorporated tibial pin, is one alternative that can permit early patient mobilization, but poses some difficulties with maintenance of reduction. A snugly molded cast-brace applied with the leg in traction, wedging the thigh plaster as needed, and using an abduction hip hinge may prevent loss of alignment. Internal fixation of femoral shaft fractures with plates or open intramedullary nailing have high complication rates compared with closed intramedullary nail fixation, which I prefer for most such injuries. In multiply injured patients, this should be done as soon as possible, preferably during the first anesthetic. The risk of infection in open fractures is probably decreased by initial irrigation and debridement, with skeletal traction through delayed primary wound closure and early soft tissue healing. Closed intramedullary nailing is then done 10 to 14 days after the initial injury. If the femoral shaft fracture is comminuted, an intramedullary nail alone may not prevent rotation or shortening. The former is readily controlled with a light single spica cast. Circumferentially comminuted fractures will shorten without postoperative traction, supplementary internal fixation, or a modified, "interlocking" nail, with proximal and distal screw transfixion. Another valuable alternative to traction for badly comminuted fractures and those with severe soft tissue damage is external skeletal fixation with the Wagner "leg-lengthening" device.

KNEE INJURIES

Mobility, trustworthy stability, and absence of pain are necessary for normal knee function. To regain these after injury, bone and articular cartilage anatomy, ligament function, and muscle strength must all be restored. Depending on the specific injuries, this may require fracture reduction, ligament and/or tendon repair, repair or excision of a damaged meniscus, and rehabilitation to regain motion, strength, and agility. It must always be remembered that high-energy knee injuries—dislocations and badly displaced fractures—may damage the popliteal artery, with amputation the potential complication.

Fractures of the distal femur can seriously compromise knee function. If displaced or angulated, they require accurate reduction. ORIF may be necessary. Properly selected fractures can be managed in traction or with cast-brace and early motion. If articular surface displacement cannot be corrected, ORIF is indicated if the condition of the patient and soft tissues permits. These procedures may be demanding. I prefer a wide anterolateral exposure and use a 95-degree blade plate or condylar buttress plate, depending on the extent of comminution. Bone grafting is often advisable.

Patellar fractures that are displaced require repair to restore quadriceps continuity. If the articular surface can be reconstructed, ORIF is done with K-wires and tension band, interfragmentary wiring, or screws. If comminution prevents ORIF, a partial or total patellectomy is indicated with repair of the quadriceps mechanism, including torn retinacular expansions.

Meniscus tears may be either peripheral or within the substance of the semilunar fibrocartilage. The former should be reattached. The latter may require partial or possibly total meniscectomy. But in the absence of other indications for arthrotomy, treatment can be postponed until it is clear that the patient is symptomatic. Diagnostic and surgical arthroscopy are playing an increasing role in the evaluation and treatment of acute knee injuries.

If *knee dislocation* is present, it should be reduced promptly with axial traction and manipulation as needed. Arteriograms are routinely obtained. *Penetrating injuries* of this superficial joint require arthrotomy for irrigation, removal of retained foreign material, and debridement of any osteochondral fracture fragments.

Obvious *ligamentous instability* usually needs surgical repair. Examination will reveal varus or valgus laxity in collateral ligament ruptures. Posterior cruciate ruptures often, but not always, show posterior mobility of tibia on femur. This may be produced by the force of gravity on the flexed knee and should be looked for carefully with the leg in this position. Remember that apparently stable knees with acute post-traumatic hemarthroses usually have sustained a significant injury, most often disruption of the anterior cruciate ligament. While treatment of such patients is controversial, many advocate early surgical repair of anterior cruciate ligament disruptions in young and active patients. Frequently this is done with intra-articular augmentation using local tendon grafts such as the semitendinous or a portion of the patellar ligament.

Fractures of the tibial plateau split off part of the articular surface, depress a portion of it with an impacted fracture of the underlying cancellous bone, or combine these two modes of injury. Depending on the stability of the knee to stress examination in extension and the degree of deformity of the articular surface, treatment may require open reduction, with elevation and bone grafting of any depressed area. Alternatives include traction arranged to permit early motion, cast brace, and plaster cast. For best results, treatment should permit early motion, whereas weight bearing is deferred until healing is secure.

FRACTURES OF THE TIBIA AND FIBULA

These common fractures are frequently open, may have associated nerve or vessel injuries, including compartment syndrome, and vary greatly in severity. The appropriate treatment for an isolated, minimally displaced spiral fracture of the tibia is rarely the best for a transverse, comminuted, Grade 3 open fracture in a multiply injured patient. Occasionally an open tibia fracture is so badly injured that reconstruction, even if technically possible, will take so long and offer such unpredictable results that the patient might reasonably prefer a below-knee amputation.

Although tibial shaft fractures with intact fibulae usually indicate a milder injury, they may have a higher incidence of varus deformity and delayed union. When only the fibula is fractured, it is important to evaluate both knee and ankle carefully, as this generally innocuous fracture may be associated with a collateral ligament injury of either joint.

Many treatments are advocated for tibial shaft fractures. Before choosing one, the patient, his other medical problems, and the extent of injury to the soft tissues must be considered, in addition to the fracture's radiographic appearance. Many tibial fractures can be managed perfectly adequately in a plaster cast or fracture brace, usually with early weight bearing. I prefer a long leg (knee flexed 10 to 15 degrees) plaster initially, with subsequent conversion to a "PTB" if the fracture is in the distal half or a hinged knee cast brace if it is more proximal. Healing usually requires about 4 months. Open wounds may be very difficult to care for in a cast. Windows and multiple cast changes frequently compromise wound care, fracture alignment, and patient mobilization. External skeletal fixation permits wound access and sufficient bone stability for early mobilization, but risks pin wound complications and delayed union. The former can be minimized by using half-pin fixation inserted through the subcutaneous border of the tibia instead of transfixion pins that perforate the leg muscles. Early aggressive bone grafting may be required to prevent the latter. Another approach is to discontinue external fixation as soon as the wounds are healed and manage the fracture with external support. Plate fixation of tibia fractures can be very helpful. It offers a reliable way of stabilizing a highly comminuted fracture for wound care and patient mobilization. However, weight bearing must be delayed, and wound complications, including sloughs and infections, are unfortunately common. Therefore I generally restrict the use of plates to situations in which a metaphyseal or intra-articular fracture requires anatomic reconstruction or in which an extensive wound is already present, so that further dissection is minimal, and fracture comminution prevents adequate stabilization with external fixation or intramedullary rods.

Intramedullary rodding of suitable tibial shaft fractures is a very promising technique. *Unreamed* nails should probably always be used for fresh fractures, definitely if the fracture is open. Although Lottes's nail is acceptable, I prefer two flexible, unreamed rods (Ender nails) inserted from the medial and lateral surfaces of the proximal metaphysis into corresponding positions inside the cortical bone of the distal metaphysis. Some motion may persist at the fracture, but it is well controlled, and alignment is readily maintained. A splint or cast worn initially can usually be discarded within 6 weeks, and weight bearing is generally well tolerated early after injury, a major benefit for patients with bilateral injuries or upper extremity problems that preclude crutches. I think complications are less frequent with this technique than with any other for tibial shaft fractures and I advocate it whenever skeletal fixation is needed and the fracture is neither too comminuted nor too close to either end of the bone.

ANKLE INJURIES

Congruity and stability are both required for normal function of this weight-bearing joint. Injuries are common and may be open or closed. Fractures and ligament ruptures are often combined. Additionally, important tendons, nerves, and blood vessels cross the ankle; all are at risk of injury that should be readily identifiable. AP, lateral, and mortise radiographs are essential for evaluation of ankle injuries.

Fractures of the distal tibia may involve the malleoli or may disrupt the horizontal tibial plafond. Malleolar fractures may be undisplaced and stable, minimally displaced and acceptably aligned, or significantly displaced. Whether or not the talus is normally located under the plafond is the major issue, for the contact area between the two is seriously reduced by only a slight sideways shift of the talus. Fractures disrupting the weight-bearing surface of the plafond are usually obvious and may be severe. When the condition of patient and soft tissues permits, anatomic reconstruction of the articular surface and precise realignment of the talus with the mating tibia are key steps toward recovery of normal ankle function. This can require extensive exposure, with risk of skin slough and infection. An alternative is traction via the calcaneus or fixed distraction with an external fixator or pins-and-plaster from tibia to calcaneus. If at all possible, after repair, early motion (but delayed weight-bearing) seems to improve the prognosis of severe injuries. I think movement should be delayed until the patient is able to do it comfortably, and that the ankle must be splinted in a neutral position initially to avoid development of an equinus contracture.

Ligament injuries most commonly involve the lateral collateral. Initial treatment is with a well-padded splint that holds the ankle in neutral. Severe sprains should be protected in a short leg cast for 6 weeks. The medial collateral (deltoid) ligament is rarely injured in isolation, but may be one component of a significantly unstable "bimalleolar" injury when the fibular fracture is much more obvious on x-ray examination. In addition to the status of the malleoli and collateral ligaments, it is essential to assess the syndesmotic ligaments that bind together the distal tibia and fibula. Mortise widening, permitted by syndesmosis disruption, requires temporary internal fixation of the distal fibula to the tibia.

Undisplaced malleolar ankle fractures can often be treated satisfactorily in plaster, but some of these are unstable and will lose alignment. Careful radiographic monitoring through the cast will demonstrate this and permit timely repair. Most *displaced bimalleolar injuries* can be well reduced closed. Subsequent loss of reduction in plaster is so common that I generally prefer ORIF for these patients. An additional benefit is the ability to avoid a long leg cast, and often to permit earlier weight bearing.

When soft tissue condition, multiple injuries, or other factors contraindicate ORIF of very unstable malleolar fractures, a helpful maneuver is transfixion of the joint with a stout Steinmann pin, inserted from the sole of the foot through calcaneus, talus, and well into the tibia. The foot and ankle must be held reduced and in neutral.

Dislocations of the talus require prompt reduction, usually open, as do its displaced fractures.

FOOT INJURIES

The ability to walk normally can be significantly compromised by residua of foot injuries. Their early recognition prevents complications. Prompt treatment is often more effective than that postponed "until he's over the other injuries." Foot trauma may appear relatively insignificant, but it must not be ignored.

Subtalar dislocations require prompt reduction to avoid skin slough. Closed reduction is usually possible, but a general anesthetic is often needed. Manual traction with correction of deformity (inversion or eversion) is effective.

Calcaneal fractures are often severe bursting injuries that signify major damage to the heel. Associated vertebral fractures are not unusual. Swelling may be marked, occasionally to the point of delayed skin slough. Bed rest, leg elevation, and a well-padded splint to hold the foot in neutral are advisable. While some advocate ORIF, the results seem little better than closed treatment, which might include manipulation to correct gross deformity, but emphasizes maintenance of a plantigrade foot and ankle mobilization rather than restoration of normal anatomy.

Midtarsal and tarsometatarsal joint disruptions may be obvious radiographically or may be minimally displaced, with small avulsion fractures and slight deformity the only indication of the gross instability obvious on physical examination.

These severe injuries may include damage to skin and neurovascular structures and place the patient at risk of amputation. Open reduction may be required, but closed manipulation usually suffices. Because of marked swelling, position is hard to maintain in plaster. Therefore percutaneous pinning is helpful if closed reduction is acceptable. A normally shaped foot with its sole perpendicular to the leg is the primary goal.

Metatarsal and phalangeal fractures may be displaced enough to interfere with normal weight bearing. If they are, reduction, usually closed, is required. Small Kirschner wires usually hold an unstable reduction. A well-padded splint is advisable to hold foot and ankle in neutral during the early phases of recovery. As soon as foot and other injuries permit, weight bearing begins in a well-molded plaster.

REHABILITATION FOLLOWING MUSCULOSKELETAL TRAUMA

Unlike most trauma to other organ systems, the ultimate result of musculoskeletal injuries does not depend exclusively on the effectiveness of the initial therapy. In fact, several months of well-directed rehabilitation often contribute more to the outcome than whatever "definitive fracture treatment" is chosen. Although early aggressive fracture stabilization can greatly facilitate the initial management of a multiply injured patient, it does not guarantee a satisfactory recovery. Injured bones usually heal, and deformity is generally preventable, but joint injuries always present the challenges of impaired mobility, instability, and pain. Muscles, weakened by injury and inactivity, require sustained use to regain their strength. The injured patient's cardiorespiratory reserve diminishes rapidly while his activity is limited and is restored only by prolonged aerobic reconditioning.

Whenever possible, motion—passive, active, or both—should begin promptly for all injured joints. This is especially crucial for the shoulder, hand, and knee. If early movement is not appropriate, immobilization must be in a functional position. Mobilization is vital for mild injuries as well. For example, in an older patient with a flail chest, a contused shoulder may stiffen irreversibly unless assisted range-of-motion exercises are begun promptly, even while the patient is on a respirator in the intensive care unit.

Rehabilitation begins simultaneously with diagnosis and early treatment of injuries. It must continue until maximal recovery is achieved. Follow-up supervision is thus required until the patient has clearly reached an acceptable plateau.

BURNS

Juris Bunkis, M.D.
Robert L. Walton, M.D.

Given the ubiquitous nature of thermal injuries, it behooves all physicians to understand the basic physiologic alterations occurring as a result of thermal injuries and to at least possess the ability to provide first aid to the burn victim. At least two million people in the United States annually sustain burns serious enough to warrant medical attention, but most require little more than first aid treatment for relief of pain. A quarter of a million patients with minor burns can be adequately managed on an outpatient basis. Approximately 100,000 patients annually will sustain burns severe enough to warrant hospitalization, and of these approximately 12,000 will die as a result of their injuries. Such statistics exemplify the importance of thermal injury as a disease entity. The economic effects are magnified when one considers the number of working years lost due to the fact that the majority of burn patients are males under the age of 40. Half of all burns serious enough to require hospitalization occur in the home, and of these at least two thirds are considered preventable. The cause of burns varies from one part of the world to another. Numerically, flame and scald victims constitute the largest percentage of patients sustaining thermal injuries. In the United States, approximately 75 percent of burns are due to flame injuries, 13 percent to scalds, 5 percent to contact burns, 3 percent to electrical burns, 1 percent to chemical burns, and less than 1 percent to radiation injuries. Whether produced by flame, scald, chemical, contact, or electricity, many of the pathophysiologic mechanisms of hyperthermic injuries are similar—extensive tissue destruction is accompanied by an increased capillary permeability and massive extravascular fluid loss.

PATHOPHYSIOLOGY

Cutaneous Response

An understanding of the basic physiologic responses to burn injury is essential in caring for the burn patient. Thermal injury results in injury to the skin. One must remember, however, that a severe burn causes alteration of virtually every organ system in the body.

The skin is one of the largest organs of the body and constitutes 15 percent of total body weight. The average adult has a skin surface area of 4.7 sq. meters. The skin is a vital organ, loss of substantial areas of which impairs the homeostatic mechanism and exposes the body to the damaging elements of the environment. If the lost skin is not replaced by the patient's own skin, death may result. Destruction of the protective layers of the skin eliminates the normal vapor barrier and allows body water to evaporate through areas of injury at the same rate as it would from an open pan. The average insensible water loss through intact skin is approximately 15 ml/m^2/hr (700 to 1,000 ml/day), but water loss through areas of full-thickness burn may reach 200 ml/m^2/hr. Slightly less water loss will be experienced with partial-thickness burns. The evaporative water loss is accompanied by a 560-kilocalorie heat loss with the evaporation of each liter of water. With major burns, total energy expenditures associated with the increased evaporative water loss may result in a 7,000-kilocalorie per day deficit. This energy expenditure will be accompanied by a significant rise in oxygen consumption and basal metabolic rate.

The second major protective function of skin is the prevention of invasive infection. Subsequent to thermal injury, surface microorganisms persisting in the skin appendages begin to multiply, reaching quantitative bacteriologic counts as high as 10^8 organisms per gram of tissue by the second or third post-burn day. The predominant bacteria constituting this initial proliferation are gram-positive staphylococci, but by the fifth to seventh post-burn day, gram-negative bacilli, particularly *Pseudomonas aeruginosa*, are dominant. With partial-thickness injuries, some protection against invasive sepsis persists. All burns are contaminated, but every effort must be made to prevent burn wound sepsis (defined quantitatively as a burn wound containing more than 10^5 microorganisms per gram of tissue). Following partial-thickness injuries, infection may cause a conversion of the wound to a full-thickness injury. Wound cultures obtained by swabbing the surface and visual inspection of the wound provide little information about the degree of infection; every unit providing care of the seriously burned patient should have the capability to monitor wound bacteriologic status with frequent quantitative cultures.

With full-thickness injuries, cell death occurs as a result of coagulation necrosis. Thermal injury may result in interference with cell metabolism, denaturation of cell protein, and secondary interference with vascular supply. A decrease in the severity of injury is noted vertically from the surface to the depth of the wound and peripherally in all directions from the central point of injury. Three concentric zones of injury directly related to the intensity of the thermal stimulus have been described. The central "zone of coagulation" contains permanently irreversible coagulation and lacks capillary blood flow. Tissue in this area is irreversibly damaged from the outset. Surrounding the necrotic tissue is a "zone of stasis" characterized by a sluggish capillary blood flow. Any further injury (e.g., secondary to desiccation or infection) may result in total cessation of blood flow and necrosis with enlargement of the "zone of coagulation." A peripheral "zone of hyperemia" constitutes the third concentric zone of thermal injury. The hyperemia results from the usual inflammatory response of healthy tissue to nonlethal injury and, unless complicating factors develop, this injury is usually healed by the seventh day.

Cardiovascular and Metabolic Response

Immediately following a burn, the most striking physiologic alteration is related to the circulatory system. Increased capillary permeability allows water, electrolytes, and protein to escape from vascular compartments into the burn wound. Following minor burns, this immediate and reversible vascular response to burning is confined to the burned area, but with involvement of more than 30 percent of the body surface area, increased capillary permeability is systemic. The most significant loss from the vascular compartment is the loss of serum (i.e., the saline component). In-

creased capillary permeability is accompanied by a sudden marked decrease in cardiac output concomitant with increased pulse rate, decreased stroke volume, and a marked rise in peripheral vascular resistance. Within 3 hours following major thermal injury, 50 percent of the total plasma volume can be lost through the open wound. Appropriate fluid resuscitation must be undertaken to prevent hypovolemic shock, progression of burn injury, and acute renal tubular necrosis secondary to hypovolemia.

The initial loss of large volumes of protein-rich fluid presents the same physiologic threat to life as acute external hemorrhage. Marked loss of plasma results in hemoconcentration with subsequent sludging and the possibility of a further decrease in peripheral tissue perfusion and oxygenation, and then cell death, particularly in the "zone of stasis."

Plasma volume reduction is accompanied by hemoconcentration, blood cell agglutination, and sludging of the microcirculation. A variable amount of red blood cell destruction takes place in the burn area, but due to the relatively more significant loss of plasma with resultant hemoconcentration, transfusion of whole blood is rarely necessary during the first 72 hours.

Serum protein levels may drop precipitously in the first 4 days following burn injury, with protein losses equalling twice the total plasma pool. Approximately half of this protein is lost through the wound, but the remainder may lie sequestered in the extravascular space for as long as 3 weeks before being returned to the vascular compartment. In addition, catabolism of all proteins proceeds at twice the normal rate.

The increased capillary permeability in response to burning is greatest within the first 12 hours post-burn, although additional loss at a much slower rate may continue for another 6 to 24 hours. Capillary permeability returns to normal 48 hours after injury and the resorption of edema fluid begins. This process is expressed clinically as a diuresis. The subacute phase following shock phase is manifested clinically by diuresis and mobilization of sodium. Anemia generally becomes manifest as the clinical edema subsides and blood transfusions may be necessary.

Immediately following a burn, the metabolically active zones of the wound are flooded with fluid, plasma proteins, and polymorphonuclear leukocytes. As with any major injury, the patient experiences an increased basal metabolic rate, increased secretion of multiple hormones (e.g., catecholamines, cortisol, renin–angiotensin, antidiuretic hormone, aldosterone), negative potassium and phosphorous balance, disturbed carbohydrate utilization, fat mobilization, salt and water retention, alteration in the metabolism of certain vitamins, and a negative nitrogen balance with resultant weight loss. The severity of these alterations generally parallels the extent of injury. Fluid loss, hypermetabolism, and caloric requirements may be decreased by the application of biological dressings and by placing the burned victim in a warm humidified environment. It is difficult, however, to obtain a positive nitrogen balance prior to closure of the wound. Following wound closure, the anabolic phase of injury is entered.

Pulmonary Response

Pulmonary changes are noted even in the absence of "inhalation injury." Initial depression of arterial oxygen tension is noted, but normal levels return by the end of the first week unless complications supervene. With burns involving more than 40 per cent of the body surface area, increased minute ventilation occurs by the third post-burn day, peaks by the fifth day, and gradually declines. Airway resistance, however, does not appear to be significantly increased except in the presence of inhalation injury. Interestingly, increased pulmonary capillary permeability is not believed to occur, even with extensive burns, in the absence of inhalation injury. Pulmonary edema, when it occurs, is thought to be the result of overaggressive resuscitation and not of increased capillary permeability.

It is impossible to produce a thermal injury below the larynx by inhalation of hot air. Steam, however, has a heat-carrying capacity four thousand times that of air, and can cause an actual burn of the pulmonary tree. Most patients with inhalation injuries damage the tracheobronchial mucosa as a result of the inhalation of the noxious products of combustion. Severe inflammation, congestion of the submucosal blood vessels, and marked edema of the mucosa occur. These changes classically occur 24 hours post-burn. With severe injuries, sloughing of the entire trachobronchial mucosa can occur. Most deaths following burn injuries today are due to accompanying inhalation injuries or the result of complicating pulmonary infections.

Gastrointestinal Response

An adynamic intestinal ileus develops in all patients with burns involving more than 30 percent body surface area. This generally subsides in 48 to 72 hours, following which the gastrointestinal tract may be employed for nutritional purposes.

In the past, 25 percent of hospitalized burn patients developed massive melena or hematemesis due to "Curling's ulcers." Now that all major burn victims are treated with antacids or histamine blockers, clinically significant GI bleeding is rarely encountered. Colonic mucosal ulcerations may also cause lower gastrointestinal bleeding, but these are rarely encountered.

Immunologic Response

The immune system is depressed by thermal injury. Impaired cellular immunity is demonstrated by lymphocytopenia, delayed rejection of allografts, and anergy to common antigens.

Humoral defects are characterized by a depression of immunoglobulins, specifically IgG, IgA, and IgM. Serum immunoglobulin levels are maximally depressed 2 to 5 days after injury. Complement titers also decrease following burn injury, but this may be due to protein leakage from permeable capillaries.

Burn patients are more susceptible to infection. These infections are frequently refractory to treatment with antibiotics. It has been shown experimentally that neutrophil phagocytosis progresses normally, but the efficiency of intracellular killing is diminished. Impaired chemotaxis delays neutrophil migration. An overall deficit in host-defense mechanisms results.

PATIENT EVALUATION

The severity of burn injury is related to the depth of the burn, the total body surface area involved, the patient's age, the severity of associated injuries, and the pre-injury state of health of the victim. Information regarding each of these categories must be sought in order to establish therapeutic priorities, devise a treatment plan, and determine the eventual prognosis.

History

A thorough history provides the surgeon with clues as to the magnitude of the burn, as well as information regarding associated injuries and pre-existing medical conditions. When, where, and how the injury occurred must be established. The patient—as well as other family members, firemen, policemen, emergency medical technicians, and other eye witnesses—may provide illuminating details of the accident. Most patients, even following extensive burns, are alert immediately following the accident, thus allowing a full history to be obtained while the examination is being performed and treatment initiated.

Burns result from the application of an energy source to the skin, with energy transfer occurring directly by contact or indirectly by radiance. The depth of the burn varies with the intensity and duration of the applied heat as well as the conductivity of the involved tissues. The speed with which the transfer takes place is much more important than the total amount of heat transferred. As the rate of heat transfer exceeds the body's ability to dissipate the energy, heat damage occurs. Tissue conductivity is influenced by water content, surface oils and secretions, insulating material such as the cornified keratin layer of the skin, and the density of local pigmentation. A 0.54-second exposure of human skin to 3.9 cal/cm^2/sec of radiant heat results in a second-degree burn; increasing the heat delivered to 4.8 cal/cm^2/sec would lead to a third-degree injury. Cell damage rarely occurs with a heat source below 45°C, but with temperatures greater than 50°C, denaturation of various protein elements begins, although the damage may be reversible. Above 65°C, protein denaturation is usually complete, and cell death results from protein coagulation. Knowledge of these facts, combined with an appreciation of the mechanism of thermal injury, may have a predictive value clinically in determining the depth of injury. Therefore, one can predict that a brief flash burn or spill scald will result in partial-thickness burns, whereas flame burns and immersion scalds, owing to prolonged contact with the heat source, are more likely to produce a full-thickness burn injury. Immersion injuries expose the tissue to uniform intensity of heat for a prolonged duration and result in homogeneous tissue destruction. Flame burns, on the other hand, are more likely to expose the skin to varying intensities of exposure and frequently produce a patchy distribution of full-thick-ness and partial-thickness destruction. Flash and scald burns are unlikely to produce inhalation injury, but flame burns sustained within an enclosed space or steam burns may be associated with an inhalation injury.

The patient's age is closely linked to the predicted mortality for the burn injury. For any given extent of burn, patients under the age of 2 and those over the age of 65 have a higher predicted mortality. The very young and the very old may have a greater susceptibility to infection owing to incompletely developed or depressed immune systems. The very young (immature dermal papillae) and the very old (atrophic dermal papillae) also have thinner skin than do people between these extremes of age and thus develop deeper burns from the same heat intensity. In addition, cardiac disease, diabetes, or chronic obstructive pulmonary disease may significantly worsen the prognosis in the elderly. Information regarding antecedent illnesses, allergies, and medications is useful in the planning of management of the burn patient. Chronically administered cardiac, hormonal, and anticonvulsant medications must be continued during the hospitalization.

A thorough history—including the setting and events leading to the burn, the alleged mechanism of injury, and the appropriateness of parental response—must all be evaluated to rule out the possibility of child abuse or neglect. Evidence of a suicide attempt is a signal for early psychiatric intervention to prevent a repeat performance and to minimize problems in social adjustment to the injury.

Physical Examination

A rapid preliminary evaluation to assess the magnitude of injury and to establish the priorities for treatment must precede the recording of a detailed history and physical examination. Most pertinent aspects of the history can usually be obtained and the initial evaluation performed while the patient is being undressed and placed on the examining table. Following severe burns, it is necessary to establish an airway and to initiate the resuscitation concurrently during the initial evaluation.

As with any major trauma patient, a thorough physical examination must be performed. This requires removal of all clothing, dressings, makeup, jewelry, and dentures. The presence of asso-

TABLE 1 Predicted Mortality Following Burn Injury

Age (Years)	% BSA Burned									
	10	20	30	40	50	60	70	80	90	100
10	0	4	14	37	60	78	91	97	99	100
20	0	3	13	35	59	77	90	97	99	100
30	0	4	16	39	62	79	92	97	99	100
40	1	7	22	47	69	84	94	98	100	
50	3	13	35	59	77	90	96	99	100	
60	9	27	53	72	87	96	99	100		
70	24	49	70	85	95	99	100			
80	51	71	86	95	99	100				
90	75	89	97	99	100					

ciated injuries must be determined. Hyperemic oral or nasal mucosal surfaces, singed nasal hairs, or the presence of intranasal or intraoral soot may herald a significant inhalation injury. The patient's age, extent and depth of burn, as well as the presence of pre-existing or associated injuries will influence prognosis and immediate therapeutic decisions.

Extent of Burn. The age of the patient and the extent of the burn are the two most important factors in predicting the prognosis of the burn victim (Table 1). Extent of a burn is expressed as a percentage of the total body surface area (percent BSA) injured. A careful calculation of the percent BSA of involvement forms the basis for predicting the amount of fluid required for resuscitation, forms the basis of the American Burn Association severity index, and allows the surgeon to prognosticate with regard to final outcome. Knowledge of the extent, depth, and location of burn; the presence of associated injuries; and pre-existing medical conditions allows the surgeon to classify the burn as mild, moderate, or severe, thus forming the basis of initial triage decisions and allowing determination of the initial treatment protocol (Table 2).

The palmar surface of each hand equals approximately 1¼ percent BSA. The extent of small burns can be calculated rapidly by comparing the size of the burned area to multiples of the area of the hand; thus, a burn the size of two hands would be equivalent to 2.5 percent BSA. For larger burns, the percent BSA involved can be calculated rapidly and accurately by application of the "Rule of Nines." This rule divides the body surface into areas representing multiples of 9 percent. In the adult, approximately 9 percent is allowed for each upper extremity, 18 percent for the anterior thorax

TABLE 2 American Burn Association Burn Severity Categorization

Burn Classification	Characteristics	Implications for Treatment
Minor burn injury	1° burns 2° burn < 15% BSA in adults 2° burn < 5% in children/aged 3° burn < 2% BSA	These patients may qualify for outpatient therapy.
Moderate burn injury	2° burn 15–25% BSA in adults 2° burn 10–20% BSA in children/aged 3° burn < 10% BSA	Hospitalization is required. Given adequate staff and facilities, a community hospital may suffice.
Major burn injury	2° burn > 25% BSA in adults 2° burn > 20% BSA in children/aged 3° burn > 10% BSA Burns involving hands, face, eyes, ears, feet, or perineum Most patients with inhalation injury, electrical injury, concomitant major trauma, or significant pre-existing diseases	Care in a specialized burn center is indicated.

and abdomen, 18 percent for the back and buttocks, 18 percent for each lower extremity, and the remaining 1 percent for the neck. In the child, the relatively larger BSA of the head and proportionally smaller BSA of each lower extremity must be taken into consideration. The age-related charts modified by Lund and Brower provide a more accurate determination of the extent of burn. Each emergency room and burn unit should have these charts available and one should be filled out initially for every burn victim.

Depth of Burn. Frequently, the most difficult aspect of burn wound evaluation involves determining the depth of the burn. Several classifications have been employed to differentiate various depths of injury. The simplest and most useful divides burn wounds into two basic categories: partial-thickness injuries (those which under ideal circumstances will epithelialize spontaneously from retained skin appendages) versus full-thickness injuries (those in which the entire thickness of skin has been destroyed, thus relying on wound contraction, migration of epithelial cells from the periphery, or surgical intervention to produce healing).

Traditionally, burn wounds have been divided into three categories by degree. The first-degree wound is characterized by erythema, which blanches on pressure, and tenderness and edema of the skin (probably related to the release of various amines from reversibly injured cells). The damage is confined to the epidermal layer, although dermal blood vessels are dilated and congested. Most first-degree burns are the result of prolonged exposure to the sun or of minor scalding injuries. Pain normally subsides after 48 to 72 hours and healing takes place uneventfully. As the involved epithelium peels off within 5 to 10 days, it is replaced by new cells from the basal layer of the epidermis. Owing to the superficial nature of the injury, the protective barrier of the skin is retained, thus minimizing fluid loss and any danger of infection. The burned area usually heals without residual scarring.

Second-degree injuries involve the epidermis and varying depths of the dermis, while leaving viable dermis containing skin appendages (hair follicles, sweat or sebaceous glands) from which epidermal repopulation can occur. Such burns are characterized by vesicle formation due to detachment of the epidermis from the underlying dermis. The presence of intact bullae is usually a good sign that circulation in the deeper areas of the dermis

has been preserved, and that spontaneous healing can be expected. More superficial wounds are erythematous, progressing to a waxy, white coloration with increasing depth. With deeper injuries, waxy, insensitive skin may be difficult to differentiate from full-thickness injury. The burn surface appears moist, owing to the loss of the protective barrier function of the skin and subsequent serous fluid loss. Varying degrees of thrombosis of the dermal vessels and wound edema are seen. Such burns are likely to be painful. The rate of healing of a second-degree burn is directly proportional to the depth of injury. Superficial second-degree wounds can be expected to heal uneventfully within 7 to 10 days unless infection supervenes. Deep partial-thickness injuries may require a month for epithelial regeneration from the remaining glands and hair follicles. Minimal scarring results from healing of a superficial second-degree burn, but prominent scarring with unstable overlying epithelium can be expected following healing of deep partial-thickness injuries. Fluid loss and metabolic derangements likewise are progressively more severe as the depth and extent of burn injury increases. Any partial-thickness wound can be converted to a full-thickness injury by infection, desiccation, or maceration.

Third-degree burn wounds are characterized by destruction of the entire thickness of dermis along with all the contained skin appendages, and by thrombosis of the subdermal vascular plexis. Following third-degree flame, electrical, or chemical burns, the skin appears dry, hard, insensate, inelastic, waxy, and white. With full-thickness scald burns, the epidermal layer frequently sloughs immediately following the injury, and the patient presents with a lobster-red, insensate coagulated dermis. Such burn wounds are insensate owing to the destruction of terminal, sensory nerve endings in the dermis. In addition, one may suspect third-degree injury if hair shafts can be pulled from their follicles easily and painlessly. Increased capillary permeability and wound edema are more severe than in second-degree injuries. In the untreated burn wound, the coagulated collagenous eschar can be expected to begin separating in 10 to 14 days, partially as a result of autolysis and leukocyte digestion accompanied by suppuration, revealing a granulating tissue bed. Since such wounds lack epidermal appendages, healing can only occur by wound contraction (frequently complicated by severe contractures), by migration of epithelial cells from the periphery, or by surgical intervention. Chronic open wounds, or those with unstable epithelium, are at an increased risk of undergoing malignant degeneration many years later.

Tissue fluorometry can distinguish between deep-partial and full-thickness burns for diagnostic purposes. Practically speaking, however, better results, both functionally and aesthetically, are obtained by treating deep dermal and full-thickness wounds in a similar fashion by early excision and grafting, thus obviating the necessity to distinguish clinically between the two levels of injury prior to the initiation of therapy.

TREATMENT

First Aid

At the scene of the accident, the first priority is to remove the victim from the heat source. Burn victims should be moved to well-ventilated areas away from flaming material to minimize the possibility of continued inhalation injury. A burning patient should be placed in a horizontal position and the flames smothered by rolling the patient in a blanket, rug, or large garment, or the flames can be extinguished by water. Frequently, a patient whose clothes are on fire may instinctively begin to run, but this should be avoided as running only fans the flames. Similarly, maintaining the erect position allows clothing and hair to burn more vigorously in a wick-like fashion, thus once again stressing the importance of assuming the horizontal position in order to allow the flames to be extinguished rapidly.

Following electrical injury, power should be shut off if possible and the patient removed from the source of electricity. The rescuer must not touch the patient who is still in contact with a live electric wire lest he be electrocuted or sustain a similar electrical burn injury. Following contact with a noxious chemical, the burned area should be washed with copious quantities of water. Following inadvertent contact with hot tar or molten metals, the involved part should be cooled with water, but efforts to remove the tar or metal should not be started at the scene of the accident.

All burned parts should be cooled with water as soon as possible following a burn. Although the beneficial effects of cooling remain controversial, we believe that application of cold water (4°C) minimizes progression of the burn injury in the zone-of-stasis. Experimentally, retention of intact blisters has been shown to prevent dehydration necrosis in the zone of stasis much more effectively than does cooling. Cooling does, however, appear to have a beneficial effect on the dermal microvascular circulation at the burn site. In addition, the use of ice compresses brings almost immediate relief from burn pain. Cold compresses are applied to the burned areas for 30 minutes following the injury.

Clean, moist dressings should be applied to the burn wound to minimize wound contamination and to maximize patient comfort. Any clean sheet, towel, or cloth may be used as an emergency dressing. Frequently, the lay person applies topical first-aid medications or home remedies such as butter, petroleum jelly, or antibiotic creams before seeking professional assistance. Public education efforts should discourage use of such medications, as there is no evidence of a beneficial effect from such remedies and they may be difficult to remove later. Following application of the clean dressings, the patient should be positioned for comfort and, if appropriate, the burned areas elevated to minimize subsequent edema.

Burn patients may develop an ileus with the subsequent risk of aspiration. Oral fluids should be avoided initially; alcoholic beverages should definitely be prohibited.

All burn victims with full-thickness burns, partial-thickness burns involving more than 5% BSA, burns involving vital body parts (such as the hand, face or perineum), significant associated injuries, or pre-existing diseases should be evaluated by a physician. Arrangements must be made to transport the patient to a medical facility as soon as possible following the burn injury. Most communities are served by well-trained emergency medical technicians and suitable transportation vehicles that are available for transport of the seriously injured burn patient to the emergency room. Following minor burns, the patient may be brought to the emergency room by any appropriate available means.

Outpatient Burn Therapy

"Minor burns," as defined by the American Burn Association severity categorization index, may be treated on an outpatient basis provided the patient and/or his parents are considered reliable and other complicating factors are absent (see Table 2). The majority of burn patients presenting to an emergency room can be treated in this way.

Following any burn injury, the initial evaluation must include a determination of the extent, depth, and location of the burn as well as the patient's age, the presence of pre-existing illness, and associated injuries. The extent of the burn must be diagrammed in the medical record, and if there is any question of legal implications, photographs should be obtained for further documentation. Vital signs must be determined and a complete physical examination performed. Social factors must be considered. Only then can the decision be made to treat the patient on an outpatient basis. Occasionally, hospitalization of a patient with a minor burn may be indicated for the first day or two while the patient or his family are educated in dressing changes and wound care. Criteria for admission to the hospital are frequently liberalized when dealing with the pediatric and geriatric populations.

Severe anxiety and pain frequently accompany a burn injury. A calm and reassuring approach by the physician is of prime importance in minimizing the patient's anxiety and apprehension. The requirement for sedation is usually inversely proportional to the depth of the initial thermal injury. Relatively minor injuries treated on an outpatient basis can, therefore, be quite painful. Narcotics and other vasodilating agents must not be administered to the hypotensive or hypovolemic patient. Once the vital signs have stabilized, a full therapeutic dose of parenteral narcotic (up to 1.5 mg/kg body weight of meperidine or 0.2 mg/kg of morphine sulfate) may be necessary to provide initial pain control. The narcotic must be given in small increments, however, to minimize complications that could result from vasodilation or respiratory depression. Most minor burns do not require continued narcotic support following initial debridement and application of dressings. Topical analgesics, while quite effective, should be avoided in all but small burns to avoid absorption of the potentially semi-toxic medications.

Partial-thickness wounds should be washed gently but thoroughly with balanced salt solutions to remove all surface contaminants. Irritating soaps and antiseptics should be avoided, as these produce further tissue injury. Ruptured blisters should be debrided, but the temptation to aspirate or debride intact blisters definitely should be avoided. Blister fluid provides the most physiologic microenvironment for rapid wound healing.

In general, dressings are recommended for all burns treated on an outpatient basis, except for second-degree burns of the face. A well-applied occlusive dressing minimizes pain and contamination and frequently allows the patient to continue usual activities. A layer of nonadherent petrolatum gauze can be placed against the superficial partial-thickness burn and incorporated in a bulky, comfortable dressing. Furacin mesh gauze may be employed as an alternative to the petrolatum gauze. Topical antimicrobial agents generally are not necessary for the treatment of small burns. Such agents diminish the rate of epithelialization and thus wound healing. In areas subject to excessive contamination (e.g., perineum, groin) and in the treatment of deep partial-thickness burns, however, topical antimicrobial agents (e.g., silver sulfadiazine) minimize the possibility of infection. Allografts, xenografts, and synthetic biological dressings are occasionally advocated, but are prohibitively expensive and usually unnecessary for small wounds typically handled on an outpatient basis. It is difficult to keep a tidy facial dressing in place, and for this reason, partial-thickness facial injuries are best managed by frequent application of moist compresses followed by application of neosporin or bacitracin antibiotic ointment to avoid desiccation.

Prophylactic antibiotics are not indicated in the treatment of uncomplicated burns. Should peripheral erythema, tenderness, or fever suggest streptococcal infection, however, cultures must be obtained and appropriate antibiotic therapy instituted. In addition, tetanus prophylaxis must be considered in all patients with burn injuries.

Limited deep dermal or full-thickness burns involving nonvital areas can be excised and closed primarily by approximation of the wound edges or covered by a split-thickness skin graft in an outpatient surgical facility. This is usually performed within the first 48 hours following the burn injury to minimize the possibility of wound infection and graft loss. Patients suitable for outpatient burn surgery must be selected carefully to avoid complications involving donor sites or the grafted wounds.

At least initially, the patient should be seen in the outpatient burn clinic or physician's office on a daily basis for wound re-evaluation and redressing. Burn wound classification is not static and, particularly if a partial-thickness wound becomes infected, conversion to a full-thickness injury may result, with the accompanying need for hospitalization. As the wound begins to show signs of epithelialization, outpatient visits may become less frequent, until total wound healing has been achieved. All patients with partial-thickness burn injuries should be followed closely until the wounds are completely epithelialized. Subsequently, the patient should be re-examined every 1 to 3 months for evidence of scar hypertrophy. Pressure garments, special exercises, and splints may be indicated to avoid or minimize hypertrophic scarring. The patient must be instructed to avoid excessive exposure to sunlight for at least a one-year period to minimize scar or graft hyperpigmentation.

Burns usually result in damage to the normal lubricating mechanism of the skin. Following epithelialization or grafting, healing areas may benefit from a mild lanolin lotion to decrease dryness. Pruritus in particular is a common complaint following burn injury. An antihistamine, such as diphenhydramine hydrochloride (i.e., Benadryl), may provide symptomatic relief.

Appropriate rehabilitation—physical, psychological and social—must be directed by the physician. Optimal patient care is provided by specialized personnel trained in the management of the burn patient; outpatients with burns should be seen in the same area as those who have been discharged from a burn unit and are returning for follow-up care. The superior results can be attributed to the specialized training and facilities and the personal interest expressed by the burn clinic personnel.

Hospital Burn Care

Criteria for inpatient care of the burn patient must be individualized to take into consideration general medical and social factors. Generally, adult patients sustaining partial-thickness burns exceeding 15 percent BSA (10 percent in children) or full-thickness burns exceeding 2% BSA require hospitalization. In addition, patients with burns involving the hands, face, eyes, ears, feet, or perineum; inhalation or electrical injury; major associated injuries; or serious pre-existing illnesses should be admitted for treatment of their injuries.

Care of a patient with a major burn proceeds more smoothly if a pre-established protocol is followed. Such a protocol is particularly helpful to physicians who do not deal with acutely burned patients on a daily basis. Such a protocol should include information regarding the following categories:

1. Patient evaluation including required laboratory data.
2. Establishment of airway and maintenance of breathing.
3. Insertion of indwelling intravenous lines and initiation of resuscitation.
4. Insertion of indwelling bladder catheter +/− CVP line for patient monitoring.
5. Confirmation of peripheral circulation, escharotomies PRN.
6. Initiation of nasogastric suctioning.
7. Sedation.
8. Initiation of tetanus and antibiotic prophylaxis.
9. Burn wound care.
10. General supportive measures.

Patient Evaluation. Rapid preliminary evaluation will allow determination of the magnitude of injury and the establishment of treatment priorities. A quick history, determination of the extent and depth of burn, drawing of blood samples for baseline laboratory tests and crossmatching, a portable chest roentgenogram, and an electrocardiogram can be obtained while resuscitation is being initiated. Charting of the depth and extent of the burn wound should also be delayed until resuscitation is underway and the patient is in stable condition, but should definitely be performed before dressings are applied to the burned areas.

Establishment of Airway and Maintenance of Breathing. The patient's history and physical examination are helpful in raising the suspicion of an inhalation injury. The most sensitive indicators of the degree of pulmonary injury are provided by arterial blood gas and carboxyhemoglobin determination. A patient with a suspected inhalation injury should be initially treated with a mask providing humidified air with high oxygen content and meticulous tracheobronchial toilet. If bronchospasm and wheezing are present, bronchodilators and mucolytic agents may be helpful. Flexible bronchoscopy may be employed to assess the degree of damage and to remove carbonaceous sputum plugs, but routine repeated bronchoscopy has not been shown to be significantly helpful. Indications for intubation and respiratory support are the same as those for any patient following major trauma. If hypoxemia (PaO_2 < 60 mm Hg) or hypercarbia ($PaCO_2$ > 55 mm Hg) persists following the application of an oxygen mask, the patient should be intubated to ensure an adequate airway and respiration. Any patient who demonstrates marginal respiratory status during the initial evaluation should be intubated immediately. Gas exchange predictably deteriorates during the first few days following an inhalation injury. In addition, massive edema during the resuscitative phase can be expected to further compromise the airway and make intubation difficult later. Generally, patients requiring prolonged ventilatory support tolerate nasotracheal intubation better than orotracheal tubes. In burned victims, a formal tracheostomy is accompanied by a markedly increased complication rate and thus tracheostomy should be avoided unless absolutely necessary. Antibiotics should be reserved for treatment of documented infections. Prophylactic steroid therapy likewise has not been shown to be beneficial in the treatment of inhalation injury.

Circumferential burns involving the chest or neck may interfere with ventilation. A thick, unyielding circumferential eschar may prevent normal chest excursion during respiration. A leathery, circumferential eschar around the neck may prevent external swelling during the resuscitative phase; internal fluid shifts can result in a sufficient pressure elevation to occlude the neck veins or to compromise the airway. If the patient presents with circumferential chest or neck eschar, prophylactic escharotomies are indicated. The longitudinal decompression incisions must be extended beyond the constricting eschar proximally and distally. As many incisions as necessary to relieve the compression should be made under sterile conditions, but anesthesia is not required as the full-thickness burn wound is insensate.

Fluid Resuscitation. Resuscitation of burn shock by aggressive intravenous fluid administration is of paramount importance during the initial phase following injury. The goals of fluid resuscitation are to replace and maintain effective plasma volume during the period of increased capillary permeability and evaporated surface losses, as well as to provide maintenance fluid during the immediate post-burn period associated with intestinal ileus. Intravenous fluid resuscitation is generally required if burns exceed 20 percent BSA in adults and 10 to 15 percent BSA in children or the elderly.

A large-bore intravenous cannula must be inserted to allow administration of the large quantities of fluid required for resuscitation. Suppurative thrombophlebitis remains a possibility during the entire treatment period. Antibiotic ointment and a sterile dressing are applied around the catheter entry site to minimize the incidence of phle-

bitis. Frequently, finding adequate intravenous access is difficult, especially following burns involving all four extremities. If at all possible, intravenous lines, whether inserted by percutaneous puncture or cutdown, should not be placed through burned tissue to avoid the almost certain occurrence of subsequent phlebitis. During the resuscitative phase, however, reliability of venous access is more important than violation of the burn wound. Similarly, use of the upper extremities for vascular access is preferable to use of lower extremities because of the lesser incidence of phlebitis. Central venous lines occasionally provide the only reasonable route for fluid administration, but owing to potentially lethal infectious complications, the placement of central lines solely for the purpose of fluid administration should be avoided if peripheral alternatives are available.

Most burn formulas are based on the patient's body weight and the percent BSA burned. Always remember to calculate fluid requirements from the time of burn injury, not from the time the patient is first seen in the emergency room. All burn formulas, however, should be treated as mere guidelines for the calculation of fluid deficits during the initiation of resuscitation. Each patient must be monitored continuously and therapy modified according to the individual patient's responses.

A number of formulas have been proposed to help the surgeon determine the amount of electrolyte solution, colloid solution, and free water necessary to effect the resuscitation. The most commonly recommended formulas guiding resuscitation are the Brooke, Evans, and Baxter formulas (Table 3). Analysis of these formulas reveals that the total volume and the total sodium load recommended for the initial 48-hour period vary little, the major differences being in the timing of the colloid administration. Colloid administration within the first 24 hours post-burn is of little benefit as osmotic pressure cannot be maintained over freely permeable capillary membranes. During the initial 24 hours following the burn, the colloid leaks into the extravascular space and actually augments extravascular fluid retention. Therefore, most major burn centers no longer provide a colloid component during the initial 24 hours of fluid resuscitation and rely instead on a sodium-containing electrolyte solution. Measurements of cardiac output, plasma volume, and extracellular fluid have demonstrated that plasma volume replacement during the first 24 hours post-burn is dependent only upon the rate, not the type, of fluid administered. The

TABLE 3 Fluid Replacement Formulas for Initial 48 Hours

Burn Formula	1st 24 Hours				2nd 24 Hours		
	Colloid	Electrolyte	Water	Rate of Administration	Colloid	Electrolyte	Water
Evans	1 ml/kg/% BSA burn	1 ml/kg/% BSA burn (up to 50% max.)	2,000 ml	½ first 8 hr ¼ second 8 hr ¼ third 8 hr	0.5 ml/kg/% BSA burn	0.5 ml/kg/% BSA burn	2,000 ml
Brooke	0.5 ml/kg/% BSA burn	1.5 ml/kg/% BSA burn (up to 50% max.)	2,000 ml	½ first 8 hr ¼ second 8 hr ¼ third 8 hr	0.5 ml/kg/% BSA burn	0.75 ml/kg/% BSA burn	2,000 ml
Revised Brooke (1979)	—	2–3 ml/kg/% BSA burn (no upper limit)	—		Sufficient to replace vascular volume and maintain normal urine output	—	Sufficient to maintain normal serum sodium concentration
Baxter	—	4 ml/kg/% BSA burn (no upper limit)	—	½ first 8 hr ¼ second 8 hr ¼ third 8 hr	Sufficient to replace vascular volume and to maintain normal urine output		

sodium load administered during the resuscitation is a prime determinant of the return of cardiac function. For these reasons, the Baxter formula is the most frequently employed in the United States today. Electrolyte solutions during the first 24 hours restore plasma volume. During the second 24 hours, maintenance fluid is given as free water to maintain serum sodium near 140 mEq/L, and sufficient colloid solutions are administered to maintain normal plasma volume. One must appreciate, however, that very little difference exists between the different formulas. For this reason, physicians should select a single resuscitation method and learn to use it well instead of attempting to mix the several approaches found in the current literature.

Certain investigators have advocated hypertonic salt solutions for burn shock resuscitation in order to inhibit weight gain and wound edema. Hypertonic solution resuscitation allows adequate vascular volume restoration by inducing extracellular movement of intracellular water. The argument of isotonic versus hypertonic fluids for resuscitation becomes one of whether it is more physiologic to have a normal serum sodium concentration with extensive edema or an elevated sodium serum concentration with cellular dehydration. Each theory has its proponents, but definitive studies demonstrating the superiority of one method over the other are lacking.

Patient Monitoring. Response to resuscitation can be measured by several criteria including clinical observation (e.g., vital signs, mental status, central venous pressure, urine output) and laboratory data (e.g., hematocrit, electrolytes, osmolalities). During the early post-burn period, however, the blood pressure and pulse are unreliable guides to the adequacy of resuscitation. Hematocrit, electrolyte, and protein levels should be determined initially and followed throughout the hospitalization. These laboratory values likewise do not provide a reliable guide to the adequacy of initial fluid resuscitation.

An adequate urine output (1.0 ml/kg/hr) is the best single guide to the adequacy of fluid replacement. An indwelling bladder catheter should be inserted immediately upon the patient's admission to the emergency room and urine output monitored closely. If urine output drops below 30 ml/hr in the average adult patient, the rate of fluid administration should be increased. Similarly, if the urine output exceeds 100 ml/hr, the patient should be re-evaluated to ascertain that fluid requirements

have not been overestimated. A low urine output unresponsive to a fluid challenge may herald acute renal insufficiency.

The adequacy of resuscitation can be determined by following the urinary output in most burned patients. Patients failing to respond to an apparently adequate fluid challenge and those with pre-existing pulmonary or cardiac abnormalities may benefit from monitoring of central pressures. The best indicator of adequate fluid replacement is left ventricular end diastolic filling pressure, but in most patients determination of right-sided central venous pressure will suffice. CVP less than 7 cm of water indicates a need for more vigorous fluid resuscitation. Caution should be exercised if the CVP rises above 15 cm of water and the need for prophylactic digitalization considered.

Circulation. With burns involving the extremities, peripheral circulation may be compromised by the circumferential, thick leathery eschar. Internal fluid shifts occur beneath the unyielding eschar, and tissue pressures may rise sufficiently to threaten limb viability. The inelastic eschar acts as a limb tourniquet; as tissue pressure increases, lymphatic, venous, and arterial flow are interrupted in a sequential manner. The extremity may appear pale, cool, and pulseless. If the circumferential burn is isolated to a proximal segment of the extremity, the spared area distal to the eschar may develop severe edema and may similarly become pulseless.

Escharotomies must be performed early to prevent irreversible ischemic insult. Following obvious full-thickness circumferential extremity burns, prophylactic escharotomies are performed in the emergency room. With circumferential extremity burns of indeterminate depth, clinical re-evaluation must be performed frequently to determine the necessity for escharotomies. The onset of neurologic signs such as paresthesia, anesthesia, or deep tissue pain mandates immediate decompressing escharotomies. Absent, severely delayed, or extremely rapid nail bed capillary filling may provide a useful clinical sign indicating compromised peripheral circulation due to the constricting eschar. One must remember that arterial occlusion occurs later than venous obstruction.

Longitudinal escharotomies, which extend beyond the limits of the burn, are performed under sterile conditions. The decompression must extend down into the subcutaneous tissue, but care must be taken to avoid injury to the underlying veins, lymphatics, and cutaneous nerves. The incisions must be carried just deep enough to allow the wound edges to separate. Except during treatment of electrical injury, fasciotomies usually are not required. Following severe hand burns, the escharotomies must be carried along the midaxial lines of the digits to the fingertips, care being taken to avoid injury to the underlying neurovascular structures. All involved digits must be released bilaterally with the incisions joining within the web spaces. In addition, multiple dorsal incisions may be necessary to fully decompress the hand. Due to the thicker nature of the palmar skin, full-thickness burns of the volar surface of the hand are most unusual, and palmar escharotomies are rarely indicated.

Enzymatic debridement can provide a non-surgical decompression of burned extremities. When decompressing circumferential eschar, we limit the use of Sutilains ointment (Travase), which contains a proteolytic enzyme derived from *Bacillus subtilis,* to extremities that are well-perfused at the time of admission. If the extremity is cold and pulseless initially—or if it becomes so subsequently, immediate surgical escharotomies must be performed.

Burned extremities should be elevated to minimize edema. With lower extremity burns, the foot of the bed should be elevated. Elevation of the upper extremities is facilitated by the use of stockinettes. The hand is maintained in the protective position by applying splints and comfortable bulky dressings. The wrist should be extended 15 or 20 degrees, the thumb maintained in abduction, the metacarpal phalangeal joints flexed maximally, and the interphalangeal joints fully extended.

Although patients with severe burns spend considerable amounts of time in bed and are hypercoagulable, clinical deep vein thrombophlebitis or pulmonary emboli are rarely seen. Prophylactic anticoagulation is not indicated.

Nasogastric Suctioning. Adynamic ileus frequently accompanies extensive burns. Initial therapy of major burns should include nasogastric intubation for at least the first 24 to 72 hours. Burn patients frequently experience an intense thirst, but oral solutions should be avoided. Given unlimited access to oral fluids, such patients may develop acute gastric dilatation and the subsequent risk of aspiration. Oral and nasogastric feedings should be avoided until peristalsis returns. Although of little consequence in itself, the effect of ileus may be detrimental to the patient in that it prevents enteral alimentation during a time that large amounts of fluid and calories are required. If the ileus persists beyond the resuscitative phase, consideration should be given to total parenteral nutrition. Ileus that persists or develops following the resuscitative phase is generally indicative of a complication such as burn wound sepsis or gastrointestinal tract perforation.

The nasogastric tube also allows sampling of gastric secretions to permit accurate titration of the gastric pH with antacids. Administration of cimetidine (Tagamet, 400 mg IV q. 4 h.), however, is technically simpler and better tolerated by the patient than frequent administration of large quantities of antacids. The nasogastric tube is particularly useful in patients with altered levels of consciousness to prevent regurgitation and vomiting with possible aspiration. A nasogastric tube must be inserted in all patients during the initial evaluation prior to transfer to a major burn center to prevent a catastrophe en route.

Sedation. All conscious burn patients exhibit severe anxiety and experience pain requiring sedation and analgesia. The patient must not, however, be reflexly given a large dose of narcotics by a sympathetic physician or nurse. Cold compresses may be applied to the wounds initially to provide relief while the patient is being evaluated. Narcotics should be withheld while the patient is in profound shock. One must also remember that agitation may not be a sign of discomfort, but of cerebral hypoxia, a state that might be aggravated by the administration of narcotics. All sedatives and analgesics administered during the acute period should be given intravenously and in small doses to provide prompt pain relief. Intramuscular or subcutaneous administration during this period of hemodynamic instability results in variable absorption and may allow drug accumulation with later sudden absorption leading to fatal apnea. In the adult patient, a small dose of morphine sulfate, 1 to 3 mg intravenously, usually provides satisfactory sedation and analgesia. This dose may be repeated every 1 to 3 hours as needed, but the patient must be carefully observed for signs of respiratory depression. Inadvertent narcotic overdosage is treated by intravenous administration of the specific antagonist, naloxone. A small dose of diazepam (Valium), 2 to 5 mg intravenously, provides satisfactory sedation in the extremely anxious patient. In addition, diazepam provides an extremely beneficial amnesic effect, which is particularly helpful during subsequent dressing changes.

Subsequent dressing changes are usually anticipated by the burn patient with great anxiety. Judicious doses of appropriately timed analgesics usually are sufficient, but occasionally, particularly in children, additional sedation is required. In such cases, intravenous diazepam (0.1 mg/kg), followed by a subanesthetic dose of intravenous ketamine (Ketalar 0.5 mg/kg), will allow the dressings to be changed without inflicting further psychologic trauma. If such a regimen is to be used, an anesthesiologist should be available, resuscitative equipment present, and the patient must have an empty stomach to prevent aspiration. Long-term analgesia for a patient with extensive burns presents a difficult clinical problem. Every effort must be made to provide the patient satisfactory pain relief while avoiding drug addiction. Hypnosis has been of value in the long-term management of patients with chronic pain.

Tetanus and Antibiotic Therapy. Intensive use of prophylactic antibiotics has been ineffective in decreasing the incidence of infectious complications following burn injury. Traditionally, prophylactic penicillin therapy has been recommended during the early post-burn period to prevent group A beta hemolytic streptococcal cellulitis. Should streptococcal cellulitis occur in a patient who had not been treated prophylactically with antibiotics, the infection will be very sensitive to intravenous penicillin therapy. Prophylactic penicillin therapy, however, hastens the emergence of antibiotic-resistant gram-negative organisms. Burn wound sepsis and other infectious complications occasionally seen in the burn victim are not prevented by prophylactic antibiotic therapy. The risks of prophylactic antibiotic therapy are outweighed by any possible benefits, and therefore we agree with the general principle that systemic antibiotics are not indicated on a prophylactic basis for the burn victim.

The majority of pathogenic bacteria gain entrance to the burn surface from foci within the nasopharynx and hands of burn unit personnel, from other patients, from various pieces of hospital equipment, and from the patient's own respiratory and alimentary tracts. Gross contamination of the wounds should be minimized by isolation techniques and meticulous handwashing. Surface cultures of the wounds, nares, throat, urine, and sputum should be obtained at the time of admission and at regular intervals thereafter. Bacteriologic data dictate the need for specific antibiotic coverage of infectious complications.

Intact burn eschar provides initial protection from burn wound sepsis. Following successful re-suscitation, however, consideration should be given to excising the eschar and grafting the wounds before the onset of clinical infection. All open wounds quickly become contaminated and yield a variety of organisms by qualitative surface swab cultures. Surface cultures demonstrate the presence of bacteria, but yield little information regarding the magnitude of risk of burn wound sepsis. The presence of burn wound sepsis can only be definitively confirmed by quantitative wound biopsy assays; burn wounds containing more than 10^5 organisms per gram of tissue by definition represent burn wound sepsis. Histologic examination of a portion of the biopsy specimen will demonstrate the depth of bacterial invasion. *Pseudomonas aeruginosa* and *Staphylococcus aureus* are the organisms most commonly implicated in burn wound sepsis. Quantitative cultures demonstrating burn wound sepsis or consistently positive blood cultures require wound debridement, systemic antibiotic therapy, and a probable change of topical antimicrobial agents. Subeschar antibiotic injections may serve as a temporizing maneuver, but total wound excision and appropriate antibiotic coverage—systemic and topical—are more efficacious.

The avascular nature of the burn eschar and the sluggish blood flow in the surrounding zone of stasis contribute to the inability of parenterally administered antibiotics to reach the burn wound, to modify the bacterial flora, or to influence the mortality rate in the burn population. Topical chemotherapeutic agents, however, have been efficacious in the prevention of burn wound sepsis with resultant improvement in mortality rates. Ideally, the topical antimicrobial agent should be effective against the organisms proliferating in the burn wound, lack local and systemic toxicity, be readily available and easily applied, rapidly excreted or easily metabolized, and should not interfere with wound healing. No single agent satisfies all these requirements, but several excellent topical preparations have met most of these requirements. These include 0.5 percent silver nitrate solution, mafenide acetate (Sulfamylon), and silver sulfadiazine (Silvadene) creams. Advantages and disadvantages of these agents are summarized in Table 4. Topical antimicrobial agents, applied in solution or as water-soluble creams, markedly reduce evaporative water loss, and thus caloric demands. Reduced wound bacterial levels also result in lessened caloric requirements.

Tetanus prophylaxis is indicated for all patients with injuries resulting in a break in epithelial

TABLE 4 Topical Antimicrobial Agents

Agent	Composition	Application	Bacterial Spectrum	Resistance	Advantages	Disadvantages
Silver nitrate	0.5% solution of the inorganic silver salt $AgNO_3$, in distilled water	Moist compresses changed b.i.d. and saturated q.4h. Painless	Bacteriostatic to entire spectrum	None	No sensitivities Not inactivated by specific antagonists	Does not penetrate eschar well Dilutional hyponatremia and hypokalemia due to leaching of electrolytes into wound Discolors wound, unburned skin, and environment Hypochloremia due to AgCl precipitation
Mafenide acetate	Methylated sulfonamide, 11.1% suspension in a water dispersible cream base	Applied topically b.i.d. as a cream; medication washed off daily Painful for 20–30 minutes following application to 2° burn	Bacteriostatic to entire spectrum, but minimally effective against staphylococci and fungi	Occasionally to staphylococci	Penetrates eschar well	Potent carbonic anhydrase inhibitor Tends to produce acidosis Sensitivity in 5 percent, manifested by a maculopopular rash
Silver sulfadiazine	1% suspension in a hydrophilic cream base	Applied topically b.i.d. as a cream; medication washed off daily	Bacteriostatic to entire spectrum	Occasionally to Pseudomonas and Enterobacter	No significant effect on fluids or electrolytes	Penetrates eschar poorly Can cause granulocytosis

integrity. All second- and third-degree burns result in necrotic tissue, thus providing an ideal milieu for tetanus infection. Although this disease is rare, tetanus in the burn victim is almost always fatal. The prior immunization status of the patient determines the need for tetanus prophylaxis (see Table 3 in chapter on *Wound Management*).

Wound Care. The principal aims of wound care are to allow survival of any remaining viable tissue, to prevent infection, and to provide suitable circumstances to allow the best possible functional and aesthetic results to occur as the wounds heal. The use of topical antimicrobial agents has resulted in a dramatic improvement in survival from major burns, but 70 percent of all burn deaths are still the result of burn wound sepsis. Sterile techniques must be employed when burn wounds are handled. This includes wearing a cap, mask, sterile gown, and gloves whenever handling the burn victim or his wounds.

The burn victim must first be undressed and the wounds inspected while the history is being obtained, physical examination performed, and resuscitation initiated. Immediate cooling by immersion in ice water or by application of ice compresses for 20 minutes diminishes pain, subsequent edema, and progression of the burn injury. Cooling should be limited to patients with burns involving less than 30 percent BSA to avoid complications stemming from hypothermia.

The surface of all burn wounds should be cleansed with a mild antiseptic solution. Intact blisters protect the wound and therefore should be left undisturbed. Loose necrotic tissue may be debrided after the patient has been placed in the hydrotherapy tank. Vigorous mechanical debridement may further damage the injured tissue and should be avoided initially. Since discomfort is aggravated by air currents over the burn wound, the wounds are covered with a topical antimicrobial agent and dressed. Silver sulfadiazine and mafenide acetate creams are the most commonly employed topical antimicrobial agents. Subsequently, the burn wound should be bathed daily to remove necrotic debris and the topical antimicrobial agent; the burn wound should be inspected, the cream reapplied, and the wound redressed. Silver sulfadiazine is employed most frequently because it causes little pain, is easy to apply, and has an effective antibacterial spectrum. Mafenide acetate has better eschar penetrating ability and therefore is the agent of choice for burns with thick eschar or those infected with anaerobic or gram-negative organisms. The topical antimicrobial agents may be applied to areas of partial-thickness and full-thickness burns. Superficial partial-thickness burns should heal in 7 to 14 days. Deeper burns generally require removal of the eschar and skin grafting to obtain wound coverage. One must remember that topical antimicrobial agents do not sterilize the burn wound, but only reduce the number of bacteria present, thus minimizing the incidence of invasive infection.

Following application of the topical antimicrobial agent, a single layer of fine mesh gauze is placed next to the wound. Several layers of multiple-ply, coarse-mesh gauze without cotton filling are next applied. The outer layer consists of bias stockinette. Splints are incorporated into the dressing between the coarse mesh gauze and the outer wrap in extremity burns to immobilize joints in the positions of function. Extremities should be elevated to minimize edema. At each dressing change, joints should be put through active and passive range of motion exercises. The splints may be discarded after the wounds have healed. During the resuscitative phase, occlusive extremity dressings must be modified to allow monitoring of blood supply in order to determine the need for escharotomies.

Partial-thickness burns of the face and neck are more easily treated by the open technique. The wound is rinsed gently twice a day with a sterile physiologic saline solution. This is followed by application of an antibiotic ointment (e.g., Bacitracin, Neomycin) or standard topical antimicrobial agents.

The full-thickness burn wound must be free of eschar before skin grafts can be applied. Different options for obtaining a satisfactory bed for grafting include waiting for spontaneous separation of eschar, enzymatic debridement, total burn wound excision to fascia, or tangential debridement.

Spontaneous separation of eschar begins between the tenth and fourteenth post-burn days in the untreated wound. This separation of the eschar from the underlying burn wound results from bacterial growth and autolysis of necrotic tissue. Treatment with topical antimicrobial agents will delay eschar separation. Following eschar separation, a granulating bed is usually present which may require minor debridement in preparation for grafting. Unfortunately, however, the burn wound remains susceptible to invasive sepsis during this entire phase. For this reason, enzymatic or surgical debridement of the eschar and early skin grafting are now practiced in most major burn centers.

Enzymatic debridement has proved to be particularly effective for debridement of burned hands. Sutilains ointment (Travase), applied three times daily, effectively dissolves an eschar in 24 to 36 hours. Twenty-four hours following initiation of enzymatic therapy, the wound can be debrided with the edge of a scalpel handle, scraping rather than cutting, to expose underlying viable tissue which will accept a skin graft. The operative time is short and simple. Blood loss is negligible and long-term function results are excellent. Proteolytic enzymes, however, allow bacterial proliferation; when they are used alone, cellulitis and even evasive burn wound sepsis can occur. To lessen the possibility of infection during this phase, the Sutilains ointment is combined with silver sulfadiazine ointment prior to application to the burn wound. This method is effective when applied to small, localized wounds such as those occurring on the dorsum of the hand.

More extensive deep-dermal and full-thickness burn wounds require surgical debridement. This may take the form of early, total excision of the burn wound down to the underlying fascia or tangential debridement to bleeding tissue. Excision of the entire burn wound down to underlying fascia can be performed rapidly by means of the cutting current of the electrocautery unit, produces minimal blood loss, and results in a satisfactory bed for immediate skin grafting. Burn wound excision to fascia, however, removes subcutaneous tissue and can result in a significant contour deformity. Tangential escharectomy is more tedious, is accompanied by significant blood loss, and, with full-thickness burns, results in a poorly vascularized, adipose tissue bed for subsequent skin grafting. Hemostasis is simpler to obtain following fascial than tangential escharectomy. Following tangential escharectomy, delayed skin grafting (24 hours later, prior to the onset of significant bacterial proliferation) may be necessary if perfect hemostasis cannot be achieved initially. The method employed to rid the patient of the necrotic eschar in preparation for skin grafting is not as important as the timing of the debridement. Debridement must be individualized according to patients' needs. Every effort should be made, however, to remove all necrotic tissue and to close the wound with skin grafts before significant bacterial proliferation occurs. Except in unusual circumstances (e.g., a concomitant brain injury or myo-

cardial infarction), escharectomies are performed within 48 hours of the burn injury and wound closure begun. Should a delay be necessary, quantitative bacterial assays must be employed to insure that wound bacterial counts are less than 10^5 bacteria per gram of tissue before grafts are applied.

A free hand knife or any of the standard dermatomes can be employed to obtain the skin grafts. The thighs and buttocks are the most common donor sites for split-thickness skin grafts. Following injury to these sites or in the presence of extensive burn, skin grafts may be obtained from any unburned site. It is rarely possible to skin graft areas larger than 30 percent BSA at any one time. Following extensive burns, sufficient donor sites may not be available initially to provide total wound coverage. In these instances, the entire eschar is initially removed, the available autografts are applied, and biological dressings employed to cover the remaining open wounds. In such instances, the initial autografts are usually applied to the hands or other joint areas (in order to allow early restoration of function), or to aesthetically important sites such as the face. Temporary biological dressings reduce fluid and protein exudation from the wound, promote patient comfort, and preserve bacteriologic control of the wound until donor sites have had the opportunity to re-epithelialize prior to reharvesting. A variety of biological dressings have been proposed, including cadaver allografts, amniotic membranes, xenografts, and synthetic biocomposite wound dressings (e.g., Biobrane).

Donor sites may be dressed with an impregnated fine mesh gauze dressing. Op-Site, a recently introduced hypoallergenic, moisture vapor permeable synthetic membrane, allows rapid epithelialization of the donor site, is easy to use, and promotes patient comfort. If thin grafts are harvested, donor site re-epithelialization can be expected in 10 to 14 days and the donor sites may be reused every 2 to 3 weeks. Donor site infection delays re-epithelialization and may even result in loss of remaining dermal and epidermal elements with conversion to a full-thickness wound.

Sheet grafts are employed to cover small wounds and aesthetically important areas such as the face. Grafts can be meshed (allowing expansion from 1.5 to 9 times the original size). Although theoretically sheet and mesh grafts should display a similar incidence of take, clinically mesh grafts appear to do better over extremity and trunk wounds. The mesh grafts allow egress of serum and better contouring of the graft to an irregular bed, and they increase the area covered per graft. The remaining raw interstices epithelialize rapidly and the final aesthetic result is usually acceptable.

Complete immobilization of the graft on its bed is essential to allow the graft to take. Grafts may be immobilized by any combination including sutures, surgical staples, adhesive tapes, or conforming dressings. Staples provide the most rapid method of graft fixation. Staples are removed on the fifth day following grafting. Grafted extremities are dressed with immobilizing, conforming, circumferential dressings. A single layer of Furacin-impregnated fine mesh gauze is applied directly to the skin grafts. Coarse mesh gauze, prefabricated orthoplast splints, and bias stockinette complete the extremity dressing. Furacin solution is employed to keep the dressings moist until the first dressing change 48 to 36 hours following grafting. It is much more difficult to apply an effective dressing over trunk or facial skin grafts. Respiratory or normal facial movements beneath a dressing may cause shearing between the skin graft and its bed. Following grafting of trunk or facial wounds, a sheet graft may be left exposed to allow constant observation, but a single layer of Xeroform gauze should be applied to meshed grafts to prevent desiccation. These patients frequently require sedation, and occasionally even restraints, to minimize patient motion in order to enhance graft take during the initial postoperative period. Rarely, in the well-selected patient, it may be necessary to paralyze and mechanically ventilate the patient for a few days following application of crucial split-thickness skin grafts.

External splints and percutaneous pins serve two main functions. First, splints and pins can be employed to immobilized extremities during the post-grafting phase to allow successful vascularization of the skin grafts. Second, pins and splints can be employed to maintain joints in the position of function to minimize joint contractures and to facilitate subsequent rehabilitation. This is particularly important following burns to the hand, but other joints should not be forgotten. Interphalangeal joints should be held in extension, metacarpal phalangeal joints maximally flexed, the thumb abducted, the wrist slightly extended, the elbow almost completely extended, the shoulder abducted, the knee almost completely extended, and the ankle in neutral position. External splints may also be designed to keep the neck extended. This aspect

of burn wound care is frequently performed by physical therapists, occupational therapists, or burn unit nurses. The patient's physician, however, must have a thorough understanding of basic principles of physical medicine and maintain a leadership role in the patient's rehabilitation.

Burn wounds that have been skin grafted or have healed secondarily are frequently unsightly, particularly during the early hypertrophic phase. The patient must take special care of the skin during this period. The patient should be fitted with custom-made pressure garments (Jobst garments) prior to discharge from the hospital in order to minimize scar hypertrophy and keloid formation. Topical or intralesional steroids may be employed to reduce hypertrophic scars but their use is confined to small areas. Patients with healing wounds frequently complain of pruritus and dryness, which can be helped by lanolin creams. Lanolin ointment and gentle massage facilitate scar maturation and improve patient comfort. Exposure of the burned areas to sunlight must be avoided. Ultraviolet radiation may further damage the scarred skin and produce permanent hyperpigmentation. The patients must be educated in the use of sun-screening agents—these should be applied to all exposed areas whenever the patient anticipates outdoor activity.

In spite of optimal wound care, severe scarring may dictate the need for subsequent reconstructive surgery in order to return the burn victim to a reasonable social situation. The most common procedures include release of burn scar contractures and resurfacing of unacceptable areas, preferably in aesthetic units.

Supportive Measures

One of the most significant advances in the management of burn patients during the past few decades has been the increasing realization of the need for adequate nutrition and the development of means to provide it. Negative nitrogen balance and increased metabolic needs begin abruptly at the time of injury and continue until the wound is closed. Protein loss into the wound, loss of muscle from disuse, and increased metabolic rate from evaporative water loss all contribute to the negative nitrogen balance. An increased secretion of catabolic hormones such as glucocorticoids, catecholamines, and glucagon occurs concomitantly with an impaired secretion of the anabolic hormone insulin, contributing to the hypermetabolic, negative nitrogen balance state. The duration and magnitude of the negative nitrogen balance are influenced by the severity of the burn and the nutritional regimen employed. The basal metabolic rate and oxygen consumption increase in a linear fashion parallel with the extent of the burn injury up to a maximum level corresponding with a 40 to 50 percent BSA maximum. Energy expenditures seem to peak toward the end of the first week, but nitrogen balance does not return to normal (3 to 4 g of nitrogen per meter^2/day) until wound closure has been achieved. Malnutrition increases the incidence of infection and reduces the efficiency of wound healing in the nutritionally depleted burn patient. Therefore, every effort must be made to maintain nutritional status during this period of hypermetabolism.

Oral feeding is preferred whenever possible. By the second day following extensive burns, the obligatory intestinal hypoperistalsis has usually resolved and oral feedings may be started. It is preferable to start oral intake with limited amounts of fluids at frequent intervals, but the diet may progress as tolerated by the patient. A lack of appetite frequently occurs in the post-burn patient. Attention should be directed toward attractively presented and tastefully prepared meals. Total caloric needs may be calculated employing the "Curreri formula" (caloric requirement = 25 Kcal/kg + 40 Kcal/percent burn). Nitrogen requirements can be met by supplying 1 protein/150 Kcal. Most patients find it difficult to consume sufficient quantities of protein and calories during regular mealtimes. A high-protein, high-caloric liquid supplement can be given between meals via a nasogastric feeding tube. Such supplements usually consist of a concentrated protein and milk formula and are well tolerated by the majority of burn patients, but occasionally, particularly in black adults, a galactase deficiency may produce intolerance of milk feedings. Provision of adequate protein and calories does not return metabolism to preinjury levels, but does reduce nitrogen loss, promote healing, and hasten the patient's recovery.

In addition to protein and calories, routine vitamin supplements are recommended as follows: ascorbic acid, 1500 mg; thiamine, 50 mg; riboflavin, 50 mg; and nicotinamide, 500 mg daily. The vitamin supplements and increased caloric diet should be continued until burn wounds are healed.

It is imperative not to fall behind caloric requirements in the burn patient. Should the gastrointestinal tract be unavailable for feedings, total parenteral nutrition must be instituted promptly, employing the same guidelines used for any other seriously injured patient.

Periodic transfusions and therapeutic administration of albumin or gamma globulin may be necessary in patients with extreme emaciation and hypoproteinemia following delayed referral to a burn center.

Finally, total rehabilitation of the burn patient necessitates a return to adequate social function. This requires the cooperation of a large number of individuals including not only physicians, nurses, nutritionists, and physical therapists, but also psychologic and social support teams. All burn unit personnel must contribute to a supportive environment during the patient's recovery. Skin is man's outer cover. Burn injury induces severe anxiety, an altered body image, and a physical and possibly a social handicap. A burn injury may produce devastating emotional and social consequences. Initially, the patient is apprehensive for his life, but later is plagued by fear of permanent disability and disfigurement. Patients frequently develop a mild depression when preparing to leave the hospital and to face the potentially hostile community environment. Specific psychologic support eases the transition to the outside world. Although all burn patients may benefit from psychologic intervention, studies have indicated that the success of therapy depends more on the patient's pre-burn personality than on any single factor.

Burned children are particularly apt to have difficulties with psychosocial adjustment following hospitalization for their injuries. Parents of burned children frequently require psychiatric counseling to alleviate feelings of guilt regarding their responsibility for the child's accident. Psychologic counseling may also be required for spouses and other relatives of burn victims. Despite relative marital satisfaction, studies have demonstrated dissatisfaction in sexual relations involving rehabilitated burn injured patients. A number of regional and national support groups consisting of rehabilitated burn victims have been organized. Such peer groups can provide the burn victim much needed support. In the presence of an effective rehabilitative team, better than 95 percent of burn victims are able to return to their pre-burn socioeconomic status.

ELECTRICAL INJURIES

Damage due to electrical injury is frequently referred to as an electrical burn. The intensity of current, the duration of contact, the resistance at points of contact, the efficiency of grounding, and the pathway of the current through the body determine the extent of injury. Higher voltage and prolonged contact increase the severity of injury. Thin skin and surface moisture decrease resistance to the electrical current, whereas thick skin and surface oil increase it. A larger area of grounding will encourage greater current flow and consequently increase the degree of injury. The current flows in a direct line between the points of grounding. Cardiac or respiratory arrest may occur if the pathway of the current includes the heart or brain. The current rarely causes irreversible damage to the heart or lungs; prompt cardiopulmonary resuscitation should allow return of vital functions to an unimpaired level and residual cardiopulmonary disease is rarely encountered in these patients. Direct current produces muscular spasms only at the start and stop of current flow, whereas alternating current produces muscular contraction and relaxation with each cycle. Thus, low-voltage direct current is less dangerous than the alternating variety.

The electric current produces tissue disruption by thermal necrosis. Treatment of electrical injury should be modified considerably from that of thermal injury because tissue damage is much deeper. The amount of heat generated is directly proportional to the resistance to current flow. The lowest resistances are offered by nerves, followed by blood vessels, muscle, skin, tendons, fat, and bone. Thus, tissues located near the center of the limb may be injured while more superficial tissues may be spared. In many aspects, an electrical injury more nearly simulates crush injury than it does a thermal burn. More tissue is always destroyed by an electrical injury than is apparent at first inspection.

Three types of skin damage are associated with electrical injuries: (1) contact burns (entry and exit sites), (2) arc burns, and (3) flame burns resulting from the ignition of clothing by electrical sparks. Initial treatment of electrical and thermal burns is similar, but a high-voltage electrical injury must be treated more like a crush injury. The current may cause thrombosis, even at some distance from the original injury. Peripheral perfusion must be monitored and a fasciotomy performed at the first sign of vascular compromise. Viability of tissues in patients with high-voltage electrical injuries can be determined only by direct visualization, and early exploration of such tissues is mandatory. Obvious necrotic tissue must be excised and daily debridement performed to extirpate remaining nonviable tissue to prevent sepsis and minimize the need for amputations. An excessive release of myoglobin into the circulation may produce renal damage, and therefore massive replacement fluid therapy is essential. Frequently, an osmotic diuretic also is indicated.

Failure to remove extensively damaged muscle may lead to anaerobic clostridial infections and death. Anticlostridial prophylaxis with large doses of penicillin and tetanus prophylaxis are necessary. Mafenide acetate cream is preferred to other topical antimicrobials for its ability to penetrate into the deeper tissues.

Fractures due to severe muscular contractions must be suspected in patients following electrical injury. Such patients must also be observed for spontaneous vascular rupture (false aneurysms), visceral injury, and vascular thrombosis.

Physical therapy is of paramount importance in the rehabilitation of the patient following electrical injury. Prosthetic training is frequently required due to the high incidence of amputations.

Unattended children frequently bite electrical cords and sustain low intensity electrical burns of the oral commissures. Such injuries are caused by the heat of the arc and are true thermal injuries without distal sequelae. Classically, children with electrical burns of the lips were admitted to the hospital for wound care and observation during the 7 to 21 days required for secondary healing. Potential hemorrhage from the labial arteries following separation of eschar provided the rationale for hospitalization. Outpatient management of children with electrical burns of the lip in conjunction with parental education, however, is in most cases safe and cost effective. Parents can be taught to control hemorrhage by direct pressure and to immediately bring the child to an emergency facility should bleeding occur. Such wounds are kept clean by frequent cleansing with physiologic saline, and antibiotic ointments are applied until secondary healing is obtained. Splinting of the oral commissures following electrical injury of the lips to prevent contracture has become increasingly accepted in the past several years. Good results have been reported utilizing intraoral splints constructed from acrylic and fixed to the teeth by the pediorthodontist. Secondary surgery may be required for microstomia.

CHEMICAL INJURY

Chemical burns tend to be progressive as long as the active agent remains in contact with the skin. Tissue destruction ceases only when the offending agent has been removed or neutralized. Initial therapy, irrespective of the causative agent, should consist of copious irrigation of the affected part with physiologic saline or water, removal of clothing, and repeated irrigation. Attempting to identify the offending agent and to locate the proper neutralizing agent will only result in delay of treatment and a progression of tissue destruction. Most chemical burns result from contact with acid or alkali. A careful search should be made for retained foreign material, particularly following contact with white phosphorus since in situ re-ignition may occur if particles are allowed to remain. Burns known to be due to white phosphorus may be washed with a 1 percent copper sulfate solution (0.5 ml/cm^2 of burn), which coats the particles with black cupric phosphide, thus impeding oxidation and allowing easy identification. Ten percent calcium gluconate solution may be injected into wounds caused by hydrofluoric acid to limit progression of tissue destruction. All wounds caused by chemical burns should be observed frequently, and if progressive tissue destruction occurs despite copious irrigation, the involved areas may require surgical excision.

Following initial management, the basic principles described for thermal injury are applicable. Tangential escharectomy may be employed to debride wounds of uncertain depth. All deep dermal and full-thickness burns should be debrided and wounds closed with skin grafts as soon as feasible.

SPECIAL PROBLEMS
Frank R. Lewis, M.D.

ACCIDENTAL HYPOTHERMIA

Accidental hypothermia has been reported with a number of preexistent medical conditions, but for practical purposes is seen in the urban setting principally in three conditions: outdoor exposure while intoxicated, prolonged unconsciousness due to drug overdosage, and cold water immersion or near drowning. Under normal circumstances, exposure in cold climates results in profound cutaneous vasoconstriction, so that little heat is lost through the skin to the air. Although it is possible, in cold climates, for hypothermia to develop in a normal person who is inadequately clothed and insulated (backpackers, mountain climbers), such an occurrence is uncommon. Hypothermia is seen most commonly in urban areas with relatively moderate or cool temperatures (30 to 60° F) in patients who are acutely intoxicated and unable to vasoconstrict effectively, and who are inadequately clothed. In such patients hypothermia typically develops over several hours. Ingestion of drugs that produce sedation or unconsciousness, such as barbiturates and other tranquilizer/hypnotics, may also result in hypothermia. These drugs generally have mild vasodilatory properties, so that heat is lost more freely, but the sedated patient fails to awaken in response to cooling.

Much less commonly, hypothermia is seen after cold water immersion following boating accidents. Because water has a greater heat capacity and penetrates most clothing, cooling occurs far more rapidly in water. Thus exposure for more than one hour to water that is cooler than 50° F is usually fatal, and even at 50 to 60° F, exposure for more than 2 hours is commonly fatal. In addition to cutaneous exposure, immersion may result in aspiration of cold water, and this produces the most rapid cooling of all, with core temperature reduced into the 80 to 90° F range within a few minutes. It has recently been shown that this is the result of cooling via the lung, with its extensive surface area for heat exchange. It has also become clear that successful resuscitation of drowning victims in cardiac arrest, even after documented periods of arrest of 15 to 25 minutes are due to this "instant hypothermia." It produces a rapid decrease in oxygen consumption and metabolic requirements, so that the arrested hypothermia victim can be successfully resuscitated well beyond the limits that are normally thought to be irreversible.

For purposes of prognosis, hypothermia to levels no lower than 90 to 92° F is rarely fatal and is usually easily treated. Most cases that result in severe complications or death have reached temperatures below 90° F, but are usually above 75° F. Survival when cooling below 75° F has occurred is quite rare, although one patient has been reported to survive with a body temperature of 67° F. It seems likely that both the degree of hypothermia and the length of time the patient remains at low temperature levels will govern the magnitude and severity of complications seen, but these relationships have not been clearly documented in the literature. In general, mortality of 50 percent is seen with hypothermia in the 75 to 90° F range.

The clinical signs of hypothermia are not specific, but one is usually led to think of it as soon as he lays hand on the patient to examine him. Normal clinical thermometers are inadequate to measure temperatures below 94° F, and either laboratory thermometers, or electric thermometers, which are commonly available, must be used. The core temperature should be monitored continuously during treatment until normothermia is attained. The cerebral signs of hypothermia are those of decreased cortical function, but they are not localized. They are progressive with decreasing temperature below approximately 94° F, to the point where coma usually is present at temperatures below 80° F. With milder degrees of cooling the patient may be apathetic, confused, or noncommunicative. As the level of cooling progresses, mental processes become more deranged, and the patient may be disoriented, somnolent, uncooperative, or totally withdrawn. Muscular rigidity and difficulty with movement and coordination are progressive with cooling below 90 ° F.

The acute metabolic effects that accompany hypothermia are multiple and produce complex changes in the cardiopulmonary system. Oxygen consumption decreases rapidly with cooling, and cardiac output falls in proportion to oxygen consumption. Patients who are cooled below 90° F typically have cardiac outputs of less than 2 liters/minute; with more profound cooling, cardiac output decreases below 1 liter/minute. Blood viscosity is increased and, in conjunction with peripheral vasoconstriction, produces marked increases in systemic vascular resistance. This tends to prevent the decreased cardiac output from causing profound hypotension, and the hypothermic patient usually has a blood pressure in the low normal to moderately hypotensive range. Diuresis accompanies severe hypothermia, but the cause has not been clearly defined. Renal tubular damage is a common sequela of moderate-to-severe hypothermia, and acute renal failure, either oliguric or non-oliguric, is common. Whether the early diuresis is a manifestation of tubular damage or a response to humoral mechanisms is unknown. It is important to recognize, however, that the hypothermic patient may be severely hypovolemic if the condition has been present for 12 hours or more, and he or she needs vigorous resuscitation and intensive cardiac monitoring. It is probable that many of the reported adverse results of rewarming from hypothermia are simply a result of failure to recognize and aggressively treat the hypovolemia that is present.

At the cellular level, the oxyhemoglobin dissociation curve is shifted to the left with hypothermia, which means that oxygen unloading peripherally is impaired. This is partially compensated by the increased amount of dissolved oxygen that is carried in the cooled plasma as well as by the decreased oxygen requirements. Thus, although peripheral hypoxia is a theoretical problem, the protective effects appear to outweigh the detrimental ones, so that overall the tissues are protected, not damaged, by cooling, at least as far as oxygenation is concerned.

Treatment of the hypothermic victim entails either passive or active rewarming, correction of metabolic and intravascular volume abnormalities, intensive cardiac and respiratory monitoring with ventilator support as needed, and close evaluation for the development of predictable complications.

The method of rewarming has evoked considerable controversy in the literature, and on one extreme there are advocates of immediate rewarming using extracorporeal bypass via the femoral vessels, while on the other extreme there are those who advocate only passive rewarming. Logically, it would seem that a rapid return of body temperature to normal is desirable, for it is clear that the hypothermic state produces significant tissue damage when present over a prolonged period of time. However, rapid rewarming by immersion of the victim in a warm tub of water or by placing heating blankets over and below him in bed has been associated, in some studies, with a greater incidence of cardiac arrhythmias or refractory hypotension. The concept has developed that rapid rewarming produces peripheral warming prior to "core" warming and, by so doing, creates vasodilation and lowered systemic resistance in excess of the ability of the heart to increase cardiac output. The actual evidence that this occurs is lacking in the literature, and it seems more likely that most of the effects attributed to it are a result of inadequate intravascular volume replacement, as was mentioned earlier. Given the rate of blood circulation between the extremities and the core, even in a profound hypothermic state, it is not possible that a significant temperature difference between them can be maintained. Despite this, the concept is often repeated in the literature and frequently governs management. It is my practice to actively rewarm all patients who have temperatures below 92° F by means of heating blankets surrounding the patient. Continuous monitoring of core temperature by esophageal or rectal probe is essential, to attain a rewarming rate of at least 1° C, and preferably 2° C, per hour. I have had no experience with the use of extracorporeal bypass for rewarming, but the reports have been favorable, and in patients with life-threatening complications such as refractory cardiac arrhythmias due to the lowered temperature, it seems indicated. In the average patient, active rewarming as described is adequate, and more aggressive means generally are not necessary.

Cardiac arrhythmias are the greatest acute threat to patients, and continuous ECG monitoring is essential. Atrial fibrillation is common, but usually resolves as normal temperature is attained and does not require treatment. If rapid ventricular response occurs and produces hypotension, conventional treatment with intravenous rapid-acting digitalis preparations is indicated. The less common but more life-threatening arrhythmias are ventricular tachycardia and fibrillation. These are treated in the conventional way with lidocaine, Pronestyl, or defibrillation, but may be difficult to convert. Least common are varying degrees of atrioventricular conduction block ranging from bundle branch blocks to complete A-V block. Only if this is severe enough to produce hypotension is treatment usually necessary.

Adequate cardiac and pulmonary monitoring of the hypothermic patient necessitates an indwelling arterial line and a central venous line for pressure measurement. Some have advocated routine placement of pulmonary artery catheters for improved definition of cardiac function, but the greater hazard of ventricular arrhythmias in this group of patients has led us to defer it until the patient's temperature is brought up to normal. A Foley catheter is placed to allow hourly monitoring of urine output, and replacement intravenous fluids are gauged by the urine output and central venous pressure. Normally we would administer balanced salt solutions rapidly until urine output is restored to 0.5 to 1 ml/kg/hr, or until the central venous pressure rises to 12 to 14 cm H_2O. Hypokalemia is a uniform occurrence in these patients, and aggressive potassium replacement is also required. Normally we have found it most effective and safest to administer potassium via intravenous drip, at the rate of 5 to 10 mEq/hr over 1 to 3 days, with close monitoring of serum potassium levels.

Acute respiratory failure and the development of interstitial infiltrates are common complications of moderate or severe hypothermia; they typically appear after rewarming is complete, usually 2 to 5 days after admission. The edema is noncardiogenic, due to permeability increases, and the cause has not been determined. In severe cases in which the patient has been comatose, aspiration pneumonia may be a cause of respiratory failure, but in many patients this seems improbable. Disseminated intravascular coagulation (DIC) is frequently present on the second to fifth day and is associated with acute respiratory failure. It is usually diagnosed by thrombocytopenia and by the presence of fibrin degradation products and soluble fibrin monomer in the blood. Whether DIC is the cause of the respiratory failure has not been determined, but it seems likely.

The frequency of respiratory problems dictates that arterial blood gas be monitored closely. If the patient develops significant hypoxemia and/or clinical respiratory failure with tachypnea and increased work of breathing, endotracheal intubation and mechanical ventilation may be needed.

We have found this to be necessary in more than 50 percent of hypothermia patients. Irreversible respiratory failure, frequently complicated by sepsis, is the most common cause of death in these patients. As a result, it should be aggressively sought and treated.

Other common complications are acute renal failure, as has been noted, and pancreatitis. If the renal failure remains nonoliguric, management is markedly simplified, as potassium management is not usually a problem, and dialysis often can be avoided. Other than early and aggressive fluid resuscitation, we know of no specific way to avoid renal failure. Its frequent occurrence should lead one to suspect it and to carry out daily creatinine clearances during the first 3 or 4 hospital days to detect it as early as possible.

Pancreatitis is often a rather subtle diagnosis, manifested by epigastric pain and tenderness with some abdominal distention, but minimal peritoneal signs of rebound tenderness. Serum amylases are frequently elevated and may confirm the clinical impression. Etiology is obscure, and treatment is supportive. In rare instances, the pancreatitis is hemorrhagic in type and produces extreme morbidity and mortality.

The final typical finding after profound hypothermia is peripheral edema that is unusually persistent and seemingly indicative of a prolonged permeability defect in the peripheral circulation. As far as I am aware, this has not been discussed in the literature, but it has been a frequent finding in my experience.

It is interesting to conjecture that most of the complications of hypothermia result from a shedding of capillary endothelial cells throughout the vascular system, and that this produces increased permeability which leads to the failure of the lung, kidney, and pancreas, as well as the peripheral edema. It also provides an explanation for the persistent DIC that is often seen, as exposure of basement membrane collagen would provide an ongoing stimulus for platelet aggregation and initiation of coagulation.

FROSTBITE

Frostbite is a cold injury of peripheral tissues in which freezing of the tissues, with ice crystal formation, occurs. It most commonly involves the feet, but also affects the hands and, on occasion, the nose and ears. The injury occurs because of direct exposure of the tissues with inadequate protection or insulation.

Tissue temperature is normally a balance between heat loss through the skin and heat inflow via the circulation. When peripheral tissues begin to cool, vasoconstriction decreases the inflow and makes the part more susceptible to the effects of environmental cooling. If external compression is present, as a result of overly tight clothing, this may further reduce inflow and predispose to freezing. Obviously, cooling is enhanced by immersion in cold water or by moisture-saturated clothing.

For frostbite to occur, the temperature of the part must decrease below 32° F, and theoretically any external temperatures below this might produce it. Practically, however, it usually does not occur unless ambient temperatures of 10 to 15° F or lower are encountered, or unless other adverse circumstances are present. The depth to which freezing in tissue occurs appears to determine the extent of the cold injury, and it may be superficial or deep. The subsequent extent of tissue loss is also principally dependent on the level to which freezing occurs, and it is usually graded as first-, second-, third-, or fourth-degree—depending, respectively, on whether the involvement is superficial, partial-thickness, full-thickness of skin, or extending into deeper structures.

The initial symptom experienced by all patients is intense coldness followed by numbness. This numbness persists as long as the part remains frozen, but after thawing occurs a number of other sensory changes are noted. The most common complaint is pain, but it is usually accompanied by paresthesias, burning, tingling, or a "pins and needles" sensation. Although these sensory disturbances are most severe in the early phases of rewarming, they tend to persist for long periods of time, and some may be permanent. Even after many years, patients may complain of pain brought on by cold and of excessive sweating. In the late phases, the extremities appear to have increased sympathetic tone, and this no doubt accounts for some of the symptoms.

If the patient is seen early, the frozen part is obviously cold, hard, and numb. More commonly, however, partial or complete thawing has occurred before the patient is seen by medical personnel, and the extent of damage may be initially underestimated. It has been well documented in the literature that prediction of extent of damage and ultimate viability is quite difficult during the early period, and only when there has been a chance for gangrene to develop into a line of demarcation can

one be sure of the extent of tissue loss. Retrospectively, the classification into first-, second-, third-, and fourth-degree tissue loss is possible, but prospectively this judgment cannot be made. Even severely injured tissue is reperfused after thawing and may be flushed and hyperemic transiently. Ultimate tissue damage and loss are due to vascular spasm and occlusion, red cell and protein extravasation with edema formation, and membrane damage.

Acute treatment, if the part has not been completely rewarmed, is to immerse it in warm water for approximately 30 minutes, until the extremity has been rewarmed to normal temperature. One method for accomplishing this has been to immerse the frozen part in progressively warmer water, starting at 20° C and increasing by 5° C at 5-minute intervals until 40° C is reached. Alternatively, water at 38 to 42° C may be used initially and maintained at that temperature throughout.

Other methods of treatment have been advocated, but relatively few have achieved any objective evidence of benefit. The one modality that seems to have value at present is intra-arterial injection of reserpine or other alpha blocking agents early after thawing, with a repeat injection at 2 to 3 days. Available evidence, both clinical and arteriographic, indicates that this may improve and maintain perfusion. Other modalities, including heparin, dextran, and indomethacin, have not been shown to have prolonged benefit. Sympathectomy has not been shown to have any value in early treatment, but in the patient who has pain and excessive sympathetic tone late after the frostbite injury, the procedure appears to produce subjective improvement with increased skin perfusion.

When tissue loss occurs, the extent of gangrene usually becomes apparent within a week or 10 days. When this is extensive, for example, extending to the ankle level, there seems little reason to temporize, and it is our practice to proceed immediately to definitive amputation. In situations in which the gangrene involves only part of a digit, it is probably better to wait and allow the part to autoamputate, so that the greatest tissue length is preserved.

SNAKEBITE

Four species of poisonous snakes are present in the United States—rattlesnakes, copperheads, water moccasins, and coral snakes. The first three are pit vipers, in the genus Crotalidae, whereas coral snakes belong to the family Elapidae. As a practical problem, pit vipers account for virtually all the snake bites seen, and coral snakes are reported to cause less than 1 percent of the total. In addition, coral snake envenomation is less frequent when a bite occurs and appears to produce fewer toxic effects, so that it is rarely a threat to life. The following discussion will therefore focus entirely on the effects of pit vipers.

Although pit vipers are present in all parts of the United States, the incidence of snake bite is most common in the southern and southwestern states. Bites usually occur in rural settings, as a result of accidental encounters with the snake, though a surprising number of people in urban areas also keep poisonous snakes for pets and are bitten while handling them. It is stated that snakes do not actively pursue humans, but when surprised or confronted they do not necessarily retreat. Snakes have poor eyesight and hearing, but a unique ability to detect prey by means of two pits on each side of the head, which are exquisitely heat-sensitive. Heat detection is thought to be the principal means by which the snake gauges the direction of strike, and even perhaps the amount of envenomation, dependent on what size the prey is thought to be. The damage inflicted by pit vipers is not strictly a bite, but rather a penetration of the skin by two fangs in the upper jaw, which are as long as 15 to 18 mm. Venom is injected through the fangs into subcutaneous tissue, where it diffuses rapidly, causing local damage. If moderate-to-large envenomations occur, systemic absorption of venom produces severe systemic effects. The quantity of venom injected is variable, dependent on the size and age of the snake as well as the size of the prey, as noted. Nearly all snakebites are on the extremities, and envenomation can occur through clothing unless it is thick, but rarely through leather boots or other protective wear.

Pit viper venom is a potent cocktail of proteolytic enzymes and other proteins that produce multiple toxic effects. The ones that are recognized to cause greatest damage are (1) hyaluronidase, which softens connective tissue and enhances spreading of venom to adjacent tissues, (2) multiple proteolytic enzymes, which digest most proteins including collagen, reticulin, and elastin, (3) procoagulants, which activate fibrinogen and result in fibrin clot formation, and (4) phospholipase A, which cleaves lecithin, releasing lysolecithin, a particularly damaging substance which destroys cell walls and membranes.

When a snakebite occurs, one should try to identify the type of snake, since the majority are nonpoisonous. The victim can sometimes identify or describe it, but if possible, the snake should be killed and examined by a knowledgeable expert. If this is not possible, the patient must be observed medically or be hospitalized until the extent of local and systemic reaction becomes evident and the need for treatment is determined.

Most of the traditionally recommended methods of snakebite treatment are without benefit and should not be practiced. Chief among these is the application of ice to the injury, since this will not inactivate the venom nor prevent its spread, but may do additional tissue damage. Incising the punctured area and sucking out the venom appears to have value only if done within the first 5 minutes of envenomation. If the victim is seen later than this, it should not be attempted. Tourniquets inflated to 50 mmHg, to impede venous and lymphatic return without producing arterial ischemia, have been recommended, but in my opinion, this measure increases local pain and accentuates swelling in the affected limb, and so its overall efficacy is questionable. Perhaps the best compromise is wrapping the entire extremity in an elastic bandage, which impedes systemic spread of the venom without increasing local edema. It is worthwhile to keep the patient as quiet as possible and keep him from using the bitten extremity if possible. Rapid transport to a medical facility is imperative so that the patient can be observed and treated as needed.

The effects of envenomation are both local and systemic. Locally, pain develops, and swelling begins within minutes to an hour or two, progressing to severe edema over several hours. The patient may report local paresthesias, and after several hours vesicles may form. Cyanosis is uncommon, but has been reported. After a day or more, ecchymoses may develop. The systemic symptoms are generalized weakness, nausea, and vomiting, and hypotension may occur. Later the signs of failure of specific organ systems are seen.

The degree of envenomation should be graded as mild if there are only local symptoms with minimal regional and no systemic involvement; moderate if local symptoms are severe and regional involvement of the entire extremity is present; and severe and life-threatening if, in addition to the aforementioned symptoms, systemic manifestations are present. The systemic organ systems that are primarily affected are cardiovascular, pulmonary, hematologic, and renal. The cardiac effects are due to fluid loss from increased capillary permeability and third space leakage of plasma, as well as vasodilatation and perhaps cardiac depression. Hypotension is common when systemic effects are present, and it requires standard methods of cardiovascular support. Pulmonary effects appear to be related primarily to interstitial edema, which in turn creates hypoxemia and decreased pulmonary compliance. Arterial blood gas monitoring is essential, and institution of ventilatory support may be necessary. The hematologic effects are similar to generalized intravascular clotting, with defibrination in severe cases. Prothrombin time and partial thromboplastin time are prolonged, and thrombocytopenia is present. Renal failure may occur if significant red cell lysis is present with hemoglobinuria, or if the patient has prolonged hypotension.

The principal care that can be given to snakebite victims is supportive when systemic manifestations are present. The usual indications and methods of cardiovascular and pulmonary support are utilized. The only specific therapy that can be administered is antivenin, which is polyvalent and effective against all pit vipers seen in the United States. When envenomation is mild, it is recommended that 50 ml (5 vials) of antivenin be used; when moderate, 100 ml, and when severe, 150 ml or more. The danger of using antivenin is that the patient may be sensitive to horse serum, from which it is made, and so sensitivity testing should precede intravenous administration. Serum sickness afterward may be anticipated in a high percentage of patients.

For severe local effects, continuous elevation and immobilization of the affected part are mandatory during the first few days, followed later by aggressive physical therapy to re-establish normal range of motion in affected parts. The edema seen is quite persistent, and if it is severe, a compartment syndrome can develop. If this occurs, fasciotomy is necessary, but this is uncommon, as the edema is usually maximal in subcutaneous tissues rather than in muscle compartments.

Overall mortality from snakebite is low, with less than 1 percent of poisonous snake bites resulting in death. The local effects, and disability from them, are far more common.

SPIDER BITES

Two spiders account for most of the severe bites seen in the United States—the black widow and the brown recluse. The black widow is usually 1 to 2 cm in size and is shiny black with a characteristic red hourglass mark on the underside of the body. This species is widely distributed in all of the continental United States as well as in South America. They tend to be found outdoors, under objects, such as rocks or logs, or in piles of rubbish or wood.

When a bite occurs, venom is injected and then absorbed into the circulation, as the principal effects are systemic. Local effects are minimal, consisting only of slight pain and swelling. The systemic effects appear to be due to a cholinergic reaction and consist of diffuse muscle cramps and spasm, with abdominal rigidity being common. Nonspecific CNS signs, such as nausea, vomiting, headache, and swelling, may be present as well. Cardiovascular or pulmonary effects appear to be minimal, although hypertension has sometimes been reported. Most patients recover after a few days. If symptoms are severe, intravenous calcium gluconate (10 ml of 10 percent solution) is used to relieve muscle cramps and spasm, and other symptoms may be treated with sedatives or analgesics as needed.

The brown recluse spider is somewhat larger than the black widow, reaching 3 to 4 cm in overall diameter. It is reddish brown with a characteristic violin-shaped mark at the anterior end of the dorsal side of the body. The venom injected by the brown recluse is a mixture of nucleases and proteases, which produce severe local tissue damage and necrosis. The initial bite may not be noticed, but after a few hours a reddish painful lesion, 1 to 3 mm in size, is noted. With time this enlarges and is surrounded by an area of vasoconstriction. After several hours extravasation of red cells may develop in a circular pattern around the central lesion. During the next few days the lesion proceeds indolently, with progressive tissue destruction and ulceration. There is local swelling, red cell extravasation, and erythema, and cellulitis may develop. The skin and subcutaneous tissue progressively necrose in the area, and debridement may be necessary. Systemic symptoms can occur in addition to the local lesions, but are not common and have been seen mainly in the pediatric population. They take the form of acute hemolytic reactions when present, with fever, chills, hemoglobinuria, and later jaundice and renal failure. If a brown recluse bite can definitely be identified, early excision of the lesion and adjacent involved tissue appears to offer the most rapid resolution.

The lesion otherwise tends to be indolent and ultimately requires sharp debridement in most cases. It is not certain that the amount of tissue loss is lessened by early debridement, but the course of the illness probably is shortened, allowing for earlier skin grafting of the area, as is usually required. Although deaths from brown recluse bites have been reported in South America, they appear to be rare in the United States, being reported only in children.

INDEX

Note: Page numbers followed by t indicate tables; those followed by f indicate figures.